OXFORD MEDICAL HANDBOOKS

Oxford Handbook of
Critical Care Nursing

Published and forthcoming Oxford Handbooks in Nursing

Oxford Handbook of Adult Nursing
George Castledine and Ann Close

Oxford Handbook of Cancer Nursing
Edited by Mike Tadman and Dave Roberts

Oxford Handbook of Cardiac Nursing, 2e
Edited by Kate Olson

Oxford Handbook of Children's and Young People's Nursing, 2e
Edited by Edward Alan Glasper, Gillian McEwing, and Jim Richardson

Oxford Handbook of Clinical Skills for Children's and Young People's Nursing
Paula Dawson, Louise Cook, Laura-Jane Holliday, and Helen Reddy

Oxford Handbook of Clinical Skills in Adult Nursing
Jacqueline Randle, Frank Coffey, and Martyn Bradbury

Oxford Handbook of Critical Care Nursing
Sheila Adam and Sue Osborne

Oxford Handbook of Dental Nursing
Kevin Seymour, Dayananda Samarawickrama, Elizabeth Boon, and Rebecca Parr

Oxford Handbook of Diabetes Nursing
Lorraine Avery and Sue Beckwith

Oxford Handbook of Emergency Nursing
Edited by Robert Crouch, Alan Charters, Mary Dawood, and Paula Bennett

Oxford Handbook of Gastrointestinal Nursing
Edited by Christine Norton, Julia Williams, Claire Taylor, Annmarie Nunwa, and Kathy Whayman

Oxford Handbook of Learning and Intellectual Disability Nursing
Edited by Bob Gates and Owen Barr

Oxford Handbook of Mental Health Nursing, 2e
Edited by Patrick Callaghan and Catherine Gamble

Oxford Handbook of Midwifery, 2e
Janet Medforth, Susan Battersby, Maggie Evans, Beverley Marsh, and Angela Walker

Oxford Handbook of Musculoskeletal Nursing
Edited by Susan Oliver

Oxford Handbook of Neuroscience Nursing
Edited by Sue Woodward and Catheryne Waterhouse

Oxford Handbook of Nursing Older People
Beverley Tabernacle, Marie Barnes, and Annette Jinks

Oxford Handbook of Orthopaedic and Trauma Nursing
Rebecca Jester, Julie Santy, and Jean Rogers

Oxford Handbook of Perioperative Practice
Suzanne Hughes and Andy Mardell

Oxford Handbook of Prescribing for Nurses and Allied Health Professionals
Sue Beckwith and Penny Franklin

Oxford Handbook of Primary Care and Community Nursing 2e
Edited by Vari Drennan and Claire Goodman

Oxford Handbook of Renal Nursing
Edited by Althea Mahon, Karen Jenkins, and Lisa Burnapp

Oxford Handbook of Respiratory Nursing
Terry Robinson and Jane Scullion

Oxford Handbook of Women's Health Nursing
Edited by Sunanda Gupta, Debra Holloway, and Ali Kubba

Oxford Handbook of Critical Care Nursing

Second Edition

Heather Baid

Fiona Creed

Jessica Hargreaves

OXFORD
UNIVERSITY PRESS

OXFORD
UNIVERSITY PRESS

Great Clarendon Street, Oxford, OX2 6DP,
United Kingdom

Oxford University Press is a department of the University of Oxford. It furthers the University's objective of excellence in research, scholarship, and education by publishing worldwide. Oxford is a registered trade mark of Oxford University Press in the UK and in certain other countries

First Edition published in 2009
Second Edition published in 2016

Published in the United States of America by Oxford University Press
198 Madison Avenue, New York, NY 10016, United States of America

British Library Cataloguing in Publication Data
Data available

Library of Congress Control Number: 2015941604

ISBN 978–0–19–870107–1

Printed and bound by
Ashford Colour Press Ltd.

Preface

Since the publication of the first edition of the *Oxford Handbook of Critical Care Nursing* there have been a number of significant changes in the management of the critically ill adult that have necessitated a review of that edition.

Therefore the second edition has been updated to reflect changes in critical care guidance for the management of a variety of conditions. Current guidance from organizations such as the National Institute for Health and Care Excellence, the British Association of Critical Care Nurses, and the Intensive Care Society has been included.

In addition to the updating of clinical guidance, the book has been restructured following extensive feedback on the previous edition. An emphasis has now been placed on nursing management, and the book is designed to help to facilitate systematic nursing assessment of the critically ill adult. New chapters focusing on changes in the delivery of critical care, systematic assessment, and end-of-life care have also been added.

It is hoped that readers will find the new structure easy to follow and helpful in clinical practice. The handbook aims to provide a quick, easy-to-follow overview of critical care nursing, and is not intended as a specialist text. Readers may need to refer to specialist critical care resources if further information is required.

It is our hope that the book will prove valuable to you in your everyday practice as a critical care nurse.

Heather Baid
Fiona Creed
Jessica Hargreaves

Acknowledgements

Firstly and foremost we would like to express our thanks to Sheila Adam and Sue Osborne for allowing us to build upon their original work.

We would also like to thank the following individuals and organizations who have contributed in various ways to the second edition of this book:

- Our work colleagues Thelma Lackey and Erika Thorne for providing expert advice and review.
- The book reviewers who all provided constructive and helpful feedback throughout the production process.
- The British Association of Critical Care Nurses (BACCN) for allowing reproduction of their material within the book.
- The National Institute for Health and Care Excellence (NICE) for allowing reproduction of their material within the book.
- The Resuscitation Council (UK) for granting permission to use their resuscitation algorithms.
- The editing team at Oxford University Press for all their support throughout the production process.

Contents

Symbols and abbreviations

↓	decreased
↑	increased
➲	cross-reference
🖱	website
ABG	arterial blood gas
ACE	angiotensin-converting enzyme
ACS	acute coronary syndrome
ACT	activated clotting time
ADH	antidiuretic hormone
AFB	acid-fast bacilli
AFE	amniotic fluid embolism
AKI	acute kidney injury
ALL	acute lymphatic leukaemia
ALS	advanced life support
ALT	alanine aminotransferase
AML	acute myeloid leukaemia
APACHE II	Acute Physiology and Chronic Health Evaluation II
APC	antigen-presenting cell
APRV	airway pressure release ventilation
APTT	activated partial thromboplastin time
ARDS	acute respiratory distress syndrome
AST	aspartate aminotransferase
ATLS	advanced trauma life support
AV	atrioventricular
AVPU	Alert Verbal Pain Unresponsive
BACCN	British Association of Critical Care Nurses
BIS	Bispectral Index
BMI	body mass index
BPAP	bi-level positive airway pressure
BPS	Behavioural Pain Scale
BSD	brainstem death
CAM-ICU	Confusion Assessment Method-ICU

CLL	chronic lymphatic leukaemia
CML	chronic myeloid leukaemia
CMV	controlled manual ventilation; cytomegalovirus
CNS	central nervous system
COPD	chronic obstructive pulmonary disease
CPAP	continuous positive airway pressure
CPP	cerebral perfusion pressure
CRP	C-reactive protein
CSF	cerebrospinal fluid
CSW	cerebral salt wasting
CT	computerized tomography
CVP	central venous pressure
CVS	cardiovascular system
CVVH	continuous venovenous haemofiltration
CVVHD	continuous venovenous haemodialysis
CVVHDF	continuous venovenous haemodiafiltration
DI	diabetes insipidus
DIC	disseminated intravascular coagulation
DIS	daily interruption of sedation
DKA	diabetic ketoacidosis
DVT	deep vein thrombosis
ECG	electrocardiogram
ECMO	extracorporeal membrane oxygenation
EEG	electroencephalogram
ERCP	endoscopic retrograde cholangiopancreatography
$ETCO_2$	end-tidal carbon dioxide
ETT	endotracheal tube
EVD	external ventricular drain
EVLW	extravascular lung water
FBC	full blood count
FFP	fresh frozen plasma
F_iO_2	fractionated inspired oxygen concentration
FRC	functional residual capacity
FTc	corrected flow time
GBS	Guillain–Barré syndrome

GCS	Glasgow Coma Scale
GEDV	global end-diastolic volume
GFR	glomerular filtration rate
GMC	General Medical Council
GRV	gastric residual volume
GTN	glyceryl trinitrate
h	hour
HADS	Hospital Anxiety and Depression Scale
Hb	haemoglobin
HELLP	haemolysis, elevated liver enzymes and low platelets
HEPA	high-efficiency particulate air
HES	hydroxyethyl starch
HHS	hyperglycaemic hyperosmolar state
HIT	heparin-induced thrombocytopenia
HIV	human immunodeficiency virus
HUS	haemolytic uraemic syndrome
ICDSC	Intensive Care Delirium Screening Checklist
ICP	intracranial pressure
ICS	Intensive Care Society
ICU	intensive care unit
IHD	intermittent haemodialysis
INR	international normalized ratio
IPPV	intermittent positive pressure ventilation
ITBV	intra-thoracic blood volume
ITP	idiopathic thrombocytopenic purpura
IV	intravenous
IVIG	intravenous immunoglobulin
JVP	jugular venous pressure
L	litre
LBBB	left bundle branch block
LFT	liver function test
LiDCO	lithium dilution cardiac output
LMWH	low-molecular-weight heparin
LOC	level of consciousness
LVF	left ventricular failure

MAP	mean arterial pressure
MC&S	microscopy, culture, and sensitivity
MI	myocardial infarction
min	minute
MODS	Multiple Organ Dysfunction Score; multi-organ dysfunction syndrome
MRI	magnetic resonance imaging
MV	minute volume
NEWS	National Early Warning Score
NICE	National Institute for Health and Care Excellence
NIV	non-invasive ventilation
NMBA	neuromuscular blocking agent
NSAID	non-steroidal anti-inflammatory drug
NSTEMI	non-ST-segment elevation myocardial infarction
PA	pulmonary artery
$PaCO_2$	partial pressure of arterial carbon dioxide
PaO_2	partial pressure of arterial oxygen
P_AO_2	partial pressure of alveolar oxygen
PAOP	pulmonary artery occlusion pressure
PAP	pulmonary artery pressure
PAWP	pulmonary artery wedge pressure
PCA	patient-controlled analgesia
PCC	prothrombin complex concentrate
PCI	percutaneous coronary intervention
PCV	packed cell volume
PE	pulmonary embolism
PEA	pulseless electrical activity
PEEP	positive end expiratory pressure
PEFR	peak expiratory flow rate
PEJ	percutaneous jejunostomy
PET	positron emission tomography
PiCCO	pulse contour cardiac output
POCT	point-of-care testing
P-PCI	primary percutaneous coronary intervention
PPH	postpartum haemorrhage

PSV	pressure support ventilation
PT	prothrombin time
PVC	polyvinyl chloride
$PvCO_2$	partial pressure of venous carbon dioxide
PvO_2	partial pressure of venous oxygen
PVR	pulmonary vascular resistance
RASS	Richmond Agitation Sedation Scale
RCN	Royal College of Nursing
REM	rapid eye movement
ROM	range of movement
RQ	respiratory quotient
RRT	renal replacement therapy
RSBI	Rapid Shallow Breathing Index
RVF	right ventricular failure
s	second
SAPS II/III	Simplified Acute Physiology Score II/III
SBAR	Situation, Background, Assessment, Recommendation
SBT	spontaneous breathing trial
SCUF	slow continuous ultrafiltration
SIADH	syndrome of inappropriate secretion of antidiuretic hormone
SIMV	synchronized intermittent mandatory ventilation
SIRS	systemic inflammatory response syndrome
SLE	systemic lupus erythematosus
SOFA	Sequential Organ Failure Assessment
SpO_2	oxygen saturation in arterial blood
STEMI	ST-segment elevation myocardial infarction
SVR	systemic vascular resistance
SVT	supraventricular tachycardia
SVV	stroke volume variation
SWS	slow-wave sleep
TB	tuberculosis
TENS	transcutaneous electrical nerve stimulation
TIA	transient ischaemic attack
TMA	thrombotic microangiopathy

tPA	tissue plasminogen activator
TPN	total parenteral nutrition
TTP	thrombotic thrombocytopenic purpura
U&E	urea and electrolytes
VAP	ventilator-associated pneumonia
VC	vital capacity
VF	ventricular fibrillation
VO_2	oxygen consumption
V/Q	ventilation/perfusion
VT	tidal volume
VT	ventricular tachycardia
VTE	venous thromboembolism
WBC	white blood cell
WBPTT	whole blood partial thromboplastin time
WFNS	World Federation of Neurosurgeons Scale

Chapter 1

Admission to critical care

Changes to the delivery of critical care

The changing face of acute nursing

The face of acute care and critical care has changed substantially over the last two decades. This change has been influenced by a number of factors, but perhaps most significantly by the increasing number of acutely ill patients within the hospital environment. A number of factors have influenced patient acuity, including:

- an ageing population with increased levels of comorbidity
- use of advanced treatment modalities and technologies
- increased complexity of patient needs.

The changes in acuity levels have meant that healthcare providers have been faced with challenges related to caring for an increasing number of acutely and critically ill patients.

Over 15 years ago the National Audit Office[1] identified a lack of provision of critical care beds, and reported that demand for critical care beds often exceeded the number of such beds available. This necessitated an urgent review of critical care provision.

The publication of *Comprehensive Critical Care: a review of adult critical care services* by the Department of Health[2] a year later helped to redevelop the provision of acute and critical care services in the UK. This document marked the end of traditional boundaries associated with critical care, and emphasized the need for a hospital-wide approach to caring for acutely and critically ill patients.

The vision of comprehensive critical care was that hospitals should meet the needs of all critically ill patients, not just those in designated critical care beds, and gave rise to the concept of 'critical care without walls.' It highlighted both the need to radically change critical care provision, and the need for the following characteristics of a modern critical care service:

- integration of services beyond the boundaries of critical care units to allow provision of acute and critical care and the optimization of resources
- the development of critical care networks to share standards and protocols and to develop future care provision
- workforce development to ensure that all staff caring for acutely and critically ill patients have sufficient knowledge and training.

Recognition of deterioration

Alongside the redevelopment of critical care services, problems with the recognition of deterioration in the patient's condition were being highlighted.

A seminal study by McQuillan and colleagues[3] first introduced the now well-recognized concept of suboptimal care for acutely ill adults. Suboptimal care relates to multifactorial issues that contribute to misdiagnosis, mismanagement, and lack of timely intervention for acutely ill deteriorating patients. Delays in treating acutely ill patients were linked to unexpected deaths and unplanned and perhaps preventable admissions to critical care units.

McQuillan and colleagues'[3] study identified that over 50% of patients encountered suboptimal management prior to admission to critical care units. Unfortunately, similar statistics are still evident despite ongoing interventions to improve the situation. The current literature often uses the term 'failure to rescue' to refer to suboptimal care.

Factors related to suboptimal care—or, more recently, 'failure to rescue'—include:

- lack of knowledge and lack of experience in dealing with acutely ill patients
- failure to appreciate the urgency of the need to treat the patient's condition
- failure to seek senior or expert advice about the patient's condition
- lack of senior medical staff involvement
- organizational failings that prevent adequate assessment and management of the deteriorating patient.

A number of initiatives have been developed to improve recognition and management of the deteriorating patient. Analysis of the literature suggests that the number of preventable deaths and unplanned critical care admissions could be reduced if deteriorating patients were identified earlier and managed in a timely manner.

References

1 National Audit Office. *Critical to Success: the place of efficient and effective critical care services within the acute hospital.* Audit Commission: London, 1999.

2 Department of Health. *Comprehensive Critical Care: a review of adult critical care services.* Department of Health: London, 2000.

3 McQuillan P et al. Confidential inquiry into quality of care before admission to intensive care. *British Medical Journal* 1998; **316**: 1853–8.

Preventing admissions to critical care

A number of initiatives have been implemented to help to prevent the admission of acutely ill patients into critical care units. These initiatives include:

- development of critical care outreach teams
- development of early warning scores
- utilization of medical emergency teams
- education initiatives.

Critical care outreach

The widespread development of critical care outreach services followed the publication of *Comprehensive Critical Care: a review of adult critical care services.*[4] Indeed, the National Institute for Health and Care Excellence (NICE)[5] identified the need to establish outreach services in all acute hospitals 24 hours a day, 7 days a week.

Outreach teams were initially established with the following key aims:

- to avert admission to critical care units
- to support staff in ward areas
- to provide education programmes for ward-based staff
- to support critical care patients following transfer from critical care, in order to avert readmissions
- to provide follow-up services on discharge from hospital, to determine the impact of critical care on the patient.

The implementation of outreach has not been consistent across acute trusts, and various teams have been developed. These include:

- critical care outreach teams
- patient at-risk teams
- rapid response teams.

Although differences exist between various configurations of critical care outreach teams, these teams are generally nurse led and have been introduced to support and help to educate ward nurses when they are caring for deteriorating and acutely ill patients. Unfortunately there is little substantive research to support the effectiveness of outreach in improving patient outcomes. Therefore more research is needed to review the effectiveness of the role of outreach.[6]

Early warning scores

These were introduced to try to help ward staff to recognize and respond to deteriorating patients on general wards. The systems use routine physiological measurements, and each measurement is given a numerical value depending on the variation from normal parameters. The individual parameter scores are added together and an aggregate score is then obtained that highlights the need for patient review. Put simply, the higher the score, the more ill the patient is. The early warning scores are linked to an escalation process.

Table 1.1 NEWS abnormal observation values

	3	2	1	1	2	3
Respiratory rate (breaths/min)	≤ 8		9–11		21–24	≥ 25
Heart rate (beats/min)	≤ 40		41–50	91–110	111–130	≥ 131
Systolic blood pressure (mmHg)	≤ 90	91–100	100–110			≥220
Temperature (°C)	≤ 35		35.1–36	38.1–39	≥ 39.1	
Oxygen saturation (%)	≤ 91	92–93	94–95			
Supplemental oxygen		Yes				
Level of consciousness						V, P, or U

Table 1.2 NEWS escalation tool

NEWS score	Frequency of monitoring	Clinical response
0	Minimum of 12-hourly	Continue routine NEWS monitoring
Total: 1–4	Minimum of 4- to 6-hourly	Inform registered nurse
Total: 5 or more or 3 in one parameter	Hourly observations	Inform medical team urgently Urgent assessment by clinician with core competencies Monitoring required
Total: 7 or more	Continuous observations	Immediately inform specialist registrar Emergency assessment by staff with critical care competencies Consider move to higher level of care

Most recently the Royal College of Physicians has been instrumental in developing a National Early Warning Score (NEWS)[7] that is in the process of being implemented throughout the UK.

This tool has been developed to provide standardization of assessment and escalation processes throughout NHS trusts. The NEWS system provides values for each observation recorded (see Table 1.1). The aggregate NEWS score is then linked to a national escalation policy (see Table 1.2). It is anticipated that implementation of this system will enable consistency in detecting and responding to acutely ill patients, and help to avoid admissions to critical care by identifying deteriorating patients earlier.

Medical emergency teams and emergency response teams

Medical emergency teams have been developed in many NHS trusts to respond immediately to a medical emergency. It is thought that a rapid response to a deteriorating patient may provide the opportunity to intervene and quickly treat symptoms. This may help to avert cardiac arrests, further deterioration, and subsequent admission to critical care units.

Medical emergency teams normally consist of doctors and nurses who possess advanced life support skills. The aim of the team is to respond early to patient deterioration and provide an immediate coordinated response for the acutely ill deteriorating patient. Calls to the team may be in response to a trigger from an early warning score (see Table 1.2), or may be based on a nurse's or doctor's concern about the patient.

Although there is no significant research to support these teams yet, there is compelling evidence that the medical emergency teams may improve quality of care for seriously ill patients who are nursed outside critical care areas.

Education initiatives

Other educational initiatives have also been developed to help to provide a multidisciplinary approach to assessment and management of the acutely ill patient .The rationale of these programmes is to provide an understanding of systematic patient assessment tools (see Chapter 2) and initial management of the deteriorating patient.

Courses are either multidisciplinary or medically focused, and use a range of low- to high-fidelity simulation scenarios to teach assessment and management of the deteriorating patient. These programmes include:

- acute NHS trust in-house training days
- the Acute Life-threatening Events Recognition and Treatment (ALERT©) programme
- the Acute Illness Management (AIM) course
- Care of the Critically Ill Surgical Patient (CCrISP®)
- Ill Medical Patients Acute Care and Treatment (IMPACT).

References

4 Department of Health. *Comprehensive Critical Care: a review of adult critical care services.* Department of Health: London, 2000.

5 National Institute for Health and Care Excellence (NICE). *Acutely Ill Patients in Hospital: recognition of and response to acute illness in adults in hospital.* CG50. NICE: London, 2007. ➚ www.nice.org.uk/guidance/cg50

6 Rowan K et al. *Evaluation of Outreach Services in Critical Care.* National Intensive Care Research and Audit Committee: London, 2009.

7 Royal College of Physicians. *National Early Warning Score (NEWS): standardising the assessment of acute-illness severity in the NHS. Report of a working party.* Royal College of Physicians: London, 2012.

Levels of care

These were first devised in 2000 by the Department of Health[8] to help to replace traditional boundaries that labelled patients as critical care patients or ward patients. Linked to the concept of 'critical care without walls', these levels help to clarify the dependency levels of patients and assist in informing decision making about the management of patient care.

The initial levels were highlighted by the Department of Health (see Table 1.3.). These levels were too simplistic, and were soon superseded by levels published by the Intensive Care Society,[9] which gave further guidance about what might be appropriate patient management at each level. The Intensive Care Society levels provide specific examples (see Table 1.4). Further details of specific examples can be found on the Intensive Care Society website (www.ics.ac.uk).

Table 1.3 Levels of care[8]

Level	Descriptor
0	Patients whose needs can be met in a ward environment
1	Patients at risk of deterioration who can be managed in a ward area with additional advice and support (this includes patients recently relocated from higher levels of care)
2	Patients who require detailed observation and support of a single failing system, or complex post-operative care (again this includes patients recently relocated from higher levels of care)
3	Patients who require advanced respiratory support or basic respiratory support together with support of at least two organ systems (also includes patients with multi-organ failure)

Table 1.4 Additional guidance, adapted from Intensive Care Society levels of care[9]

	Level criteria	Selected specific examples*
Level 1	Patients recently discharged from higher level of care	Requiring a minimum of 4-hourly observations
	Patients in need of additional monitoring	Continuous oxygen, epidurals, patient-controlled analgesia (PCA), tracheostomy *in situ*
	Patients requiring critical care support	Risk of clinical deterioration, or patient has abnormal observations
Level 2	Patients requiring pre-operative optimization	CVS, respiratory, or renal optimization
	Patients requiring extended post-operative care	Major or emergency surgery, and risk of complications
	Patients stepping down from a higher level of care	Needing hourly observation and at risk of deterioration
	Patients requiring:	
	• single organ support	Non-invasive ventilation; intubated to protect airway
	• basic respiratory or CVS support	Insertion of CVP or arterial line
	• advanced CVS support	Single vasoactive drug or cardiac output monitoring
	• renal support	Renal replacement therapy
	• neurological support	CNS depression, ICP monitoring, EVD
	• dermatological support	Major skin rashes, exfoliation, burns, or complex dressings
Level 3	Patients receiving advanced respiratory support alone	Invasive mechanical ventilation or extracorporeal support
	Patients receiving support for a minimum of two organs	Ventilation plus support of at least one other failing system

*Complete list is available on ICS website (www.ics.ac.uk).

References

8 Department of Health. *Comprehensive Critical Care: a review of adult critical care services.* Department of Health: London, 2000.

9 Intensive Care Society. *Levels of Critical Care for Adult Patients.* Intensive Care Society: London, 2009.

Admission criteria

Although the number of critical care beds has increased steadily over the past decade, there are still situations in which provision of critical care beds does not meet demand for critical care admission. Recent statistical evidence from NHS England[10] has identified a critical care bed occupancy rate of 87.8%, suggesting a service that is near to full capacity. Shortages of critical care beds may have far-reaching implications in practice, including:

- reduced access to critical care beds
- enforced transfer of critically ill patients
- cancelled urgent and elective procedures.

As critical care is a limited resource, it needs to target those patients who are most likely to benefit from admission to critical care units. Although decisions relating to admission are complex and multifactorial, and it is difficult to provide clear guidance on admission criteria, it is clear that decisions relating to admission (or, more importantly, non-admission) should be based on objective, ethical, and transparent decision-making processes.[11]

The General Medical Council (GMC) provides guidance on ethical and legal aspects of decision making, but it is sometimes difficult to apply these to critical care patients for whom the level of complexity of needs and the disease trajectory are not always clear.

A number of guiding principles may be used to assist the decision-making process, and it is important to remember that admission to a critical care unit may not be an appropriate decision for all patients. It is recommended that admission criteria should be available in all critical care units. It is therefore imperative that any local admissions policies and guidelines are utilized in conjunction with the critical care admission team. The critical care consultant's decision about admission would always take precedence over the decision of other medical staff.

Guiding principles for admission

Fullerton and Perkins[11] suggest that it is useful to:

- review the patient, and establish ongoing comorbidities and responses to current treatment
- formulate a prognosis
- discuss the risks and associated burdens of treatment with the patient and their carers
- reach a consensus on the treatment plan, and agree any ceilings to treatment in advance.

In general, critical care admission is appropriate if:

- the patient's condition is potentially reversible
- the patient can reasonably be expected to survive the critical care admission
- there is reasonable doubt about the likely outcome for the patient.

Factors that may preclude admission to critical care include the following:

- the patient's condition is likely to be fatal and will not be amenable to recovery, or has progressed beyond any reasonable likelihood of recovery
- the patient's pre-existing comorbidities make the prospect of recovery very unlikely
- the patient has mental capacity and refuses to be admitted on the basis of either an advance directive or discussion with the critical care team.

References

10 NHS England. *Critical Care Bed Capacity and Urgent Operations Cancelled 2013–14 Data.* ℛ www.england.nhs.uk/statistics/statistical-work-areas/critical-care-capacity/critical-care-bed-capacity-and-urgent-operations-cancelled-2013-14-data

11 Fullerton JN and Perkins GD. Who to admit to intensive care? *Clinical Medicine* 2011; **11**: 601–4.

Organizing admission to critical care

Nursing responsibilities

It is important that the critical care nurse possesses the appropriate skills, knowledge, and attitudes to safely admit patients to the critical care unit. The Critical Care Networks-National Nurse Leads (CC3N) have recently published competencies relating to critical care nursing.[12] One of the Step 1 Competencies relates to admissions to critical care. The key responsibilities for an effective admission to critical care include:

- safe preparation of the bed area
- safe staffing levels within the intensive care area
- initial assessment and monitoring of the critically ill patient
- communication with the patient and their family or carers.

Safe preparation of the bed area

It is likely that each individual critical care unit will have an admission protocol describing in detail how to prepare adequately for admission of a patient to critical care. If such a protocol is available it should be followed. There are several guiding principles for preparing the bed area:

- Follow local guidance relating to appropriate cleaning of the area to prevent cross-contamination from the previous patient in that bed area. Personal protective equipment should be readily available at each bed area.
- Prepare any equipment that will be required for care of the patient. This should be ready to use and safety checks completed according to local protocols. Equipment that is likely to be needed for most patients includes an appropriate ventilator, intubation equipment, safety equipment, syringe drivers, infusion pumps, and trolleys for cannulation and arterial line insertion.
- Monitoring systems should be ready to use, and additional disposable equipment such as ECG electrodes should be prepared in advance. Pressure bags and transducers should be prepared and labelled according to local guidelines.
- Computerized documentation systems for patients should be ready to use. Smaller units may still utilize paper documentation, and if so this should be prepared in advance.
- The patient details should provide an indication of the severity of the patient's condition, especially in the case of an unplanned or emergency admission. It is likely that additional staff may be required to assist with admission of an unstable critically ill patient, and this should be organized prior to admission of the patient.
- Consideration should be given to providing same-sex accommodation wherever possible.[13] In situations where this is not feasible, consideration should be given to maintaining the dignity and privacy of the patient in mixed-sex accommodation.

Safe staffing levels within the intensive care area

With regard to staffing levels, the British Association of Critical Care Nurses (BACCN)[14] and the Royal College of Nursing (RCN)[15] have provided guiding principles. Many factors may affect staffing levels, and it is difficult to provide an exact guide to what represents a safe number of staff. Local policies based on the BACCN and RCN guidelines may be used to determine safe staff numbers, as staffing is affected by a number of locally determined factors, including the following:

- The acuity levels of these patients (i.e. the number of level 2 and level 3 patients). Very critically ill patients may require two nurses for periods of care.
- The design of the unit. Units where the environment and design of the unit limit the ability to overview other patients may need increased staffing ratios.
- Flexibility should be built in to allow for unplanned events such as intra-hospital transfers or sudden deterioration.

The BACCN guidelines emphasize that it is essential for all patients to have immediate access to a registered nurse with a post-registration qualification. They suggest that level 3 patients should be nursed with a ratio of 1:1, and that the ratio for care of level 2 patients should not exceed 1:2. Problems with staffing ratios should be reported and acted upon by the nurse in charge of the unit, in order to maintain patient safety.

Initial assessment of the patient

The patient's condition will need to be assessed on admission and then reassessed frequently until it has stabilized. In the case of emergency and unplanned admissions it is likely that initial patient assessment will involve several members of the critical care team so that any life-threatening problems can be quickly identified and appropriate management provided. At the very minimum the patient should be assessed by the receiving nurse and a member of medical staff from the critical care team.

The initial assessment should be thorough and systematic. Use of the ABCDE system (see Chapter 2) ensures that life-threatening problems are assessed and managed first, before other assessments are undertaken. It also ensures that a quick and robust assessment of the patient is performed.

In addition, the initial assessment should include a full physical assessment and documentation of any areas of concern (e.g. previous pressure damage, bruising or injury prior to admission). It is important that consideration is also given to assessment of mental health status, mental capacity, and any advance directives.

Assessment for previous resistant infections should be undertaken, and local protocols followed with regard to isolation of patients transferred from other areas within the hospital, and for referrals from another hospital.

Alongside these assessments you may also be required to assess other areas that will have an impact on nursing. This will be determined by local policy, but may include:

- venous thromboembolism risk
- pressure damage risk
- nutritional assessment
- falls risk
- data collection for audit purposes
- acuity and patient scoring systems information (e.g. APACHE II, SAPS II/III, MODS, and SOFA scores). Some of these data may be obtained from electronic patient record systems.

All of the information that is obtained during the initial assessment should be either documented electronically on computerized systems or recorded on paper. This will ensure ongoing effective documented assessment and identification of the patient's needs. All of the information that is obtained at the initial assessment can then be utilized to plan effective care for the patient. Assessment findings should be communicated effectively to other members of the multidisciplinary teams, as this has been shown to improve patient safety by ensuring continuity of appropriate care.

Communication with the patient and their family or carers

Admission to the critical care environment can be a frightening experience for the patient and their family or carers, and it is vital that effective communication and psychological support are provided for all of these individuals.

It is universally accepted that communication with the patient is vital irrespective of whether they are conscious or unconscious on admission to the critical care unit. If the patient is conscious and has mental capacity, it is important that they are communicated with effectively and actively involved in decision making about their treatment and ongoing care. Family members may be able to provide insight into the patient's wishes if the patient lacks mental capacity or is unconscious.

Most critical care units provide printed booklets containing information for patients and relatives. Such information is also available from the Intensive Care Society[16] and ICUSteps[17].

Effective communication with families and carers is important, especially in the early stages of admission, as it is unlikely that they will be able to see the patient during the initial stages of assessment and treatment, or until the patient's condition has been stabilized. Effective communication about the need to stabilize and assess the patient first is vital for helping to establish trusting relationships with families and carers. The provision of honest, realistic information in a form that can be easily understood is essential both during the initial period of care and subsequently.

References

12 Critical Care Networks-National Nurse Leads (CC3N). *National Competency Framework for Adult Critical Care Nurses*. CC3N, 2013. ✆ www.cc3n.org.uk/competency-framework/4577977310

13 Department of Health. *Impact Assessment of Delivering Same Sex Accommodation*. Department of Health: London, 2009.

14 Bray K et al. *Standards for Nurse Staffing in Critical Care*. British Association of Critical Care Nurses (BACCN), Critical Care Networks-National Nurse Leads, and Royal College of Nursing Critical Care Forum: Newcastle upon Tyne, 2010.

15 Galley K and O'Riordan B. *Guidance for Nurse Staffing in Critical Care*. Royal College of Nursing: London, 2007. ✆ www.rcn.org.uk/__data/assets/pdf_file/0008/78560/001976.pdf

16 Intensive Care Society. *Patient Information Booklets*. Intensive Care Society: London. ✆ http://www.ics.ac.uk/icf/patients-and-relatives/patient-information-booklets/

17 ICUSteps. *Intensive care: a guide for patients and families*. ICUSteps: Milton-Keynes, 2010. ✆ http://icusteps.org/guide

Further reading

British Association of Critical Care Nurses (BACCN). ✆ www.baccn.org

Faculty of Intensive Care Medicine. ✆ http://www.ficm.ac.uk/

Gibson V and Hill K. Admitting a critically ill patient. In: Mallett J, Albarran JW, and Richardson A (eds) *Critical Care Manual of Clinical Procedures and Competencies*. John Wiley & Sons, Ltd.: Chichester, 2013. pp. 59–62.

Intensive Care Society. ✆ www.ics.ac.uk

Royal College of Physicians. ✆ www.rcplondon.ac.uk

Chapter 2

Systematic assessment

Assessment principles and strategies

A systematic assessment of the patient is required in order to optimize patient care and management. At the very minimum a patient assessment should be conducted on admission and at the start of each nursing handover. Additional assessments will be prompted by changes in the patient's status. Depending on the severity of the patient's condition, the assessment may need to be conducted rapidly.

The assessment process consists of a review of the patient's past medical history, the reason for their admission to the critical care unit and/or the problems currently being experienced by the patient, and the findings of the physical assessment of the patient.

Principles of history taking

History taking is an important element of the assessment of a patient, as it identifies contemporary and past illnesses, indicates how the patient and their family are affected by the illness, introduces the patient to the nurse and the care setting, and will inform the clinical diagnosis.

- Put the patient at ease to enable full disclosure of their health history.
- Start with broad questions and then move on to system-specific questions.
- Identify the primary signs and symptoms of the problem that is being experienced by the patient (e.g. chronology, severity, duration, triggers, relievers).
- Include questions about the patient's past medical, medication, family, and social history.

Principles of physical assessment

The physical assessment involves a 'look, listen, and feel' approach that corresponds to the following more formal medical terms:

- inspection
- palpation
- percussion
- auscultation.

All assessment findings should be documented in an agreed format and communicated to the multidisciplinary team and the patient as appropriate. Document the resuscitation status of the patient and the maximum level of care offered in the event of further deterioration.

Common assessment strategies include:

- ABCDE assessment
- head-to-toe assessment
- focused assessment (e.g. by body system) (see Chapters 4, 6, 8, 9, and 10).

Further reading

Cox C *Physical Assessment for Nurses.*, 2nd ed. Wiley-Blackwell: Chichester, 2009.

Douglas G, Nicol F and Robertson C (eds). *Macleod's Clinical Examination*, 13th ed. Churchill Livingstone: Edinburgh, 2013.

Hogan-Quigley B, Palm ML and Bickley LS. *Bates' Nursing Guide to Physical Examination and History Taking*. Lippincott Williams & Wilkins: Philadelphia, PA, 2011.

Ranson M, Abbott H and Braithwaite W (eds). *Clinical Examination Skills for Healthcare Professionals*. M&K Update: Keswick UK, 2014.

ABCDE assessment

This approach assesses the A[illegible] of airway, Breathing, Circulation, Disability, and Exposure. This assessment strategy is commonly used in [illegible] and is particularly suited to the [illegible] assessment of a patient.

Airway

Indicators of airway compromise (see Box 2.1):

- Look for [illegible] of [illegible] accessory muscles [illegible] (see [illegible] and [illegible]) [illegible]
- Listen for the [illegible]
- Feel for movement [illegible]

Breathing

Indicators of respiratory compromise:

- Look for signs of increased [illegible] accessory muscles [illegible] breathing [illegible]
- Listen for [illegible] breath sounds [illegible]
- Feel for [illegible]
- Record [illegible]

For specialist respiratory assessment [illegible] see Chapter 4.

Box 2.1 Airway obstruction

- [illegible]

ABCDE assessment

This consists of assessment of Airway, Breathing, Circulation, Disability, and Exposure. This assessment strategy is commonly used in a critical care context, and is particularly suited to the rapid or emergency assessment of a patient.

Airway

Indicators of airway compromise (see Box 2.1)

- **Look** for altered or increased respiratory effort, use of accessory muscles (sternocleidomastoid, trapezius, and internal intercostals), paradoxical chest and abdominal movements 'see-saw respiration', drooling (inability of the patient to swallow their own saliva), and bleeding from the nose, mouth or tracheostomy.
- **Listen** for hoarseness, stridor, snoring, gurgling, and inability to speak.
- **Feel** for movement of expired air from the mouth or nose, and for sweaty or clammy skin.

Breathing

Indicators of respiratory compromise

- **Look** for altered or increased respiratory effort, use of accessory muscles (sternocleidomastoid, trapezius, and internal intercostals), nasal flaring, pursed-lip breathing, inability to lie flat, central cyanosis, depth of breathing, pattern of breathing, unilateral chest expansion, chest and/or spinal deformity, presence and patency of chest drains, chest surgery (past or present), trauma, bruising, bleeding, and flail chest.
- **Listen** for inability to complete full sentences, audible breath sounds, and abnormal breath sounds via auscultation of the anterior, lateral, and posterior surfaces of the chest (unilateral, inspiratory and/or expiratory wheeze, crackles, pleural rub, and bronchial, decreased, or absent breath sounds).
- **Feel** for tracheal deviation, subcutaneous emphysema, crepitus, thoracic tenderness, and abnormal resonance via percussion (hyper-resonance or dullness).
- **Record** the respiratory rate (normal range, 12–20 breaths/min) and oxygen saturations (normal range, 97–100%).

For specialized respiratory assessment and monitoring, see Chapter 4.

Box 2.1 Airway obstruction

- In **complete airway obstruction** there is no air entry, with absent breath sounds and paradoxical chest and abdominal movements.
- In **partial airway obstruction** there is decreased air entry, with abnormal breath sounds and altered or increased respiratory effort.

Circulation

Indicators of circulatory compromise

- **Look** for pallor, cyanosis (peripheral and central), chest deformity, jugular venous distension, cardiac devices (pacemaker or implantable defibrillator), bruising, and haemorrhage.
- **Listen** for reduced level of consciousness due to poor cardiac output (confusion, drowsiness), complaints of chest pain, and abnormal heart sounds via auscultation (S3, S4, murmurs, pericardial rub).
- **Feel** for pulse rhythm and strength, capillary refill time (normal value ≤ 3 s), limb temperature, and sweaty, clammy, warm, or cool skin.
- **Record** heart rate (normal range, 60–100 beats/min), blood pressure (normal range, mean arterial pressure ≥ 65 mmHg), central venous pressure (normal range, 2–10 mmHg), urine output (normal range, ≥ 0.5 mL/kg/h), and core temperature (normal range, 36–37.5°C).

For specialized cardiac assessment and monitoring, see Chapter 6.

Disability

Indicators of neurological compromise

- **Look** for pupil size, equality, and reaction to light, as well as head trauma and cerebrospinal fluid leakage (otorrhoea, rhinorrhoea).
- **Listen** for reduced level of consciousness due to poor neurological function (confusion, drowsiness), and complaints of pain.
- **Record** the blood glucose concentration (normal range, 4–8 mmol/L), Alert Verbal Pain Unresponsive (AVPU) response (normal response, Alert), and Glasgow Coma Scale (GCS) score (normal score, 15/15) (see Table 2.1).

For specialized neurological assessment and monitoring, see Chapter 8.

Exposure

Indicators of physiological compromise

- **Look** for bleeding, bruising, burns, rashes, swelling, inflammation, infection, and wounds on the body.
- **Listen** for complaints of pain, pruritus, heat, and cold.
- **Feel** for venous thromboembolism and oedema.

Table 2.1 Glasgow Coma Scale (GCS)

Eye response		Verbal response		Motor response	
Spontaneous	4	Orientated	5	Obeys commands	6
To speech	3	Confused	4	Localizes to pain	5
To pain	2	Inappropriate words	3	Flexion to pain	4
No response	1	Incomprehensible sounds	2	Abnormal flexion	3
		No response	1	Extension	2
				No response	1

Head-to-toe assessment

This assessment strategy is best used in combination with the ABCDE assessment. It also focuses on physical assessment and observations, but is suitable for the routine assessment of a critically ill patient.

Head

In addition to the Disability section of the ABCDE assessment:

Assess pain

- Assess every 4 hours or as necessary.
- If the patient is able to self-report, use a numerical rating scale (e.g. scale of 0 to 10 where 0 = no pain and 10 = worst pain ever experienced). Ask the patient to score their pain from 0 to 10, and ensure that pain is assessed on movement (e.g. when the patient coughs).
- If the patient is unable to self-report, use the Behavioural Pain Scale (BPS) (score in the range 3–12) (see Table 2.2).

Assess delirium

- Assess every shift or as necessary (see Box 2.2).
- Use a delirium screening tool—e.g. the Confusion Assessment Method-ICU (CAM-ICU) (see Figure 2.1) or the Intensive Care Delirium Screening Checklist (ICDSC) (0–12) (see Figure 2.2).

Delirium is an acute event that develops over hours or days, and has a medical rather than psychiatric cause. Delirium subtypes are as follows:

- **hypoactive patient**—withdrawn, lethargic, apathetic, or may even be unresponsive
- **hyperactive patient**—extremely agitated, emotionally labile, exhibiting disruptive behaviours such as refusing care, shouting, violence, removing cannulae, and attempting to self-discharge.

Table 2.2 Behavioural Pain Scale (BPS)

Item	Description	Score
Facial expression	Relaxed	1
	Partially tightened (e.g. brow lowering)	2
	Fully tightened (e.g. eyelid closing)	3
	Grimacing	4
Upper limbs	No movement	1
	Partially flexed	2
	Fully flexed with finger flexion	3
	Permanently retracted	4
Compliance with ventilation	Tolerating ventilation	1
	Coughing but tolerating ventilation	2
	Fighting ventilator	3
	Unable to control ventilation	4

Box 2.2 Features of delirium

- Acute change or fluctuating course of mental status *and*
- inattention *and*
- altered level of consciousness *or*
- disorganized thinking.

Feature 1: Acute onset or fluctuating course	Score	Check here if Present
Is the patient different than his/her baseline mental status? OR Has the patient had any fluctuation in mental status in the past 24 hours as evidenced by fluctuation on a sedation/level of consciousness scale (i.e., RASS/SAS), GCS, or previous delirium assessment?	Either question Yes →	☐
Feature 2: Inattention		
Letters Attention Test (See training manual for alternative **pictures**) Directions: Say to the patient, *"I am going to read you a series of 10 letters. Whenever you hear the letter 'A,' indicate by squeezing my hand."* Read letters from the following letter list in a normal tone 3 seconds apart. **S A V E A H A A R T** or **C A S A B L A N C A** or **A B A D B A D A A Y** **Errors are counted when patient fails to squeeze on the letter "A" and when the patient squeezes on any letter other than "A."**	Number of errors >2 →	☐
Feature 3: Altered level of consciousness		
Present if the Actual RASS score is anything other than alert and calm (zero)	RASS anything other than zero →	☐
Feature 4: Disorganized thinking		
Yes/No questions (See training manual for alternate set of questions) 1. Will a stone float on water? 2. Are there fish in the sea? 3. Does one pound weigh more than two pounds? 4. Can you use a hammer to pound a nail? **Errors are counted when the patient incorrectly answers a question.** Command Say to patient: "Hold up this many fingers" (Hold 2 fingers in front of patient) "Now do the same thing with the other hand" (Do not repeat number of fingers) *If the patient is unable to move both arms, for 2nd part of command ask patient to "Add one more finger" **An error is counted if patient is unable to complete the entire command.**	Combined number of errors >1→	☐

Overall CAM-ICU **Feature 1 plus 2 and either 3 or 4 present = CAM-ICU positive**	**Criteria met →**	☐ **CAM-ICU positive (delirium present)**
	Criteria not met →	☐ **CAM-ICU negative (no delirium)**

Figure 2.1 Confusion Assessment Method-ICU (CAM-ICU) worksheet. (Reproduced with permission from Vanderbilt Medical University. Copyright © 2013, E. Wesley Ely, MD, MPH and Vanderbilt University, all rights reserved.)

Tufts Medical Center

Intensive Care Delirium Screening Checklist Worksheet (ICDSC)

- Score your patient over the entire shift. Components don't all need to be present at the same time.
- Components #1 through #4 require a focused bedside patient assessment. This cannot be completed when the patient is deeply sedated or comatose (ie. SAS = 1 or 2; RASS = –4 or –5).
- Components #5 through #8 are based on observations throughout the entire shift. Information from the prior 24 hrs (i.e. from prior 1-2 nursing shifts) should be obtained for components #7 and #8.

1. Altered level of consciousness — NO 0 1 Yes

Deep sedation/coma over entire shift [SAS = 1, 2; RASS = –4,–5]	= Not assessable
Agitation [SAS = 5, 6, or 7; RASS = 1-4] at any point	= 1 point
Normal wakefulness [SAS = 4; RASS = 0] over the entire shift	= 0 points
Light sedation [SAS = 3; RASS = –1, –2, –3]:	= 1 point (if no recent sedatives) = 0 points (if recent sedatives)

2. Inattention — NO 0 1 Yes

Difficulty following instructions or conversation, patient easily distracted by external stimuli.
Will not reliably squeeze hands to spoken letter A: **S A V E A H A A R T**

3. Disorientation — NO 0 1 Yes

In addition to name, place, and date, does the patient recognize ICU caregivers?
Does patient know what kind of place they are in?
(list examples: dentist's office, home, work, hospital)

4. Hallucination, delusion, or psychosis — NO 0 1 Yes

Ask the patient if they are having hallucinations or delusions
(e.g. trying to catch an object that isn't there).
Are they afraid of the people or things around them?

5. Psychomotor agitation or retardation — NO 0 1 Yes

Either: (a) Hyperactivity requiring the use of sedative drugs or restraints in order to control potentially dangerous behavior (e.g. pulling IV lines out or hitting staff)
OR (b) Hypoactive or clinically noticeable psychomotor slowing or retardation

6. Inappropriate speech or mood — NO 0 1 Yes

Patient displays: inappropriate emotion; disorganized or incoherent speech; sexual or inappropriate interactions; is either apathetic or overly demanding

7. Sleep–wake cycle disturbance — NO 0 1 Yes

Either: frequent awakening/< 4 hours sleep at night OR sleeping during much of the day

8. Symptom fluctuation — NO 0 1 Yes

Fluctuation of any of the above symptoms over a 24–hr period.

TOTAL SHIFT SCORE: ______ **(0–8)**

Score	Classification
0	Normal
1–3	Subsyndromal delirium
4–8	Delirium

Adapted from: Bergeron et al. Intensive Care Medicine 2001; 27 :859–64; Oulmet et al. Intensive Care Medicine 2007; 33: 1007–13.

Figure 2.2 Intensive Care Delirium Screening Checklist (ICDSC). (Reproduced with permission from Vanderbilt Medical University. Copyright © 2013, E. Wesley Ely, MD, MPH and Vanderbilt University, all rights reserved.)

Table 2.3 lists the risk factors that predispose critical care patients to delirium.

Assess sedation

- Assess every 24 h or as necessary.
- Use a sedation scoring system—for example, the Richmond Agitation Sedation Scale (RASS) (see Box 2.3 for sedation goals).

Table 2.3 Risk factors for delirium

All critical care patients	Critical care patients over 80 years of age
History of: • hypertension • smoking • sensory impairment • malnutrition	History of: • depression • cognitive impairment • dementia
Raised bilirubin level	Raised urea:creatinine ratio
Treatments: • epidural, urinary catheter, physical restraint	
Medications • benzodiazepines, opioids	
Severity of illness	

Box 2.3 Goals of sedation

- Rouse easily.
- Maintain diurnal rhythm.
- Relieve anxiety and discomfort.
- Facilitate treatments.
- Minimize harmful physiological responses (e.g. increased oxygenation, increased ICP).

Respiratory and ventilation

In addition to the Airway and Breathing sections of the ABCDE assessment:

Assess airway adjunct

- Every shift or as necessary.
- If an endotracheal tube is in place, note the tube lip level and check that it is fixed securely, and also check the patency of the tubing and the heat and moisture exchanger (HME) filter (if used). Confirm the cuff pressure (normal range, 20–30 cmH_2O).
- For a tracheostomy tube, perform the same checks (except for lip level), and check the patency of the inner cannula. Replace or check 4-hourly or as necessary.

Assess mechanical ventilation

- Every shift or as necessary.
- Check the ventilator settings (tidal volume, minute volume, peak and plateau pressures) and alarm limits. Check patient compliance and comfort with mechanical ventilation.

Assess oropharyngeal and tracheal secretions

- Every shift or as necessary.
- Check quantity—frequency of suctions, single or multiple passes.
- Check quality—mucoid or purulent, consistency (normal or loose), colour (clear is normal).
- Check whether the patient coughs on suctioning.

Circulation

In addition to the Circulation section of the ABCDE assessment:

Assess cardiac rhythm

- Every shift and as necessary.
- Use routine 3- or 5-lead ECG monitoring and a 12-lead ECG to check for ischaemic changes, infarction, or abnormal rhythms.

Assess fluid status

- Every shift or as necessary.
- Check blood pressure, heart rate, and urine output ≥ 0.5 mL/kg/h.
- Calculate and review cumulative fluid balance.
- Note the use of crystalloid and/or colloid.
- Note the fluid challenge response.
- Note insensible losses (e.g. diaphoresis, tachypnoea, diarrhoea).
- Check the indications, route, risks, benefits, and goals of fluid therapy support.
- Check the mucous membranes and axillae (note whether moist or dry, and with pink colour or pallor).
- Check for peripheral and pulmonary oedema, capillary refill, and jugular venous distension.
- Check the patient's weight weekly.
- Review laboratory results (e.g. FBC, U&E, and lactate).
- Review cardiac output monitoring (see ➲ p. 226).

Exposure

In addition to the Exposure section of the ABCDE assessment:

Assess the integument

- Every shift and as necessary.
- Check the patient's pressure areas for pressure ulcers.
- Note the date of insertion and location of vascular access devices, catheters, and drains.

Abdomen and nutrition

In addition to the ABCDE assessment:

Assess the abdomen

- Every shift or as necessary.
- Conduct a physical assessment of the abdomen.
- If surgical drains are present, note collection volumes.
- For specialized abdominal assessment and monitoring, see ➲ pp. 296 and 300.

Assess nutrition and elimination

- Every shift or as necessary.
- Screen for malnutrition using a recognised screening tool such as the Malnutrition Universal Screening Tool (MUST)[1] or the NUTrition Risk in the Critically ill score (NUTRIC)[2,3]. (see ➲ p. 57).
- Consider refeeding syndrome (poor diet before admission) (see ➲ p. 324).
- Check nasogastric tube position (see ➲ p. 63) and gastric residual volume (if using enteral feeding) see ➲ p. 308.
- Check the indications, route, risks, benefits, and goals of nutrition support (20–30 kcal/kg/day) (see ➲ p. 58).

- Check the patient's weight weekly.
- Check the swallowing assessment (this may fall within the remit of the speech and language therapist).
- Document nutritional intake (oral, enteral, and parenteral) (see ➔ p. 57).
- Check blood pressure and heart rate, and that urine output is ≥ 0.5mL/kg/h.
- Check blood glucose and insulin therapy (maintain blood glucose concentration ≤ 10 mmol/L).
- Review laboratory results (e.g. FBC, U&E, and lactate).
- Urinalysis.
- Check bowel output, frequency, and type using the Bristol Stool Chart (see Figure 2.3) (see ➔ pp. 304 and 306).

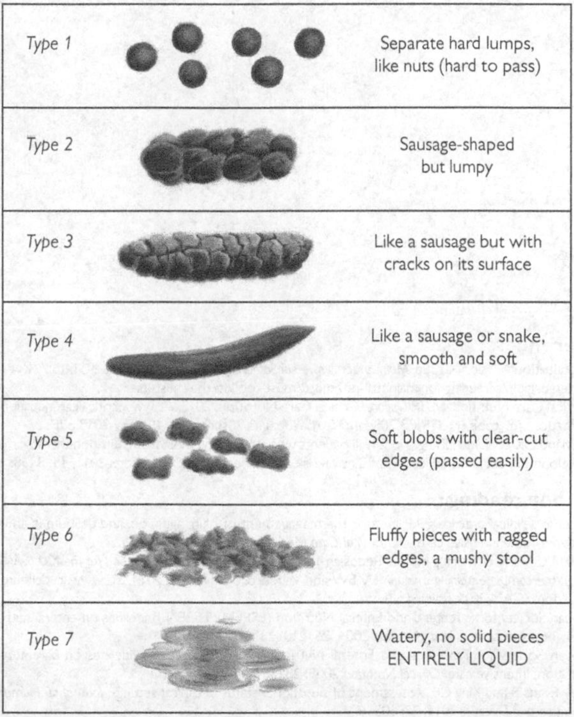

Type 1
Separate hard lumps, like nuts (hard to pass)
Type 2
Sausage-shaped but lumpy
Type 3
Like a sausage but with cracks on its surface
Type 4
Like a sausage or snake, smooth and soft
Type 5
Soft blobs with clear-cut edges (passed easily)
Type 6
Fluffy pieces with ragged edges, a mushy stool
Type 7
Watery, no solid pieces ENTIRELY LIQUID

Figure 2.3 Bristol Stool Chart. (Reproduced by kind permission of Dr K. W. Heaton, Reader in Medicine at the University of Bristol © 2000 Norgine Pharmaceuticals Ltd.)

References

1 Malnutrition Advsiory Group. *Malnutrition Universal Screening Tool*. BAPEN, 2011. http://www.bapen.org.uk/screening-for-malnutrition/must/must-toolkit/the-must-itself

2 Critical Care Nutrition. *NUTRIC score*. Critical Care Nutrition, 2013. www.criticalcarenutrition.com/docs/qi_tools/NUTRIC%20Score%201%20page%20summary_19March2013.pdf

3 Heyland DK et al. Identifying critically ill patients who benefit the most from nutrition therapy: the development and initial validation of a novel risk assessment tool. *Critical Care*. 2011; **15**: R268.

Further reading

Barr J et al. Clinical practice guidelines for the management of pain, agitation, and delirium in adult patients in the intensive care unit. *Critical Care Medicine* 2013; **41**: 263–306.

The 2014 CAM-ICU Training Manual Redesign Team. *Confusion assessment method for the ICU (CAM-ICU): the complete training manual*. Ely EW and Vanderbilt University, 2014. www.icudelirium.org/docs/CAM_ICU_training.pdf

European Society for Parenteral and Enteral Nutrition (ESPEN). ESPEN guidelines on enteral nutrition: intensive care. *Clinical Nutrition* 2006; **25**: 210–23.

European Society for Parenteral and Enteral Nutrition (ESPEN). ESPEN guidelines on parenteral nutrition: intensive care. *Clinical Nutrition* 2009; **28**: 387–400.

Langley-Evans S and King CR. Assessment of nutritional status in clinical settings. *Journal of Human Nutrition and Dietetics* 2014; **27**: 105–6.

National Institute for Health and Care Excellence (NICE). *Intravenous Fluid Therapy in Adults in Hospital*. CG174. NICE: London, 2013. www.nice.org.uk/guidance/cg174

Schneider A et al. Estimation of fluid status changes in critically ill patients: fluid balance chart or electronic bed weight? *Journal of Critical Care* 2012; **27**: 745e7–12.

Mental health assessment

Assessment of mental health and well-being is integral to the holistic care of a critically ill patient. The assessment has a twofold purpose—first, to identify the impact of physical illness or injury on the patient's mental health, and second, to establish the effect, if any, of mental ill health on the patient's physical health and recovery. In addition, nurses should be familiar with the principles and functions of mental capacity assessment.

During the mental health assessment, it may become apparent that the patient is at risk. This should prompt immediate referral to mental health services. Box 2.4 lists the physical signs and symptoms that may be attributable to mental disorders and/or medication prescribed for a mental disorder.

ABC mental health assessment

This involves rapid assessment of mental health status within three domains.

Affective domain

This domain focuses on observation of the patient's emotional state and expressed feelings. It involves objective interpretation by the nurse of the patient's non-verbal communication, and documentation of the patient's mood, which is a subjective finding.

Behaviour domain

This domain focuses on observation of the patient's behaviour. It involves subjective interpretation by the nurse of the patient's behaviour and appearance. Caution is needed when interpreting the patient's behaviour as a sign of mental disorder (e.g. inability to maintain eye contact can be a sign of depression, but this behaviour can also be due to a social or cultural convention).

Box 2.4 Physical signs and symptoms that may be caused by mental disorders and/or medication prescribed for such disorders

- Sleep disturbance
- Dizziness
- Poor memory
- Impaired speech
- Seizures
- Muscle weakness
- Sensory disturbance—vision, hearing, smell, taste, and touch
- Hyperventilation
- Tachycardia or bradycardia
- Palpitations
- Nausea and vomiting
- Increased or decreased appetite
- Weight gain or loss
- Amenorrhoea

Cognition domain

This domain focuses on evaluation of the patient's cognitive function. Within this domain there is overlap with neurological assessment (see ➲ p. 242). It involves objective interpretation by the nurse of the patient's orientation to person, place, and time, and observation of any signs of confusion or change in alertness.

Mental capacity assessment

The five key principles

- Every adult has the right to make their own decisions (i.e. a patient is assumed to have capacity unless proven otherwise).
- A person must be given as much help as is practicable before anyone treats them as not being able to make their own decisions.
- If an individual makes what might be seen as an unwise decision, they should not be treated as lacking capacity to make that decision.
- Anything that is done or any decision that is made on behalf of a person who lacks capacity must be done or decided in their best interests.
- Anything that is done for or on behalf of a person who lacks capacity should be minimally restrictive of their basic rights and freedoms.

Mental capacity assessment applies to situations where a person may be unable to make a particular decision at a particular time. It does not mean an inability to make general decisions or that a loss of capacity is permanent.

Assessment of mental capacity

- Identify the specific decision to be made.
  - The assessment of capacity relates to a particular decision made at a particular time, and is not about a range of decisions (see Box 2.5).
- Functional test of capacity.
  - Is there an impairment of, or disturbance in, the functioning of the person's mind or brain (this may be either permanent or temporary)?
  - If the answer is yes, does the impairment or disturbance result in the person being unable to make the particular decision?

The person will be unable to make the particular decision if, after all appropriate help and support has been given to them, they cannot:

- understand the information relevant to that decision, including the likely consequences of making or not making the decision
- retain that information
- use or weigh that information as part of the decision-making process
- communicate their decision (either verbally or non-verbally).

Box 2.5 Decisions about serious medical treatment

- New treatment
- Stopping current treatment
- Withholding treatment
- Treatment that has potentially serious consequences

Mental capacity terminology

- **Lasting power of attorney (LPA)**—a legal document that allows decisions to be made by an identified person (the attorney) on behalf of a person who lacks mental capacity (the donor). The document is only considered legal if it is registered with the Office of the Public Guardian.
- **Court of Protection**— a specialist court that arbitrates over issues specifically related to mental capacity. The Court of Protection will appoint a Deputy when decisions need to be made on behalf of a person who lacks mental capacity.
- **Deprivation of liberty safeguards (DOLS)**—decision making on behalf of a person who lacks capacity can potentially deprive them of their personal freedom and choice (deprivation of liberty). Safeguards now exist to ensure that decisions are made in the best interests of the person, and that the process is legal and open to challenge.
- **Independent Mental Capacity Advocate (IMCA)**—an IMCA is appointed if a person who lacks capacity has no one other than paid staff to assist them with decision making about serious medical treatment.
- **Advance decisions**—an advance decision allows a person to refuse pre-specified medical treatment at a time when they may no longer be capable of consenting to or refusing treatment. The person must have capacity at the time of making the decision, and must clearly identify which treatments would be refused and under what circumstances. Until an advance decision has been identified and confirmed as valid, the healthcare professionals must continue to act in the person's best interests.

Factors that affect the mental health and well-being of critically ill patients

- Communication barriers:
  - endotracheal tube or tracheostomy
  - sedation
  - cognitive dysfunction
  - muscle weakness.
- Confusion:
  - may be linked to the patient's past medical history (e.g. mental disorder, dementia)
  - may be the reason for their admission (e.g. neurological injury, sepsis)
  - may be caused by their treatment (e.g. post-sedation delirium).
- Environment:
  - noise levels
  - activity levels and intensity
  - privacy and dignity
  - unfamiliar surroundings
  - transfer and discharge.

Further reading

Crews M et al. Deprivation of liberty in intensive care. *Journal of the Intensive Care Society* 2014; 15: 320–4.

Menon DK and Chatfield DA. *A guide for critical care settings: Mental Capacity Act 2005*. Version 6. Intensive Care Society: London, 2011.

Mental Capacity Act 2005. http://www.legislation.gov.uk/ukpga/2005/9/contents

White SM and Baldwin TJ. 2006. The Mental Capacity Act 2005—implications for anaesthesia and critical care. *Anaesthesia* 61 (4): 381–389.

Blood gas analysis

Blood gas analysis is used to [illegible] ventilation and oxygenation [illegible] and gives a single [illegible] acid–base balance of the patient. [illegible] any venous blood gas [illegible] (see Table 2.[illegible]).

- [illegible] measure of how [illegible] blood is [illegible] [illegible] whereas [illegible] [illegible].
- $PaCO_2$—partial pressure of carbon dioxide (CO_2) [illegible] cellular respiration. CO_2 dissolves in water (H_2O) to form carbonic acid [illegible] HCO_3^- ions. This process is speeded up in the presence of the enzyme carbonic anhydrase.
- HCO_3^-—[illegible] buffer found in the [illegible] pH [illegible] HCO_3^- ions and H^+ ions [illegible] produced by the liver and kidneys.
- Buffering [illegible] Compensation is also required [illegible] kidneys [illegible] lungs [illegible] minutes [illegible] hours [illegible] period of days.
- Base excess (BE)—[illegible] amount of acid [illegible]
  - Negative BE indicates [illegible]
  - Positive BE indicates [illegible] to be added [illegible] alkalosis.

Table 2.[illegible] [illegible]

[illegible]	[illegible]
[illegible]	[illegible]
[illegible]	[illegible]
[illegible]	[illegible]
[illegible]	[illegible]
[illegible]	[illegible]
[illegible]	[illegible]

Blood gas analysis

Blood gas analysis is used to direct ventilation and oxygenation strategies and act as a guide to the acid–base balance of the patient. Normal arterial and venous blood gas values are listed in Table 2.4.

- **pH**—this is a measure of how acid or alkaline the blood is in the presence of H^+ ions. A low pH is acidotic (more H^+ ions), whereas a high pH is alkalotic (fewer H^+ ions).
- **$PaCO_2$**—partial pressure of arterial carbon dioxide (CO_2), which is the primary metabolite of cellular respiration. CO_2 dissolves in water (H_2O) to form carbonic acid, which dissociates into H^+ and HCO_3^- ions. This process is speeded up in the presence of the enzyme carbonic anhydrase.
- **HCO_3^-**—bicarbonate is a buffer found in the plasma, which resists changes in pH by retaining or releasing H^+ ions. If there are more HCO_3^- ions than H^+ ions, the blood is more alkalotic. Bicarbonate is produced in the liver and kidneys.
- Buffering is the first line of correction of pH, but the HCO_3^- supply will fall, so H^+ ion elimination is also required. Excess H^+ ions are removed from the circulation by the kidneys, which excrete H^+ ions in the urine and reabsorb HCO_3^- ions in the proximal tubule of the nephron, or by the lungs, which excrete H^+ ions in H_2O. Removal from the lungs occurs within minutes or hours, whereas removal from the kidneys occurs over a period of days.
- **Base excess (BE)**—this refers to the amount of acid required to return 1 L of blood to pH 7.4 at a PCO_2 of 5.3 kPa. It reflects the metabolic component of a pH imbalance.
  - *Negative BE* indicates the amount of acid that needs to be removed in order to return the pH to normal (i.e. as a result of a metabolic acidosis).
  - *Positive BE* indicates the amount of acid that needs to be retained or added in order to return the pH to normal (i.e. as a result of a metabolic alkalosis).

Table 2.4 Normal arterial and venous blood gas values

Normal arterial values		Normal venous values	
pH	7.35–7.45	pH	7.35–7.45
$PaCO_2$	4.6–6.0 kPa	$PvCO_2$	4.5–6.0 kPa
HCO_3^-	22–26 mmol/L	HCO_3^-	22–28 mmol/L
Base excess	+2 to –2 mmol/L	Base excess	+2 to –2 mmol/L
Lactate	0.5–1.5 mmol/L	Lactate	0.5–2.2 mmol/L
PaO_2	10.0–13.3 kPa	PvO_2	11–13 kPa
SaO_2	> 95%	SvO_2	65–75%

- **Lactate (or lactic acid)**—this chemical is produced in anaerobic metabolism, and it is an indicator that increased metabolic demand is exceeding the supply of oxygen available. A raised lactate concentration is associated with acidosis.
- PaO_2—partial pressure of arterial oxygen. Oxygen is the primary substrate for cellular respiration. It binds to haemoglobin to form oxyhaemoglobin. Different physical conditions will affect the affinity of haemoglobin for oxygen. These include pH, PCO_2, temperature, and 2,3-diphosphoglycerate (2,3-DPG).
- SaO_2—Oxygen saturation is a measure of how much oxygen is bound to haemoglobin. The higher the partial pressure of oxygen (PO_2), the higher the oxygen saturation will be.

Values are corrected for the patient's specific body temperature, and fractionated inspired oxygen concentration (FiO_2) is entered. The standard bicarbonate ($stdHCO_3^-$) and the standard base excess (stdBE) values are given with the respiratory component of the acid–base disturbance removed. Therefore if the $stdHCO_3^-$ is lower than HCO_3^-, the acidosis is metabolic in origin.

Arterial blood gas analysis

Check whether the pH is within the normal range

- If the pH is below the normal range this is acidosis.
- If the pH is above the normal range this is alkalosis.
- If the pH is within the normal range, check whether the PCO_2 and the HCO_3^- are also within the normal range.

Check the cause of the acidosis (low pH)

- If the PCO_2 is above the normal range this is respiratory acidosis.
- If the HCO_3^- is below the normal range this is metabolic acidosis.
- If the PCO_2 is above the normal range and the HCO_3^- is below the normal range this is mixed acidosis.

Check the cause of the alkalosis (high pH)

- If the PCO_2 is below the normal range this is respiratory alkalosis.
- If the HCO_3^- is above the normal range this is metabolic alkalosis.
- If the PCO_2 is below the normal range and the HCO_3^- is above the normal range this is mixed alkalosis.

Check for compensation

- If the pH is not within the normal range this is not compensated.
- If the pH is within the normal range and the PCO_2 and the HCO_3^- are outside the normal range but in opposite directions (i.e. either high PCO_2 and low HCO_3^-, or low PCO_2 and high HCO_3^-) this is compensated.

Check whether the PO_2 is within the normal range

- If the PO_2 is below the normal range this is hypoxaemia.
- If the PO_2 is above the normal range this is hyperoxaemia.

Table 2.5 summarizes the different arterial blood gas results.

Table 2.5 Representation of acidosis and alkalosis values

	pH	PCO_2	HCO_3^-
Respiratory acidosis	↓	↑	Normal
Respiratory alkalosis	↑	↓	Normal
Metabolic acidosis	↓	Normal	↓
Metabolic alkalosis	↑	Normal	↑
Respiratory and metabolic acidosis	↓	↑	↓
Respiratory and metabolic alkalosis	↑	↓	↑

Acid–base disturbances

- **Respiratory acidosis**—increased production and/or decreased excretion of CO_2. Causes include:
  - obstructive lung disease
  - respiratory depression (over-sedation, brain injury, neuromuscular disorders)
  - hypoventilation (error in non-invasive or mechanical ventilation, chest deformities, or pain restricting ventilation).
- **Respiratory alkalosis**—increased excretion of CO_2. Causes include:
  - restrictive lung disease
  - pulmonary embolus
  - hyperventilation (error in non-invasive or mechanical ventilation, hypoxia, anxiety).
- **Metabolic acidosis**—increased production or retention of acid and/or increased excretion of base/alkali. Causes include:
  - uraemia
  - acid ingestion (aspirin, ethylene glycol)
  - acid from abnormal metabolism (ketoacidosis)
  - hyperchloraemia (due to excess intravenous infusions)
  - lactic acidosis (due to exercise, shock, hypoxia, liver failure, or trauma)
  - loss of alkali (due to diarrhoea, bowel fistula, or renal tubular necrosis).
- **Metabolic alkalosis**—increased production or retention of base/alkali and/or increased excretion of acid. Causes include:
  - alkali ingestion
  - excess bicarbonate or buffer infusions
  - renal disorders
  - hypokalaemia
  - drugs (diuretics, ingestion of alkali)
  - loss of acid (due to gastric aspirates or vomiting).

Hypoxaemia

This is defined as a low oxygen concentration in the blood:

- < 8.0 kPa when breathing air
- < 11.0 kPa when breathing > 0.4 F_iO_2.

Acute compensation can occur to avoid tissue hypoxia (e.g. increasing cardiac output or increasing oxygen extraction by the tissues).

Chronic compensation by increasing red blood cell numbers and haemoglobin levels is seen in chronic obstructive pulmonary disease (COPD) and in populations who live at high altitudes.

Causes of hypoxaemia

- **Ventilatory inadequacy**—for example, mechanical defects (including airway obstruction), neuromuscular dysfunction, central nervous system depression.
- **Ventilation/perfusion mismatch**—for example, pulmonary embolus, poor right cardiac function, acute respiratory distress syndrome (ARDS).
- **Shunt**—for example, atelectasis, pneumonia.
- **Diffusion limitation**—for example, ARDS, fibrosing alveolitis, pulmonary oedema.

Tissue hypoxia

This is defined as inadequate oxygen to support cell metabolism. It is extremely difficult to monitor directly, and hypoxaemia is commonly used as a marker of possible hypoxia.

There are four categories of hypoxia.

- **Hypoxic hypoxia**—hypoxaemia results in inadequate oxygen delivery to the cells.
- **Anaemic hypoxia**—arterial oxygen is normal, but oxygen-carrying capacity is inadequate due to either low Hb or dysfunctional Hb (e.g. in carbon monoxide poisoning).
- **Circulatory hypoxia**—oxygen delivery is insufficient to meet cell needs or does not reach the cells due to shunt.
- **Histotoxic hypoxia**—the ability of the cells to utilize oxygen is impaired (e.g. in cyanide poisoning, which blocks mitochondrial electron transport).

Laboratory investigations

Critical care patients require ongoing measurement of renal function, electrolytes, and haematology indices. Blood cultures and other microbiology samples should be taken as required (in the event of inflammation, infection, or pyrexia) (see Table 2.6).

Table 2.6 Normal values for common blood tests. (Reproduced from Longmore M, Wilkinson I, Baldwin A and Wallin E, *Oxford Handbook of Clinical Medicine*, Ninth Edition, 2014, with permission from Oxford University Press.)

Measurement	Reference interval	Your hospital
White cell count (WCC)	4.0–11.0 × 10^9/L	
Red cell count	♂ 4.5–6.5 × 10^{12}/L ♀ 3.9–5.6 × 10^{12}/L	
Haemoglobin	♂ 130–180 g/L ♀ 115–160 g/L	
Packed red cell volume (PCV) or haematocrit	♂ 0.4–0.54 L/L ♀ 0.37–0.47 L/L	
Mean cell volume (MCV)	76–96 fL	
Mean cell haemoglobin (MCH)	27–32 pg	
Mean cell haemoglobin concentration (MCHC)	300–360 g/L	
Red cell distribution width (RCDW, RDW)	11.6–14.6%	
Neutrophils	2.0–7.5 × 10^9/L; 40–75% WCC	
Lymphocytes	1.3–3.5 × 10^9/L; 20–45% WCC	
Eosinophils	0.04–0.44 × 10^9/L; 1–6% WCC	
Basophils	0.0-0.10 × 10^9/L; 0–1% WCC	
Monocytes	0.2–0.8 × 10^9/L; 2–10% WCC	
Platelet count	150–400 × 10^9/L	
Reticulocyte count	0.8–2.0%[1] 25–100 × 10^9/L	
Erythrocyte sedimentation rate	Depends on age	
Prothrombin time (citrated bottle) (factors I, II, VII, X)	10–14 s	

Table 2.6 (*Contd.*)

Measurement	Reference interval	Your hospital
Activated partial thromboplastin time (VIII, IX, XI, XII)	35–45 s	
D-dimer[1] (citrated bottle, as for INR)	< 0.5 mg/L	

Drugs (and other substances) may interfere with any chemical method; as these effects may be method dependent, it is difficult for the clinician to be aware of all the possibilities. If in doubt, discuss with the lab.

Substance	Reference interval (*labs vary, so a guide only*)	Your hospital
Adrenocorticotrophic hormone	< 80 ng/L	
Alanine aminotransferase (ALT)	5–35 U/L	
Albumin	35–50 g/L	
Aldosterone	100–500 pmol/L	
Alkaline phosphatase	30–150 U/L (adults)	
α-amylase	0–180 Somogyi U/dL	
α-fetoprotein	< 10 kU/L	
Angiotensin II	5–35 pmol/L	
Antidiuretic hormone (ADH)	0.9–4.6 pmol/L	
Aspartate transaminase	5–35 U/L	
Bicarbonate	24–30 mmol/L	
Bilirubin	3–17 μmol/L	
BNP	< 50 ng/L	
Calcitonin	< 0.1 μg/L	
Calcium (ionized)	1.0–1.25 mmol/L	
Calcium (total)	2.12–2.65 mmol/L	
Chloride	95–105 mmol/L	
Cholesterol[2]	< 5.0 mmol/L	
VLDL	0.128–0.645 mmol/L	
LDL	< 2.0 mmol/L	
HDL	0.9–1.93 mmol/L	
Cortisol	AM 450–700 nmol/L midnight 80–280 nmol/L	
Creatine kinase (CK)	♂ 25–195 U/L ♀ 25–170 U/L	
Creatinine (∝ to lean body mass)	70–150 μmol/L	
CRP C-reactive protein	< 10 mg/L	
Ferritin	12–200 μg/L	

(*continued*)

Table 2.6 (*Contd.*)

Substance	Reference interval (*labs vary, so a guide only*)	Your hospital
Folate	2.1 µg/L	
Follicle-stimulating hormone (FSH)	2–8 U/L in ♀ (luteal); > 25 U/L in menopause	
Gamma-glutamyl transpeptidase	♂ 11–51 U/L ♀ 7–33 U/L	
Glucose (fasting)	3.5–5.5 mmol/L	
Growth hormone	< 20 mu/L	
HbA_{1c} = glycosylated Hb (DCCT)	4–6%. 7% ≈ good DM control	
HbA_{1c} IFCC (more specific than DCCT)	20–42 mmol/mol; 53 ≈ good DM control	
Iron	♂ 14–31 µmol/L ♀ 11–30 µmol/L	
Lactate	Venous 0.6–2.4 mmol/L Arterial 0.6–1.8 mmol/L	
Lactate dehydrogenase (LDH)	70–250 U/L	
Lead	< 1.8 mmol/L	
Luteinizing hormone (LH) (premenopausal)	3–16 U/L (luteal)	
Magnesium	0.75–1.05 mmol/L	
Osmolality	278–305 mosmol/kg	
Parathyroid hormone (PTH)	< 0.8–8.5 pmol/L	
Potassium	3.5–5.0 mmol/L	
Prolactin	♂ < 450 U/L ♀ < 600 U/L	
Prostate specific antigen (PSA)	0–4 µg/mL, age specific, see ➲ p. 538	
Protein (total)	60–80 g/L	
Red cell folate	0.36–1.44 µmol/L (160–640 µg/L)	
Renin (erect/recumbent)	2.8–4.5/ 1.1–2.7 pmol/mL/h	
Sodium	135–145 mmol/L	
Thyroid-binding globulin (TBG)	7–17 mg/L	
Thyroid-stimulating hormone (TSH)	0.5–5.7 mU/L widens with age, p208 assays vary; 4–5 is a grey area	

Table 2.6 (*Contd.*)

Substance	Reference interval (*labs vary, so a guide only*)	Your hospital
Thyroxine (T_4)	70–140 nmol/L	
Thyroxine (free)	9–22 pmol/L	
Total iron-binding capacity	54–75 µmol/L	
Triglyceride	0.55–1.90 mmol/L	
Triiodothyronine (T_3)	1.2–3.0 nmol/L	
Troponin T (see p112)	<0.1 µg/L	
Urate	♂ 210–480 µmol/L ♀ 150–390 µmol/L	
Urea	2.5–6.7 mmol/L	
Vitamin B_{12}	0.13–0.68 nmol/L (>150 ng/L)	
Vitamin D	60–105 nmol/L	

Urine reference intervals	Reference interval	Your hospital
Cortisol (free)	< 280 nmol/24h	
Hydroxyindole acetic acid	16–73 µmol/24h	
Hydroxymethylmandelic acid (HMMA, VMA)	16–48 µmol/24h	
Metanephrines	0.03–0.69 µmol/mmol creatinine (or < 5.5 µmol/day)	
Osmolality	350–1000 mosmol/kg	
17-oxogenic steroids	♂ 28–30 µmol/24h ♀ 21–66 µmol/24h	
17-oxosteroids (neutral)	♂ 17–76 µmol/24h ♀ 14–59 µmol/24h	
Phosphate (inorganic)	15–50 mmol/24h	
Potassium	14–120 mmol/24h	
Protein	< 150 mg/24h	
Protein	creatinine ratio < 3 mg/mmol	
Sodium	100–250 mmol/24h	

1 D-dimer assay is useful for excluding thromboembolic disease if the assay is normal. The D-dimer is non-specific, therefore a raised level is unhelpful and should only be requested if the probability of thromboembolic disease is low (eg Wells score). It needs to get to the lab quickly.

2 Desired upper limit of cholesterol would be < 6 mmol/L. In some populations, 7.8 mmol/L is the top end of the distribution.

Chapter 3

Generic care of the critically ill patient

Care bundles

Definition

A care bundle is a simple tool, consisting of current, evidence-based recommendations, which helps to standardize practice to improve patient care. Lengthy clinical guidelines can be linked to actual clinical practice through a care bundle (see Figure 3.1). The actions identified in a care bundle should be very specific, and should avoid being so broad that the meaning and focus of the bundle are diluted. Box 3.1 provides an overview of the distinguishing features of a care bundle.

Examples of care bundles

- Sepsis (see ➲ p. 336).
- Pain management.
- Enteral nutrition.
- Tracheostomy care.
- Weaning from mechanical ventilation.
- High-impact interventions (see ➲ p. 46):
  - processes for key clinical procedures identified by the Department of Health[1] as making a significant contribution to reducing the risk of infection.

Challenges and criticism

Academic debate

- Elements may not satisfy all people despite research and other evidence.
- Limitations of standardized practice (e.g. discouragement of critical thinking or inability of inexperienced staff to recognize when individualized care is needed).

Industry

- Conflict of interest and other issues may arise if private companies provide funding to promote elements within the bundle.

Operational

- Some areas may lack the necessary resources to undertake each element of the care bundle.

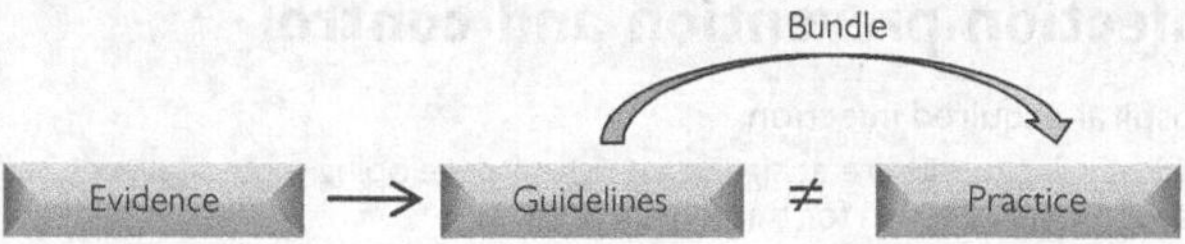

Figure 3.1 Care bundles.

Box 3.1 Summary of the elements of a care bundle

- A group of three to five (usually) evidence-based interventions related to a particular condition or event.
- In patient care, when executed together they result in a better outcome than if implemented individually.
- Each intervention should be widely accepted as good practice and widely applicable.
- They should be adhered to for every patient 100% of the time.
- They can be used to measure evidence-based practice.
- Each step is able to be audited—that is, done, not done, or subject to local exclusion.
- Audit focuses on organizational aspects of performing the intervention, rather than on how well the intervention is performed.
- Compliance with a bundle is achieved when every intervention is completed, or when a step is excluded for a pre-defined reason.

Adapted from Horner and Bellamy[2], p. 200.

References

1 Department of Health. *High Impact Interventions*. Department of Health: London, 2010. http://webarchive.nationalarchives.gov.uk/20120118164404/hcai.dh.gov.uk/whatdoido/high-impact-interventions/.

2 Horner DL and Bellamy MC. Care bundles in intensive care. *Continuing Education in Anaesthesia, Critical Care & Pain* 2012; **12**: 199–202.

Further reading

Camporota L and Brett S. Care bundles: implementing evidence or common sense? *Critical Care* 2011; **15**: 159.

Clarkson D et al. The role of 'care bundles' in healthcare. *British Journal of Healthcare Management* 2013; **19**: 63–8.

Infection prevention and control

Hospital-acquired infection

Critically ill patients are at significant risk of developing a hospital-acquired (nosocomial) infection for three main reasons:

- invasive devices, especially central venous catheters, urinary catheters, and endotracheal tubes (breaching of skin integrity and the facilitation of colonization by bypassing normal defence mechanisms)
- increased requirement for antibiotics among the critically ill, which creates resistant strains of organisms that can be transmitted rapidly from patient to patient
- lowered immune function related to sepsis or other disease processes.

Other influencing factors that may be involved in the development of hospital-acquired infections include genetic predisposition, the presence of nasogastric tubes for enteral nutrition increasing the risk of tracheal reflux and aspiration, and supine body positioning. Levels of nurse staffing that are less than 1:1 can also increase cross-infection. Prevention of the development of infections in the critical care setting should take into consideration the following factors:[3]

- hand hygiene (the single most important factor)
- environmental cleaning
- patient isolation
- fomite elimination
- decolonization
- device insertion and care
- antimicrobial stewardship (appropriate use of antibiotics)
- prophylactic antibiotics
- chlorhexidine bathing.

Hand hygiene

Poor hand hygiene is the most important and persistent source of cross-infection in patients. Hand washing is time-consuming (requiring approximately 2 min in total), and despite the use of gel-based alcohol products to supplement hand washing, staff compliance can be poor, at around 50–60%.[4] Box 3.2 lists some of the factors that have a negative impact on hand hygiene compliance among staff.

Infection prevention and control measures

Critical care units should develop policies that cover standard precautions, cleaning schedules, antibiotic-prescribing practice, and evidence-based preventive measures for specific risks such as ventilator-associated pneumonia. Standard infection control precautions should apply to care of all patients (see Table 3.1).

Box 3.2 Factors that have a negative impact on hand hygiene compliance

- Increased workload and bed occupancy.
- Increased patient acuity and other priorities of care.
- Poor staffing levels.
- Poor availability of hand-washing facilities (hand basins, soap dispensers, towels).
- Lack of availability of alcohol-based hand rubs.
- Poor training and policing of hand hygiene.
- Lack of senior role models and emphasis on hand hygiene.

Table 3.1 Standard infection control precautions

Hand hygiene	After contact with body fluids, after removing gloves, and between patient contacts
Gloves	For anticipated contact with body fluids, mucous membranes, non-intact skin, and irritants
Masks, eye protection, face shield	To protect mucous membranes during procedures that are likely to splash or spray body fluids
Gowns or aprons	To protect skin and clothing during procedures that are likely to splash or spray body fluids
Handling of sharp objects	Not recapping needles, use of puncture-resistant sharps containers, and responsible disposal of sharps in sharps bin
Handling of patient care equipment	Discarding of single-use items, appropriate cleaning of reusable items, and avoidance of contamination from used equipment

References

3 Rupp ME. Environmental cleaning and disinfection: only one piece of the critical care infection control puzzle. *Critical Care Medicine* 2011; **39**: 881–2.

4 De Wandel D et al. Behavioral determinants of hand hygiene compliance in intensive care units. *American Journal of Critical Care* 2010; **19**: 230–39.

Further reading

Bion J et al. 'Matching Michigan': a 2-year stepped interventional programme to minimise central venous catheter-blood stream infections in intensive care units in England. *BMJ Quality & Safety* 2013; **22**: 110–23.

Sax H et al. Implementation of infection control best practice in intensive care units throughout Europe: a mixed-method evaluation study. *Implementation Science* 2013; **8**: 24.

High-impact interventions

The Department of Health[5] has identified the processes involved in key clinical procedures that help to reduce the risk of infection and which are presented in the form of care bundles entitled 'high-impact interventions.' Those that are relevant to the critical care setting include:

- ventilator-associated pneumonia (see ➲ p. 111)
- central venous catheter care (see Table 3.2)
- peripheral intravenous cannula care
- prevention of surgical site infection
- urinary catheter care
- *Clostridium difficile* infection
- cleaning and decontamination
- enteral feeding
- blood cultures.

Table 3.2 Central venous catheter care bundle: insertion

Catheter type	Single-lumen catheter unless otherwise indicated. Antimicrobial-impregnated catheter if duration is estimated to be 1–3 weeks and risk of catheter-related bloodstream infection is high.
Insertion site	Subclavian or internal jugular vein. Avoid femoral vein if possible.
Personal protective equipment	Maximal sterile barriers and aseptic technique, including a sterile gown, sterile gloves, and a large sterile drape. Eye and full protection is worn if there is a risk of splashing of blood or other body fluids.
Skin preparation	2% chlorhexidine gluconate in 70% isopropyl alcohol, and allow to dry for at least 30 s. If the patient has a sensitivity, use a single-patient-use povidone–iodine application.
Hand hygiene	Hands should be decontaminated immediately before and after each episode of patient contact, using the correct hand hygiene technique.
Dressing	Sterile transparent semi-permeable dressing that allows observation of the insertion site.
Safe disposal of sharps	Disposed of safely at the point of care and in line with local policy.
Documentation	Details of insertion are documented in the records (including date, location, catheter lot number, and signature and name of operator undertaking insertion).
Hand hygiene	Hands are decontaminated immediately before and after each episode of patient contact using the correct hand hygiene technique.

Table 3.2 (*Contd.*)

Site inspection	Site is inspected daily for signs of infection, and observations noted in the patient's record.
Dressing	An intact dry adherent transparent dressing is present. Insertion site should be cleaned with 2% chlorhexidine gluconate in 70% isopropyl alcohol prior to dressing change.
Catheter injection ports	Injection ports are covered by caps or valved connectors.
Catheter access	Aseptic non-touch techniques are used for all access to the line. Ports or hubs are cleaned with 2% chlorhexidine gluconate in 70% isopropyl alcohol prior to catheter access. Flush line with 0.9% sodium chloride for lumens in frequent use.
Administration of set replacement	Set is replaced immediately after administration of blood or blood products. Set is replaced after 24 h following total parenteral nutrition (if it contains lipids). Set is replaced within 72 h of all other fluid sets or within 12–24 h if medications are present.
Catheter replacement	Catheter is removed if it is no longer required, or decision not to remove it is recorded. Details of removal are documented in the records (including date, location, and signature and name of operator undertaking removal).

Reference

5 Department of Health. *High Impact Interventions*. Department of Health: London, 2010. http://webarchive.nationalarchives.gov.uk/20120118164404/hcai.dh.gov.uk/whatdoido/high-impact-interventions/

Oral hygiene

The lining of the mouth and oropharynx consists of squamous epithelial cells that are highly vulnerable to the effects of poor blood flow, malnutrition, and drug toxicity. Saliva has a strong protective antimicrobial effect. However, in intubated patients the salivary flow is greatly reduced or absent. This reduced flow of saliva along with the presence of an endotracheal tube increases the risk of:

- oral microbe colonization
- mucositis
- ventilator-associated pneumonia (VAP).

Frequent mouth assessment and oral hygiene are required in the critical care setting to prevent mouth abnormalities (see Table 3.3).

Table 3.3 Assessment and management of the mouth

Area	Normal	Abnormal	Intervention
Mucosa	Pink, moist, intact, smooth	Reddening, ulceration, other lesions	Hydration, use of neutral mouthwash solution, pain-relieving anaesthetic gels for ulcers
Tongue	Pink, moist, intact, papillae present	Coated, absence of papillae, smooth shiny appearance, debris, lesions, crusted, cracked, blackened	Hydration, frequent, neutral mouthwashes, use of a debriding agent (e.g. sodium bicarbonate) for blackened areas
Lips	Clean, intact, pink	Dry skin, cracks, reddened, encrusted, ulcerated, bleeding, oedematous	Hydration, protection using petroleum jelly or lubricant jelly
Saliva	Watery, white, or clear	Thick, viscous, absent, bloodstained	Hydration, use of artificial salivas
Gingiva	Pink, moist, firm	Receding, overgrown, oedematous, reddened, bleeding	Tooth brushing 12-hourly with small soft brush Chlorhexidine (0.1–0.2%) mouthwash
Teeth	White, firm in sockets, no debris, no decay	Discoloured, decayed, debris, wobbly	Tooth brushing 12-hourly with small soft brush Dental assessment

Prevention of VAP

- The VAP care bundle published by the Department of Health[6] recommends:
  - cleaning the mouth with chlorhexidine gluconate gel or liquid 6-hourly
  - leaving at least a 2-h gap between chlorhexidine and tooth brushing because of inactivation of chlorhexidine by toothpaste
  - brushing the teeth 12-hourly with standard toothpaste
  - see ➔ p. 111.
- Use of either chlorhexidine gel or mouthwash reduces the incidence of VAP by 40% in critically ill adults.[7]

References

6 Department of Health. *High Impact Intervention. Care bundle to reduce ventilation-associated pneumonia*. Department of Health: London, 2010. http://webarchive.nationalarchives.gov.uk/20120118164404/hcai.dh.gov.uk/whatdoido/high-impact-interventions/

7 Shi Z et al. Oral hygiene care for critically ill patients to prevent ventilator-associated pneumonia. *Cochrane Database of Systematic Reviews* 2013; Issue 8: CD008367.

Further reading

Alhazzani W et al. Toothbrushing for critically ill mechanically ventilated patients: a systematic review and meta-analysis of randomized trials evaluating ventilator-associated pneumonia. *Critical Care Medicine* 2013; **41**: 646–55.

Richards D. Oral hygiene regimes for mechanically ventilated patients that use chlorhexidine reduce ventilator-associated pneumonia. *Evidence-Based Dentistry* 2013; **14**: 91–2.

Yildiz M, Durna Z and Akin S. Assessment of oral care needs of patients treated at the intensive care unit. *Journal of Clinical Nursing* 2013; **22**: 2734–47.

Yusef H. Toothbrushing may reduce ventilator-associated pneumonia. *Evidence-Based Dentistry* 2013; **14**: 89–90.

Eye care

Normally the eyes are protected from dehydration by the tear film, which is continually replenished by the lacrimal gland at a rate of approximately 1–2 μL/min. Tears are spread over the surface of the eye by the blink reflex. Frequent eye assessment and eye care are required to keep the eyes moist, protected, and free of abnormality, particularly if the patient is sedated (see Table 3.4). The patient should be referred to specialist ophthalmology services as appropriate.

Critical care risk factors for eye abnormalities

- Reduced ability to blink.
- Dehydration affecting tear production.
- Incomplete eyelid closure.
- Drug side effects.
- Lowered immune function.
- Increased likelihood of cross-infection.
- Orbital oedema due to:
  - increased intra-thoracic pressure from mechanical ventilation
  - prone positioning.

Dry eyes

- Can be caused by a combination of critical care risk factors for eye abnormalities (see previous list).
- Result in a further increased risk of developing other eye abnormalities.

Exposure keratopathy

- Non-inflammatory corneal disease caused by incomplete lid closure.
- Damage to the corneal epithelium can lead to abrasion, ulceration, or scarring, which may result in permanent damage.

Infection and inflammation

- Keratitis—affects the cornea:
  - white/yellow areas on the cornea, redness, discharge, and excessive tear production.
- Conjunctivitis—affects the conjunctiva:
  - redness, swelling, and discharge affecting eye and inner eyelids.
- Blepharitis—affects the eyelash follicles and sebaceous glands:
  - redness, swelling, and discharge affecting eyelid and lid margins.

Table 3.4 Assessment and management of the eyes

Area	Normal	Abnormal	Intervention
Eyelid closure	Upper eyelid completely covers the eye	Eyelids do not fully meet, or corneas are swollen and extruded	Close eyelids with hydropolymer dressing, lubricating ophthalmic ointment, or moisture seal chamber
Hydration status	No fluid restriction, no signs of dehydration, corneal surface is moist	Other features of dehydration or restricted fluid intake, plus dry corneal surface	Use sterile water to cleanse the eye, and apply artificial tears (hydroxyethylcellulose or hypromellose)
Corneal surface	Moist, clear, white	Purulent, coated, crusting exudate, clouding, oedematous, haemorrhage	Swab for culture, clean with sterile water, and apply appropriate topical antibiotic as per culture result
Orbital oedema	Cornea and orbital area are not swollen or extruded	Cornea and orbital area are swollen, reddened, or extruding	Maintain a head-up position to reduce pressure; ensure that tapes securing endotracheal or tracheal tube are not too tight

Further reading

Azfar MF, Khan MF and Alzeer AH. Protocolized eye care prevents corneal complications in ventilated patients in a medical intensive care unit. *Saudi Journal of Anaesthesia* 2013; **7**: 33–6.

Marshall AP et al. Eyecare in the critically ill: clinical practice guideline. *Australian Critical Care* 2008; **21**: 97–109.

Rosenberg JB and Eisen LA. Eye care in the intensive care unit: narrative review and meta-analysis. *Critical Care Medicine* 2008; **36**: 3151–5.

Shan H and Min D. Prevention of exposure keratopathy in intensive care unit. *International Journal of Ophthalmology* 2010; **3**: 346–8.

Werli-Alvarenga A et al. Nursing interventions for adult intensive care patients with risk for corneal injury: a systematic review. *International Journal of Nursing Knowledge* 2013; **24**: 25–9.

Fluid management

See ➡ p. 24 for an overview of key principles for assessing the fluid status of a critically ill patient. It is important to consider whether there is an *effective circulating blood volume* (volume of arterial blood required to ensure that there is sufficient tissue perfusion), because a patient can have large amounts of fluid within a 'third space' but still experience relative hypovolaemia with a low intravascular volume. *Third spacing* occurs when excessive fluid accumulates in the extracellular space where the fluid is not physiologically useful or 'effective' because it is not in the vasculature or cells. Examples of third spacing include peripheral and pulmonary oedema (fluid in the interstitium), ascites (fluid in the peritoneum), pleural effusion (fluid in the pleural space), and ileus (fluid in obstructed intestine).

Critically ill patients can experience either severe fluid deficit or fluid excess depending on the clinical context and progression of the critical illness. The aim of fluid management is for the patient to achieve normovolaemia. A patient with fluid deficit requires the administration of IV fluids (see ➡ p. 54), and a patient with fluid excess requires fluid removal by means of diuretics (see ➡ p. 284) or renal replacement therapy (see ➡ pp. 286 and 290).

Goals of fluid management

The following clinical findings of normovolaemia can be used as goals to help to guide fluid management therapies:

- blood pressure: sufficient mean arterial pressure (MAP), no swing in arterial trace (see ➡ p. 219)
- urine output: > 0.5 mL/kg/h
- mucous membranes: pink and moist
- central venous pressure (CVP): 2–10 mmHg:
  - CVP monitoring (see ➡ p. 222) is routine practice in critical care, with the assumption that CVP is a direct indicator of intravascular volume and right ventricular preload, and is also an indirect indicator of left ventricular preload
  - however, a systematic review by Marik and colleagues[8] demonstrated that there is a very poor correlation between CVP as a pressure reading and actual blood volume, and showed that CVP is not a reliable way to predict responsiveness to a fluid challenge; this could possibly be due to other factors, such as venous tone, intra-thoracic pressure, and ventricular compliance, influencing pressure readings
  - CVP readings should therefore be interpreted with caution, taking into account that the absolute value of the CVP reading may not be accurate, although extreme values or the CVP trend may be clinically useful while managing the fluid status of a patient.
- stroke volume: 60–100 mL.
- other clinical findings: FTc, SVV, GEDV, ITBV, EVLW, PAWP (see ➡ p. 226 for normal values for these types of haemodynamic monitoring values, depending on the type of monitoring device used), to help to guide fluid management strategies (e.g. PiCCO, LiDCO, Doppler, or pulmonary artery catheter).

IV therapy: fluids and electrolytes

The administration of IV fluids and electrolytes requires clinical decision making about the type of solution to be given (see ➔ p. 54), the rate of delivery, and the total volume to be infused within a set period of time. The National Institute for Health and Care Excellence (NICE)[9] recommends key principles based on 'the 5 Rs'—resuscitation, routine maintenance, replacement, redistribution, and reassessment.

Resuscitation

- There is an urgent need for IV fluids if hypovolaemia causes decreased tissue perfusion (see ➔ p. 175).
- Goal-directed therapy should be used with specific end points of resuscitation identified (e.g. urine output, blood pressure, lactate, CVP) to prevent under- or over-resuscitation.
- An initial fluid-challenge bolus of 500 mL crystalloid with Na^+ in the range 130–154 mmol/L should be given, followed by further fluid challenges as required[9].
- For fluid resuscitation of trauma patients, see ➔ p. 470.

Routine maintenance

- Give 25–30 mL/kg/day of water with 1 mmol/kg/day K^+, Na^+, and Cl^-, and 50–100 g/day glucose.[9]
- Use ideal body weight for obese patients using lower-range volumes.
- Administer with caution and consider reduced doses for patients who are older or who have renal or cardiac dysfunction.
- Promote discontinuation of maintenance IV fluids if oral or enteral fluid intake can be established.

Replacement

- Non-urgent replacement of fluid and electrolyte losses (e.g. losses from gastrointestinal tract, urine, fever, or burns).
- Consider other intake from enteral nutrition and routine IV maintenance.

Redistribution

- Consider which type of IV solution is needed to help correct internal fluid shifts (e.g. third spacing) or abnormal distribution of electrolytes.
- Patients who are particularly at risk for fluid and electrolyte distribution abnormalities include those with:
  - gross oedema
  - severe sepsis
  - increased or decreased Na^+ levels
  - decreased albumin levels
  - renal, liver, or cardiac dysfunction.

References

8 Marik PE and Cavallazzi R. Does the central venous pressure predict fluid responsiveness? An updated meta-analysis and a plea for some common sense. *Critical Care Medicine* 2013; **41**: 1774–81.

9 National Institute for Health and Care Excellence (NICE). *Intravenous Fluid Therapy in Adults in Hospital*. CG174. NICE: London, 2013. www.nice.org.uk/guidance/cg174

IV fluids: crystalloids

Crystalloids are solutions that contain substances such as electrolytes and glucose. They are classified according to their osmolarity in comparison with blood tonicity (see Table 3.5).

Isotonic saline

- This consists of 0.9% NaCl, available premixed with or without K^+ added.
- Fluid is distributed throughout the extracellular space (30% as intravascular fluid and 70% as interstitial fluid). If present in large amounts it contributes to oedema.
- High Cl^- content can cause hyperchloraemic metabolic acidosis.
- High Na^+ content can cause increased intravascular Na^+ and water retention.

Indications

- Fluid resuscitation—it is the safest IV fluid to give initially for hypovolaemia, until the patient's full fluid and electrolyte status is known.
- Maintenance IV fluid therapy.

Contraindications

- Hypernatraemia.

Balanced isotonic crystalloid solutions

- Examples include:
  - Hartmann's solution (compound sodium lactate)
  - Lactated Ringer's solution.
- Fluid is distributed throughout the extracellular space. However, due to lower levels of Na^+ and Cl^-, there is less Na^+ retention, water retention, and hyperchloraemia compared with isotonic saline.
- Include K^+, Ca^{2+}, and lactate (which is converted into HCO_3^- by the liver).

Table 3.5 Crystalloid IV fluids

	Type of fluid	Content (mmol/L)	Osmolarity (mOsm/L)
0.9% NaCl	Isotonic	Na^+ 154 Cl^- 154	308
Hartmann's solution	Isotonic	Na^+ 131 Cl^- 111 K^+ 5 Ca^{2+} 2 HCO_3^- 29 (lactate)	278
Lactated Ringer's solution	Isotonic	Na^+ 130 Cl^- 109 K^+ 4 Ca^{2+} 3 HCO_3^- 28 (lactate)	273
0.18% NaCl Glucose 4%	Hypotonic	Na^+ 31 Cl^- 31 Glucose 40 g/L	284
0.45% NaCl	Hypotonic	Na^+ 77 Cl^- 77	154
Glucose 5%	Hypotonic	Glucose 50 g/L	278
3% NaCl	Hypertonic	Na^+ 513 Cl^- 513	1026

Indications

- Fluid resuscitation.
- Maintenance IV fluid therapy.

Contraindications

- Liver dysfunction (because the liver is unable to convert lactate into HCO_3^-).
- Lactic acidosis.
- Hyperkalaemia.

Hypotonic crystalloid solutions

- Examples include:
  - 0.18% NaCl/4% glucose
  - 0.45% NaCl
  - 5% glucose—isotonic in the bag, but considered to be hypotonic because glucose is quickly metabolized, leaving free water.
- Fluid is distributed across both the intracellular and extracellular (interstitial and vascular) spaces.

Indications

- Cellular dehydration.
- Hypernatraemia.

Contraindications

- Raised ICP (hypotonicity will increase cerebral oedema).
- Hypotension.
- Hyponatraemia.

Hypertonic crystalloid solutions

- Examples include 3% NaCl and 7% NaCl.
- Promote rapid intravascular volume expansion with a relatively reduced water content compared with other IV fluids.
- Should be used with caution because of the potential for heart failure due to fluid overload, hypernatraemia, and hyperchloraemia.

Indications

- Raised ICP.
- Hypovolaemia due to trauma, although further research is needed.

Contraindications

- Fluid overload.
- Hypernatraemia.

Further reading

Bauer M et al. Isotonic and hypertonic crystalloid solutions in the critically ill. *Best Practice & Research. Clinical Anaesthesiology* 2009; 23: 173–81.

Lobo DN et al. *Basic Concepts of Fluid and Electrolyte Therapy*. Bibliomed: Melsungen, Germany, 2013. http://www.bbraun.com/documents/Knowledge/Basic_Concepts_of_Fluid_and_Electrolyte_Therapy.pdf

Williams E and von Fintel N. Hypertonic saline: a change of practice. *Nursing in Critical Care* 2012; 17: 99–104.

IV fluids: colloids

Colloids are solutions that contain macromolecules (e.g. starch or protein) which increase the oncotic pressure, resulting in plasma volume expansion. There has been a recent move towards discouraging the use of colloids for fluid resuscitation of critically ill patients because of the following:

- Colloids do not improve survival and have an increased financial cost compared with crystalloids.[10]
- The CHEST trial showed that there is no significant difference in mortality between patients who receive crystalloid and those given hydroxyethyl starch (HES), and there is an increased need for renal replacement therapy with HES use.[11]
- Septic patients who receive HES (compared with crystalloid or albumin) have an increased need for renal replacement therapy and transfusion of red blood cells, and an increased risk of serious adverse events.[12]
- A significant number of publications about HES by Joachim Boldt have been withdrawn due to his fraudulent colloid research.[13]

The current literature therefore suggests that the routine use of colloids for the fluid resuscitation of critically ill patients should be avoided. However, there may be a role for albumin administration in patients with severe sepsis, or as a replacement fluid after ascites has been drained (see ➔ p. 315). Further research is needed to clarify the role of albumin as a colloid in the critical care setting.

References

10 Perel P, Roberts I and Ker K. Colloids versus crystalloids for fluid resuscitation in critically ill patients. *Cochrane Database of Systematic Reviews* 2013; Issue 2: CD000567. http://onlinelibrary.wiley.com/doi/10.1002/14651858.CD000567.pub6/pdf

11 Myburgh JA et al. Hydroxyethyl starch or saline for fluid resuscitation in intensive care. *New England Journal of Medicine* 2012; **367**: 1901–11.

12 Haase N et al. Hydroxyethyl starch 130/0.38-0.45 versus crystalloid or albumin in patients with sepsis: systematic review with meta-analysis and trial sequential analysis. *British Medical Journal* 2013; **346**: f839.

13 Wise J. Boldt: the great pretender. *British Medical Journal* 2013; **346**: f1738.

Nutrition: critical care implications

Nutrition should be given via the oral, enteral, or parenteral route as appropriate, depending on the clinical context and the type of feeding tolerated by the patient (for an overview of assessment of the nutritional status of the critically ill patient, see ➲ p. 24). Factors that influence how nutrition is delivered include:

- level of consciousness
- the presence of an endotracheal tube or tracheostomy
- the patient's ability to swallow
- the level of function of the gastrointestinal tract.

In the acute phase of critical illness, nutrition should provide sufficient calories and protein to maintain body weight and reduce nitrogen loss. The level of catabolism associated with the stressed state of critical illness does not allow the replenishment of body stores until the recovery phase, which puts critically ill patients at risk for malnutrition. It is estimated that 45% of intensive care unit patients are malnourished.[14] Table 3.6 compares malnutrition due to starvation with malnutrition of critical illness.

Consequences of malnutrition

- Decreased immune function, ventilatory drive, and respiratory muscle strength.
- Increased ventilatory dependence, infections, and morbidity and mortality.

Table 3.6 Comparison of malnutrition caused by starvation and critical illness

	Starvation	Critical Illness
Cause	Insufficient storage of essential nutrients	Abnormal processing of nutrients
Treatment	Increase in nutrient intake	Resolution of cause of critical illness, not just increased intake of nutrients

Reference

14 Racco M. Nutrition in the ICU. *RN* 2009; **72**: 26–31.

Further reading

British Association for Parenteral and Enteral Nutrition. www.bapen.org.uk
Critical Care Nutrition. www.criticalcarenutrition.com
European Society for Clinical Nutrition and Metabolism. www.espen.org
Faber P and Siervo M, eds. *Nutrition in critical care*. Cambridge University Press: Cambridge, 2014.
McClave SA et al. Feeding the critically ill patient. *Critical Care Medicine*: 2014 **42**: 2600–10.

Nutrition: daily requirements

Tables 3.7, 3.8, 3.9, and 3.10 list the recommended daily requirements for nutrients, electrolytes, trace elements, and vitamins (these tables are intended to serve as a guide, and each patient should be assessed individually).

Table 3.7 Daily nutrient requirements

Nutrient	Amount per day	Influencing factors
Protein (nitrogen)	0.7–1.0 g/kg/day (0.15–0.3 g/kg/day)	Hypermetabolism can increase protein requirements to 1.5–2.0 g/kg/day
Carbohydrate	Amount needed will depend on the patient's energy requirements, two-thirds of which are usually provided by carbohydrate, and one-third by fat A useful quick estimate of requirements is: Male: 25–30 kcal/kg/day Female: 20–25 kcal/kg/day	Patients with respiratory insufficiency or weaning after long-term ventilation may not handle the amount of carbon dioxide produced when intake exceeds requirement. Ratios of fat to carbohydrate should be changed to 50:50
Fat	Only necessary in very small amounts to prevent fatty acid deficiency. Usually the amount delivered contributes to providing energy. It represents between one-third and one-half of the total number of calories required A useful quick estimate of requirements is 0.8–1.0 g/kg/day	Tolerance of intravenous fat can be limited (see ➲ p. 66 on parenteral nutrition complications), and the amount delivered may need to be adjusted if this is the case

Table 3.8 Daily electrolyte requirements

Typical daily requirement	Additional factors
Sodium 70–100 mmol/day	More may be needed with loop diuretic therapy or during increased gastrointestinal losses (e.g. due to diarrhoea or fistulae)
	Less may be needed in oedema and hypernatraemia
Potassium 70–100 mmol/day	More may be needed during early repletion, post-obstructive diuresis, loop diuretic therapy, and increased gastrointestinal losses
	Less may be required in renal failure
Magnesium 7.5–10 mmol/day	As above
Calcium 5–10 mmol/day	—
Phosphate 20–30 mmol/day	More may be needed in early nutritional repletion, when there may be dramatic falls in serum phosphate levels (see ➲ p. 324 on refeeding syndrome)
	Less may be required with renal dysfunction

Table 3.9 Daily trace element requirements

	Recommended daily requirement		Effects of deficiency
	Enteral nutrition (µmol/L)	Parenteral nutrition (µmol/L)	
Zinc	110–145	145	Impaired cellular immunity, poor wound healing, diarrhoea
Chromium	0.5–1.0	0.2–0.4	Insulin-resistant glucose intolerance, elevated serum lipids
Copper	16–20	20	Hypochromic microcytic anaemia, neutropenia
Iodine	1–1.2	1.0	—
Selenium	0.8–0.9	0.25–0.5	Cardiomyopathy
Molybdenum	0.5–4.0	0.2–1.2	—
Manganese	30–60	5–10	CNS dysfunction
Fluoride	95–150	50	—

Table 3.10 Daily vitamin requirements

Vitamin	Recommended daily requirement	
	Enteral nutrition	Parenteral nutrition
A (retinol) 5000 (mcg)	600–1200	800–2500
B_1 (thiamine) (mg)	0.8–1.1	3–20
B_2 (riboflavin) (mg)	1.1–1.3	3–8
Niacin (mg)	2–18	40
B_6 (pyridoxine) (mg)	1.2–2.0	4.0–6.0
B_{12} (cyanocobalamin) (mcg)	1.5–3.0	5–15
C (ascorbic acid) (mg)	40–60	100
D (cholecalciferol) (mcg)	5	5
E (δ- and α-tocopherol) (mg)	10	10
Folic acid (mcg)	200–400	200–400
K (phytomenadione) (mcg/kg)	1	0.03–1.5
Pantothenic acid (mg)	3–7	10–20
Biotin (mcg)	10–200	60

Enteral nutrition

[illegible]

Types of enteral feeding tubes

[illegible]

Box [illegible] Advantages of enteral nutrition

[illegible]

Box [illegible] Disadvantages of enteral nutrition

[illegible]

Enteral nutrition

If the patient is unable to take food orally, enteral nutrition is the preferred route (its advantages and disadvantages are listed in Boxes 3.3 and 3.4). The local protocol for enteral nutrition should be followed. This typically involves initiating enteral nutrition at 30 mL/h within 24–48 h following admission, checking gastric residuals every 4 h (see ➲ p. 308), and increasing the feeds as tolerated until the target enteral feeding rate has been reached. Safe delivery of enteral feeding requires ongoing monitoring of tube placement and integrity, checking for tolerance of the feed, and ensuring that the required volumes are delivered.

Types of enteral feeding tubes

Wide-bore feeding tubes

- Sizes 12–16 Fr.
- Made from polyvinylchloride (PVC).
- Short-term use (< 10 days) because gastric acid degrades PVC.
- Also used for gastric drainage, aspiration, and decompression.

Fine-bore feeding tubes

- Sizes 8–10 Fr.
- Made from a range of materials.
  - PVC tubes should not be used for more than 14 days.
  - Polyurethane can be used for longer periods (e.g. up to 6 weeks: always check the manufacturer's guidelines), and is the material of choice for enteral feeding.
- Available with or without a guidewire and weighted tip.

Box 3.3 Advantages of enteral nutrition

- Nearer normal physiologically, using the gastrointestinal route for absorption, and stimulating normal enzyme and hormone involvement.
- Preserves gastrointestinal mucosal integrity.
- Prevents translocation of bacteria from the gastrointestinal tract to other areas of the body, because the gastric mucosa is intact.
- Reduced risk of gastrointestinal bleeding.
- Central venous access is not needed—this reduces the risk of insertion complications and infection compared with parenteral nutrition.
- May modify the immune response to stress if administered in the early stages after trauma.
- Cheaper than parenteral nutrition.

Box 3.4 Disadvantages of enteral nutrition

- May be associated with increased volumes of diarrhoea.
- Difficult to ensure that the patient receives and tolerates the volume of feed required to meet their energy and other nutritional needs.
- Requires functioning gastrointestinal tract.
- May be associated with increased risk of VAP.

Feeding tube position

Placement of all enteral tubes should be documented, including the time, date, length of insertion, and position site (see Table 3.11). It is also important to check that the feeding tube is in the correct position after the initial insertion, before commending feeds, prior to giving medications if feeds are not in progress, and if there are physical signs of possible displacement (e.g. vomiting, regurgitation, excessive coughing, or prolonged hiccupping). This checking process should follow the guidelines issued by the National Patient Safety Agency.[15]

- X-ray is the most reliable method of assessing the feeding tube position.
- pH paper:
  - Only use pH indicator paper that is made specifically for checking gastric aspirate and which is CE marked.
  - The pH of gastric content aspirates should be in the range 1–5.5.
  - pH paper is of limited use in critical care because continuous enteral feeding and proton pump inhibitors increase the gastric pH. A high pH value may then be misinterpreted as the feeding tube being placed in the small intestine or lungs when it is in fact in the stomach.

Types of enteral feeds

- Standard:
  - 1 kcal/mL with or without fibre (routine feeding).
- High energy:
  - 1.2–2 kcal/mL (fluid restriction or increased caloric requirements).
- Low energy:
  - 0.5–1 kcal/mL (long-term feeding with reduced caloric requirements).
- Elemental or peptide:
  - proteins provided as free amino acids or peptides to aid digestion (e.g. in pancreatic insufficiency or inflammatory bowel disease).
- Therapeutic:
  - tailored to specific conditions (e.g. renal, cardiac, respiratory, or immune modulating).
- Probiotic supplements:
  - may help to restore the flora of the gastrointestinal tract and decrease VAP, although further research is needed to confirm this.[16,17]

Table 3.11 Feeding tube position sites

NG	Nasogastric	Routine route for establishing enteral feeding
OG	Orogastric	Used for patients with basal skull or facial fractures
ND NJ	Nasoduodenal Nasojejunal	Post-pyloric enteral feeding
PEG	Percutaneous gastrostomy	Long-term enteral feeding
PEJ	Percutaneous jejunostomy	Long-term enteral feeding

Post-pyloric feeding

Post-pyloric feeding occurs when the tip of the feeding tube sits past the stomach through a nasoduodenal (ND), nasojejunal (NJ), or percutaneous jejunostomy (PEJ) tube. Insertion of an ND or NJ tube can be done at the bedside using prokinetics (e.g. metoclopramide, erythromycin) to aid the advancement of the tip of the feeding tube into the small intestine. Alternatively, endoscopy or fluoroscopy may be required for ND or NJ tube placement, and a PEJ tube is surgically placed for long-term feeding.

The time, cost, and expertise required for post-pyloric feeding limit its routine use, and debate continues as to its benefits compared with gastric tube feeding. However, the possible benefits of post-pyloric feeding include decreased gastric residual volume (GRV), a reduced risk of aspiration pneumonia, and increased delivery of required calories.[18,19]

Indications for post-pyloric feeding

- High GRV that is not responsive to prokinetics (see ➔ p. 308).
- Acute pancreatitis.
- Gastric outlet stenosis.
- Hyperemesis.
- Frequent pulmonary aspiration.

Complications of enteral feeding

- Mechanical (tube related):
  - Knotting of the tube can occur with increased curling in the stomach. Endoscopic or even surgical removal may be necessary.
  - Clogging or blockage can occur due to fragments of inadequately crushed tablets, adherence of feed residue, or incompatibilities between feed and medication given (e.g. phenytoin). Tablets should be crushed and dissolved well, or soluble forms of drugs used if available. The feeding tube should be flushed with 20 mL of water after drug delivery or aspiration checks.
  - Incorrect placement (usually in the bronchial tree).
  - Nasopharyngeal erosion and discomfort—the patient's nostrils should be checked for signs of pressure externally, and the tube should not be left in for longer than the recommended time.
  - Sinusitis and otitis—the tube should be changed at the recommended intervals.
  - Oesophageal reflux and oesophagitis—tube placement should be checked regularly and the patient nursed at 45°.
  - Tracheo-oesophageal fistula—the tube should be changed at the recommended intervals, and never use force when placing the tube. Consideration should be given to placing a PEG if the tube is likely to remain in for longer than 12 weeks.
- Nausea and vomiting (see ➔ p. 310).
- Pulmonary aspiration.
- Diarrhoea (see ➔ p. 304).

- Abdominal distension and/or delayed gastric emptying caused by:
  - critical illness and altered immune system
  - feed formula (associated with high density and high lipid content)
  - medications (e.g. opiates)
  - ileus
  - gastric atony
  - medical conditions (e.g. pancreatitis, diabetes, malnutrition, or post-vagotomy).
- Cramping.
- Constipation (see ➔ p. 306).
- Hyperglycaemia.
- Electrolyte and trace element abnormalities.
- Hypercapnia:
  - higher than required levels of carbohydrate in feeds can produce large amounts of CO_2 that require increased minute volumes and respiratory rate in order to be excreted
  - this may precipitate ventilatory failure in a patient with compromised respiratory function or during weaning of a patient. Accurate calculation of the patient's nutritional requirements is essential.

References

15 National Patient Safety Agency (NPSA). *Reducing the Harm Caused by Misplaced Nasogastric Feeding Tubes in Adults, Children and Infants*. NPSA: London, 2011. ℘ www.nrls.npsa.nhs.uk/EasySiteWeb/getresource.axd?AssetID=129697&

16 Morrow LE, Gogineni V, and Malesker MA. Probiotics in the intensive care unit. *Nutrition in Clinical Practice* 2012; **27**: 235–41.

17 Petrof EO et al. Probiotics in the critically ill: a systematic review of the randomized trial evidence. *Critical Care Medicine* 2012; **40**: 3290–302.

18 Jiyong J et al. Effect of gastric versus post-pyloric feeding on the incidence of pneumonia in critically ill patients: observations from traditional and Bayesian random-effects meta-analysis. *Clinical Nutrition* 2013; **32**: 8–15.

19 Zhang Z et al. Comparison of postpyloric tube feeding and gastric tube feeding in intensive care unit patients: a meta-analysis. *Nutrition in Clinical Practice* 2013; **28**: 371–80.

Further reading

Kreymann KG et al. ESPEN guidelines on enteral nutrition: intensive care. *Clinical Nutrition* 2006; **25**: 210–23. ℘ http://espen.info/documents/ENICU.pdf

Medlin S. Recent developments in enteral feeding for adults: an update. *British Journal of Nursing* 2012; **21**: 1061–7.

Simons SR and Abdallah LM. Bedside assessment of enteral tube placement: aligning practice with evidence. *American Journal of Nursing* 2012; **112**: 40–46.

Parenteral nutrition

Parenteral nutrition is indicated within 24–48 h if the following conditions are present:[20]

- oral nutrition is not expected to be given within the next 3 days
- enteral nutrition is contraindicated or not tolerated.

Boxes 3.5 and 3.6 list the advantages and disadvantages of parenteral nutrition. The parenteral feeding solution should be provided as an all-in-one, pre-mixed bag and administered through central venous access, although some solutions (e.g. < 850 mOsm/L) can be delivered via peripheral venous routes. Multiple-lumen central venous catheters can be used for parenteral nutrition delivery, so long as one lumen is dedicated solely to this. Care of the catheter must be meticulous due to the increased risk of infection. Ongoing monitoring for metabolic abnormalities (see Table 3.12) is also required while caring for a patient who is receiving parenteral nutrition.

Metabolic abnormalities

Other complications of parenteral feeding are rare, but include:

- precipitation of respiratory failure and failure of weaning due to excessive carbohydrate administration
- hyperosmolar states with an excessive osmotic diuresis
- abnormal platelet function and hypercoagulability states
- anaemia after prolonged use of IV lipids.

Clinical guidelines for the delivery of parenteral nutrition to critically ill patients have been provided by the European Society for Clinical Nutrition and Metabolism.[20] The key aspects that are relevant to critical care nursing practice are summarized here.

Box 3.5 Advantages of parenteral nutrition

- It ensures that essential nutrients are delivered.
- It allows the gastrointestinal tract to rest.

Box 3.6 Disadvantages of parenteral nutrition

- Potential risks from central venous access insertion (e.g. pneumothorax, arterial puncture, catheter misplacement).
- Potential risks from ongoing use of central venous access (e.g. infection, thrombus, air embolus).
- Increased risk of metabolic abnormalities (see Table 3.12).
- Increased risk of overfeeding.
- Gut mucosal atrophy.
- Increased financial cost and mortality compared with enteral feeding.

Table 3.12 Metabolic abnormalities associated with parenteral nutrition

Hyperglycaemia	Causes include persistent gluconeogenesis, blunted insulin response, decreased sensitivity to insulin, impaired peripheral utilization of glucose or phosphate, and chromium deficiency. Late development in a stable patient may signal a new infection or complication
Hypoglycaemia	Sudden discontinuation of total parenteral nutrition (TPN) may induce hypoglycaemia, particularly if the patient is concurrently receiving insulin. Insulin should be discontinued or reduced prior to stopping TPN. If this is not possible, 10–20% glucose may be commenced. Blood glucose should be frequently monitored
Hyperlipidaemia	Lipid clearance can be impaired in liver disease. Rapid infusion of lipid may also result in transient hyperlipidaemia
Hepatic dysfunction	Abnormal liver function tests (LFTs) and fatty infiltration of the liver can develop in carbohydrate-based parenteral nutrition. It is treated by reducing the amount of calories or increasing the proportion of fat
Acid–base disturbances	Hyperchloraemia can develop from amino acid metabolism, but the resulting acidosis is usually mild, and most amino acid preparations contain acetate as a buffer. Metabolic alkalosis can be seen with diuretic use, continuous nasogastric drainage, or corticosteroid therapy if concomitant replacement of sodium, potassium, and/or chloride ions is inadequate
Electrolyte imbalance	Generally, sodium, potassium, chloride, and bicarbonate are monitored and corrected before problems occur. However, significant body deficiencies may not be reflected by plasma levels due to the effect of pH and serum albumin levels or hormonal influences, such as aldosterone or antidiuretic hormone (ADH), which are often altered in the critically ill. Occasionally, magnesium, calcium, and phosphate may become imbalanced

Caloric requirements

- Minimize negative energy balance by providing sufficient calories as close to measured energy expenditure as possible.
- If indirect calorimetry is not available, use a target of 25 kcal/kg/day.
- Patients who are receiving enteral nutrition at less than the targeted dose for more than 2 days should have supplementary parenteral nutrition considered.

Carbohydrates

- Use a minimum of 2 g/kg/day glucose.
- Avoid hyper- and hypoglycaemia.

Lipids

- Use 0.7–1.5 g/kg over 12–24 h.
- Fish oils may have a role in parenteral nutrition of critically ill patients.

Amino acids

- Use 1.3–1.5 g/kg/day of a balanced amino acid mixture.
- Amino acid solution should include 0.2–0.4 g/kg/day of L-glutamine.

Micronutrients

- All parenteral nutrition should include daily multivitamins and trace elements.

Reference

20 Singer P et al. ESPEN guidelines on parenteral nutrition: intensive care. *Clinical Nutrition* 2009; 28: 387–400. http://espen.info/documents/0909/Intensive%20Care.pdf

Further reading

Canadian Clinical Practice Guidelines Committee. *Critical Care Nutrition. Canadian Clinical Practice Guidelines Updated in 2013.* www.criticalcarenutrition.com/index.php?option=com_content&view=category&layout=blog&id=21&Itemid=10

National Confidential Enquiry into Patient Outcome and Death (NCEPOD). *Parenteral Nutrition: a mixed bag.* NCEPOD: London, 2010. www.ncepod.org.uk/2010pn.htm

Anxiety and fear

Anxiety

Anxiety is defined as a state of disequilibrium or tension caused by apprehension of a potential [illegible] ... It is a [illegible] ... [illegible] and patients [illegible] ... or death associated [illegible] ...

Assessment of the level of anxiety depends almost wholly on subjective judgement, [illegible] ... the Hospital Anxiety and Depression Scale (HADS), are beyond the scope of ... [illegible] patients [illegible] ...

[illegible]

Interventions to reduce anxiety

- [illegible] ...

Fear

Fear is defined as a state of ... [illegible] ...

[illegible] ... and [illegible] ... relaxation [illegible] ...

- [illegible]
- [illegible]
- [illegible]
- [illegible]

[illegible] ... behavioural [illegible] ...

Anxiety and fear

Anxiety

Anxiety is defined as a state of disequilibrium or tension caused by apprehension of a potential non-specific threat. It is a natural response to the experience of critical illness and potential closeness of death associated with admission to critical care.

Assessment of the level of anxiety depends almost wholly on subjective judgement, as complex tools, such as the Hospital Anxiety and Depression Scale (HADS), are beyond the scope of critically ill patients to complete.

A recently developed facial expression scale for assessing anxiety has yet to be validated fully, but may help to identify anxiety in the critically ill.

Interventions to reduce anxiety

Nursing interventions that may be helpful are listed in Table 3.13.

Fear

Fear is defined as a state of distress and apprehension that causes sympathetic arousal.

The physiological response invoked by fear reflects the level of sympathetic stimulation, and is mediated by adrenaline (epinephrine) and noradrenaline (norepinephrine) release. Symptoms include:

- increased heart rate and blood pressure
- dilated pupils
- dry mouth
- peripheral and splanchnic vasoconstriction
- sweating.

The patient's behavioural response can be affected by their background, culture, and social conditioning.

Table 3.13 Coping mechanisms for anxiety

Patient mechanisms	Nursing interventions to enhance coping mechanism
Denial	Encouragement to verbalize fears. Recognition of the need for denial
Rationalization	Giving appropriately worded and timed information
Substituting positive thoughts for negative ones	Positive feedback for coping techniques
Retention of control of environment, timing of care, etc. (this is often via the nurse, who must facilitate this)	Facilitation of patient retention of control
Additional nursing interventions	
Use of empathetic and therapeutic touch	Access to spiritual counselling as needed
Supporting unrestricted family visiting	Amelioration of environmental stressors (e.g. noise from alarms, etc.)
Offering relaxation and/or meditation techniques	Providing appropriate background music (e.g. slow, flowing rhythms)
Speaking calmly and slowly using warm tones	If necessary, administration of anxiolytics (e.g. lorazepam)
Ensuring that pain relief is adequate	Nursing presence, attentiveness, and reassurance
Providing biofeedback (e.g. patient view of heart rate on monitor)	

Pain management

Pain is a complex phenomenon involving social, cultural, emotional, psychological, and physiological components. It is aggravated by anxiety and fear, and compounded in the critically ill by difficulties with communicating.

Due to communication barriers (e.g. confusion, intubation, or sedation), critically ill patients often have difficulty indicating that they are experiencing pain or discomfort. This leads to pain frequently being unrecognized and undertreated in the critical care setting.[21] Critical care nurses should take an active role in the ongoing assessment of pain (see ➲ p. 20) to enable the initiation of suitable pain management strategies. Relief of pain is important in order to:

- improve patient comfort, and reduce emotional stress and anxiety (see ➲ p. 70)
- reduce the physiological stress response, which can lead to increased metabolic rate and oxygen requirements, as well as increased water and sodium retention
- promote mobility to reduce the risk of DVTs
- promote deep breathing and coughing to reduce the risk of pneumonia
- prevent sleep deprivation caused by discomfort (see ➲ p. 86).

Non-pharmacological methods

- Repositioning.
- Massage.
- Relaxation techniques.
- Localized warmth for relief of aches and muscular spasms.
- Localized cooling, particularly for burn pain.
- Reassurance and communication to relieve underlying fear and anxiety.
- Transcutaneous electrical nerve stimulation (TENS)—this is more successful in reducing analgesic requirements than in providing total alleviation of pain.

Pharmacological methods

Opioids are the mainstay of analgesia in critical care. They are usually delivered intravenously, and commonly by infusion to ensure consistent analgesia. Other ways to deliver analgesia include patient-controlled analgesia (PCA) (in the conscious patient), and the epidural, oral/nasogastric, intramuscular, and rectal routes. The dose depends on age, weight, haemodynamic status, and renal and hepatic function, as well as clinical effect (see Table 3.14).

Paracetamol or non-steroidal anti-inflammatory drugs (NSAIDs) can be used for less severe pain, or in addition to opioids as a background to reduce analgesic requirements. NSAIDs should be used with caution because they have a number of serious side effects, including gastrointestinal bleeding (due to increased likelihood of gastric ulceration), general bleeding (due to platelet inhibition), renal impairment, and sodium retention. Antidepressant or anticonvulsant medications (e.g. amitriptyline, gabapentin) may be considered for neuropathic pain.

Patient-controlled analgesia

PCA has the advantage of allowing the patient to be in control of the pain management, which reduces dose requirements by avoiding excessive levels of pain, and decreases the likelihood of overdose, as a drowsy patient will not self-administer ongoing doses of pain relief. Comparison of the number of demands for analgesia made by a patient with the number of delivered doses allows effectiveness to be evaluated.

Epidural

An epidural may be indicated in the critical care setting for the pain management of non-sedated patients (e.g. post-operative, trauma, or high-dependency patients with other sources of acute pain). Contraindications for an epidural include:

- infection near the epidural insertion site
- systemic infection
- low blood pressure
- coagulopathy
- raised intracranial pressure.

Analgesia can be delivered through an epidural as intermittent boluses or as a continuous epidural infusion using an opioid, a local anaesthetic (e.g. bupivacaine), or both. Local protocols for the care of an epidural infusion should be followed, ensuring that the epidural site is monitored and the epidural pump/tubing is clearly marked as dedicated for epidural use only. The patient should also have ongoing assessment of their vital signs, pain score, sedation score, and level of motor–sensory block. Potential complications of an epidural include:

- low blood pressure, low respiratory rate, and reduced level of consciousness (LOC)
- nausea and vomiting
- pruritus
- urinary retention
- back pain
- leakage of cerebrospinal fluid
- motor–sensory dysfunction (limb weakness and/or altered sensation)
- insertion site infection or haematoma
- local anaesthetic toxicity (mouth tingling, reduced LOC, lowered blood pressure, lowered heart rate, tinnitus, seizures, or arrhythmias).

Local protocols should be followed for removal of an epidural, with particular care taken to check that the patient has not recently had an anticoagulant, and to observe the epidural site for signs of infection or bleeding. Oral analgesia should be prescribed to ensure that the patient remains comfortable after the epidural is no longer needed.

Reference

21 Alderson SM and McKechnie SR. Unrecognised, undertreated pain in ICU: causes, effects, and how to do better. *Open Journal of Nursing* 2013; **3**: 108–13.

Further reading

Barr J et al. Clinical practice guidelines for the management of pain, agitation, and delirium in adult patients in the intensive care unit. *Critical Care Medicine* 2013; **41**: 263–306.

Opioids: medication review

Opioids may be administered as an analgesic primarily for pain relief, or for their sedative properties while sedating a critically ill patient. The dosage should be titrated according to the targeted patient response, with ongoing review and adjustment to ensure that the patient is not under- or over-treated. For sedated patients, there should be a daily interruption of continuous IV analgesia, with the infusion restarted as clinically appropriate. Opioids have a synergistic effect when given simultaneously with sedative medications, which allows reduced dosages of both to be given to achieve the same effect (see Table 3.14 for doses of IV opioids, and Table 3.15 for a summary of the timing and side effects of opioids).

Patients with renal or liver dysfunction may require careful assessment to identify whether a reduced opioid dosage is needed due to metabolite accumulation, which increases both therapeutic and adverse effects. Alternatives to morphine (e.g. fentanyl, alfentanil, or remifentanil) should also be considered if there is renal impairment, or if a short-acting analgesic is required. Remifentanil differs from other opioids in that it is metabolized by blood and tissue esterases rather than by the liver. With such an extremely rapid onset, metabolism, and excretion, there is no residual analgesia after a remifentanil infusion is turned off, and therefore another analgesic needs to be provided after discontinuing remifentanil if discomfort is likely to persist.

Table 3.14 Doses for IV opioids

	Bolus dose	Infusion
Morphine	0.1–0.2 mg/kg	0.05–0.07 mg/kg/h
Diamorphine	0.05–0.1 mg/kg	0.03–0.06 mg/kg/h
Fentanyl	5–7.5 mcg/kg	5–20 mcg/kg/h
Alfentanil	15–30 mcg/kg	20–120 mcg/kg/h
Remifentanil	1 mcg/kg	0.05–2 mcg/kg/h
Pethidine	0.5 mg/kg	0.1–0.3 mg/kg/h

Table 3.15 Timing and side effects of IV opioids

	Timing	Side effects	Notes
Morphine	Onset: 5–10 min Duration: 3–4 h	↓BP, ↓RR, ↓CNS, H_2 release, ↓gut motility, nausea, ↑muscle tone	Poor GI absorption, accumulation in renal dysfunction, avoid with severe asthma
Diamorphine	Onset: 5 min Duration: 2–3 h	↓BP, ↓RR, ↓CNS, H_2 release, ↓gut motility, nausea, ↑muscle tone	Poor GI absorption, accumulation in renal dysfunction, avoid with severe asthma
Fentanyl	Onset: 1–2 min Duration: 2–4 h	↓BP, ↓RR, ↓CNS, ↓gut motility, nausea, ↑muscle tone	Muscular rigidity seen with high doses
Alfentanil	Onset: 1–2 min Duration: 30–60 min	↓BP, ↓RR, ↓CNS, ↓gut motility, nausea, ↑muscle tone	Muscular rigidity seen with high doses
Remifentanil	Onset: 1–2 min Duration: 5–10 min	↓BP, ↓RR, ↓CNS, ↓gut motility, nausea, ↑muscle tone	Ultra-short-acting, may cause rebound pain if stopped suddenly
Pethidine	Onset: 5–10 min Duration: 2–4 h	↓BP, ↓RR, ↓CNS, H_2 release, ↓gut motility, nausea, ↑muscle tone	Respiratory depression despite maintained RR, seizures with accumulation

BP, blood pressure; RR, respiratory rate; CNS, central nervous system; GI, gastrointestinal.

Further reading

Erstad BL et al. Pain management principles in the critically ill. *Chest* 2009; **135**: 1075–86.

Sedation management

Possible reasons for using sedative medications in critically ill patients include:

- alleviation of anxiety
- relief of discomfort
- promotion of sleep
- facilitation of procedures or treatment
- obtundation of detrimental physiological responses (e.g. increased FiO_2 requirements, raised intracranial pressure).

If the clinical context requires the patient to be kept continuously sedated, it is important for the nurse to ensure that an appropriate amount of sedative medication is administered to achieve the optimal sedation level required at that particular time. Ideally, the patient should be kept as lightly sedated as possible to prevent the complications of over-sedation (in particular, prolonged mechanical ventilator days and incidence of delirium, which both significantly contribute to increased ICU length of stay and patient discomfort). Table 3.16 lists the consequences of under-sedating and over-sedating patients.

Factors that influence the response to sedatives

- Kidney dysfunction.
- Liver dysfunction.
- Advanced age.
- Malnutrition, fat and muscle mass, and high total body water.
- Increased volume distribution.
- Slow metabolism.
- Underlying illness.
- Substance misuse:
  - patients with a history of alcohol and/or drug misuse may require higher doses of analgesia and sedation
  - withdrawal symptoms (e.g. raised blood pressure, tachycardia, tachypnoea) may occur with interruptions to sedation.
- Chronic medication use.
- Polypharmacy.

Table 3.16 Sedation practice

Under-sedation	Over-sedation
Problems with ventilation	Prolonged mechanical ventilation
Ventilation/perfusion (V/Q) mismatch	Weaning difficulties
Accidental extubation	Tolerance of sedatives
Catheter displacement	Withdrawal syndrome
Cardiac stress	Delirium
Anxiety	Cardiovascular depression
Post-traumatic stress disorder	Sleep disturbances

Patient-oriented goal-directed sedation

- Use a sedation scoring tool, to identify a specific target sedation level.
- The target sedation level for most patients is a calm patient who is easily aroused and who maintains a diurnal rhythm that is normal for them.
  - Specific circumstances may require deeper sedation (e.g. facilitation of 'difficult to tolerate' modes of ventilation such as inverse ratio ventilation, hypoxaemia on maximal oxygen therapy, raised intracranial pressure).
  - Patients who require pharmacological paralysis (see ➲ p. 82) must be deeply sedated prior to giving them a neuromuscular blocker.
  - Some patients will tolerate an endotracheal tube with no or minimal sedation, and patients with a tracheostomy may not need any sedatives.
- Sedative drug doses should be adjusted and infusion rates titrated according to ongoing hourly monitoring to maintain the target level of sedation.
- Bispectral index (BIS) monitoring may help with sedation assessment (see ➲ p. 254).
- Consider the need for pain relief before administering sedatives.
  - Analgesics can provide some degree of sedative effect.
  - A hypnotic or anxiolytic should then only be given if the patient needs it in order to reach the identified sedation-level goal.
- Non-pharmacological interventions that may help to alleviate discomfort, relieve anxiety, and keep the patient safe while reducing or stopping sedative infusions include:
  - frequent reassurance and reorientation by the nurse
  - physical contact and communication by the family
  - holding the patient's hands to prevent them from pulling out the endotracheal tube, intravenous lines, nasogastric tube, Foley catheter, or other drains or lines.

Daily interruption of sedation (DIS)

- Sedation target and dosage should be assessed daily in order to determine whether continuous infusions can have their rate reduced or be stopped.
- Landmark clinical trials by Kress and colleagues[22] and Girard and colleagues[23] showed that DIS resulted in:
  - a reduction in the duration of mechanical ventilation
  - an increase in spontaneous breathing while being mechanically ventilated
  - a reduction in the length of ICU stay and hospital stay .
  - a decrease in the amount of sedative medication needed to achieve the target sedation level
  - a reduced requirement to assess altered mental status using radiological studies.
- Research by Mehta and colleagues[24] did not show that DIS improved length of ICU stay, the number of ventilator days, or the incidence of delirium, and suggested that more daily sedative medication is needed because of sedation boluses required after DIS.
  - Current practice promotes minimal sedative administration and use of shorter-acting drugs, which may explain these results compared with earlier research when patients were kept deeply sedated.

- Even if DIS is not undertaken, only the minimum amount of sedation drug necessary should be used to maintain the target sedation level.
- DIS is included in the ventilation care bundle (see ➔ p. 111).
- DIS is referred to as 'spontaneous awakening trial' in the 'Wake Up and Breathe' protocol[25] (see Figure 3.2).

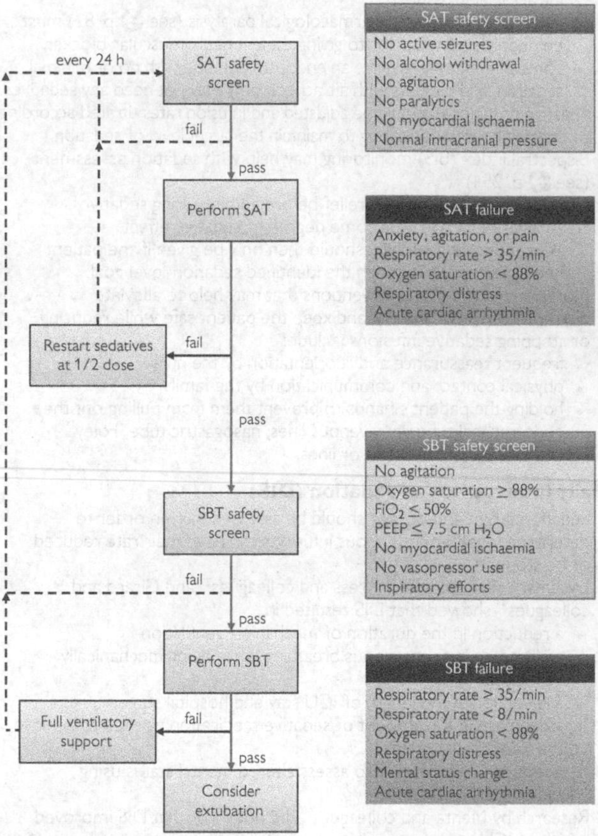

Figure 3.2 'Wake Up and Breathe' protocol. SAT, spontaneous awakening trial; SBT, spontaneous breathing trial. (Reproduced with permission of Vanderbilt University © 2008.)

References

22 Kress JP et al. Daily interruption of sedative infusions reduced duration of mechanical ventilation and intensive care unit stay in critically ill patients. *New England Journal of Medicine* 2000; **342**: 1471–7.

23 Girard TD et al. Efficacy and safety of a paired sedation and ventilator weaning protocol for mechanically ventilated patients in intensive care (Awakening and Breathing Controlled trial): a randomised controlled trial. *Lancet* 2008: **371**: 126–34.

24 Mehta S et al. Daily sedation interruption in mechanically ventilated critically ill patients cared for with a sedation protocol: a randomized controlled trial. *Journal of the American Medical Association* 2012; **308**: 1985–92.

25 Vanderbilt University. 2008. *"Wake Up and Breathe" Protocol.* www.icudelirium.org/docs/WakeUpAndBreathe.pdf

Further reading

Barr J et al. Clinical practice guidelines for the management of pain, agitation, and delirium in adult patients in the intensive care unit. *Critical Care Medicine* 2013; **41**: 263–306.

Sedatives: medication review

Table 3.17 lists the definitions of sedation-related medication properties, and Table 3.18 summarizes the classification of medications used during the sedation of critically ill patients.

Benzodiazepines

Benzodiazepines are commonly used in critical care for their multifactorial effects, which include sedative, anxiolytic, hypnotic, amnesiac, and muscle relaxant properties. They are mainly administered intravenously and in combination with analgesia. For patients with renal dysfunction, use benzodiazepines with caution—reduce the dosage, perform daily interruption to prevent over-sedation, or consider using an alternative drug.

Propofol

Developed as an anaesthetic agent, propofol is now used in lower doses for short-term sedative infusions (48–72 h). It has vasodilator and negative inotropic properties, and should be used with caution if hypovolaemia has not been fully corrected or cardiac function is poor.

There is an increased risk of propofol infusion syndrome with prolonged use at high doses along with the administration of catecholamines or steroids (see Box 3.7). Caution is needed when administering an IV infusion for more than 48 h, and there is a higher incidence of propofol infusion syndrome with children, teenagers, and head injury patients.

α2-Agonists

These act as synergistic analgesics with opiates, but cause minimal respiratory depression and the patient is easily rousable. Side effects include hypotension and bradycardia, and the patient will experience a dry mouth. Although adverse effects need to be considered and long-term outcomes are not yet known, clinical trials indicate that dexmedetomidine reduces the number of mechanical ventilator days and allows patients to communicate their pain better compared with midazolam and propofol.[26,27]

Ketamine

This is an anaesthetic agent that is also a powerful analgesic. It is associated with good airway maintenance, spontaneous respiration, bronchodilation, and cardiovascular stimulation. Side effects include hypertension and tachycardia as well as hallucinations and psychotic episodes, which usually require concurrent benzodiazepines to invoke amnesia.

Antipsychotics

Antipsychotics may have a role in the management of delirium (see ➔ p. 76). Caution is necessary, as arrhythmias and extrapyramidal disorders are associated with their use.

Table 3.17 Medication properties

Analgesic	↓ Pain and discomfort
Sedative	↓ Level of consciousness
Anxiolytic	↓ Anxiety
Hypnotic	Maintains loss of consciousness
Amnesic	Causes loss of memory
Muscle relaxant	↓ Skeletal muscle tone
Anticonvulsant	↓ Seizures

Table 3.18 Drugs used for sedated patients

Opioids	Morphine, fentanyl, alfentanil, remifentanil See ➲ p. 74
Benzodiazepines	Midazolam, lorazepam, diazepam
α_2-Agonists	Clonidine, dexmedetomidine
Anaesthetics	Propofol, ketamine, etomidate
Barbiturates	Thiopental, phenobarbital
Neuromuscular blocking agents	Suxamethonium, rocuronium, cisatracurium See ➲ p. 82
Antipsychotics	Haloperidol, olanzapine

Box 3.7 Clinical features of propofol infusion syndrome

- ↓ Heart rate.
- Heart failure.
- Rhabdomyolysis.
- Metabolic acidosis.
- Acute kidney injury.
- Hyperlipidaemia.
- Hepatomegaly.

References

26 Jakob SM et al. Dexmedetomidine vs midazolam or propofol for sedation during prolonged mechanical ventilation: two randomized controlled trials. *Journal of the American Medical Association* 2012; **307**: 1151–60.

27 Reardon DP et al. Role of dexmedetomidine in adults in the intensive care unit: an update. *American Journal of Health-System Pharmacy* 2013; **70**: 767–77.

Pharmacological paralysis

Neuromuscular blocking agents (NMBAs) are muscle relaxants that block synaptic transmission at the neuromuscular junction of skeletal muscle, causing therapeutic paralysis. Table 3.19 provides rationales for and clinical examples of paralysis of critical care patients. Ongoing paralysis should be avoided if at all possible, due to the need for concurrent deep sedation and the risk of potential complications. However, administering an NMBA as a continuous infusion during the early phase of ARDS improves patient outcomes without increasing ICU-acquired muscle weakness.[28,29]

Potential complications

- Suppression of cough and gag reflexes:
  - increased oral and pulmonary secretions
  - atelectasis
  - increased risk of pneumonia.
- Critical illness polyneuropathy and critical illness myopathy:
  - increased risk with prolonged paralysis
  - increased risk if NMBA is administered concurrently with steroids
  - respiratory muscle weakness—increased weaning duration
  - long-term muscle weakness.

Table 3.19 Indications for pharmacological paralysis

Indication	Rationale	Clinical examples
Endotracheal intubation	Relaxes vocal cords	Mechanical ventilation Airway protection
Problems with mechanical ventilation	Improves chest wall compliance ↓ Airway resistance causing high airway pressures	ARDS Severe asthma Bronchoconstriction Prone position
High ICP	↓ Cerebral oxygen requirements	Traumatic brain injury Post-operative neuro-surgery Cerebral oedema
Muscle abnormality	↓ Seizures ↓ Shivering ↓ Hypertonicity	Status epilepticus Hypothermia Tetanus
Investigations and interventions	Paralysis may be required for specific tests and procedures relevant to the critical care setting	Bronchoscopy Tracheostomy CT or MRI scan Patient transport

Nursing management

- For nursing care during endotracheal intubation, see ➔ p. 144.
- Ensure that an Ambu bag is kept at the patient's bedside in case accidental extubation occurs.
- Mechanically ventilate the patient using a controlled mode of ventilation.
- Establish deep sedation prior to paralysing the patient, and use BIS monitoring for continuous assessment of sedation level.
- For ongoing paralysis, consider stopping NMBA infusion daily to ensure that the patient remains sufficiently sedated and to assess whether there is still a need for the NMBA infusion.
- Keep the patient's eyelids closed and provide frequent eye care for corneal protection due to loss of the blink reflex (see ➔ p. 50).
- Peripheral nerve stimulator:
  - This ensures that the minimum amount of NMBA is given without over- or under-paralysing the patient.
  - Monitor the degree of blockade using the train-of-four method (see Table 3.20).
  - Titrate the NMBA to maintain 1–2 twitches.
- Perform regular head-to-toe assessment, but bear in mind that:
  - the patient will not be able to communicate or indicate if they are in pain
  - pupil reaction is the only relevant neurological assessment (GCS score and peripheral motor–sensory function tests will not be accurate)
  - NMBAs will mask muscle activity, so abnormalities such as seizures, shivering, and abdominal rigidity may go undetected.
- Stop administering the NMBA as a continuous infusion as soon as it is clinically appropriate, and restart only if necessary.
- Educate the patient's family about the need to paralyse the patient.

Table 3.20 Train-of-four assessment

Number of twitches after peripheral stimulation	Degree of blockade	Outcome
4	0–75%	Under-paralysed
3	80%	Under-paralysed
2	85%	Goal achieved
1	90%	Goal achieved
0	100%	Over-paralysed

References

28 Alhazzani W et al. Neuromuscular blocking agents in acute respiratory distress syndrome: a systematic review and meta-analysis of randomized controlled trials. *Critical Care* 2013; **17**: R43.

29 Neto AS et al. Neuromuscular blocking agents in patients with acute respiratory distress syndrome: a summary of the current evidence from three randomized controlled trials. *Annals of Intensive Care* 2012; **2**: 33.

Neuromuscular blocking agents (NMBAs): medication review

Depolarizing NMBAs

- Depolarize the plasma membrane of skeletal muscle.
- Persistent depolarization caused by the drug makes muscle fibres resistant to further stimulation by acetylcholine.
- Suxamethonium chloride (succinylcholine chloride) is the only depolarizing NMBA available (see Table 3.21).
- Commonly used for rapid sequence induction prior to endotracheal intubation.

Non-depolarizing NMBAs

- Compete with acetylcholine by binding to receptors at the neuromuscular junction to prevent acetylcholine from stimulating receptors.
- Reversed by anticholinesterases (e.g. neostigmine).
- For a comparison of various non-depolarizing NMBAs, see Table 3.22.

Aminosteroids: rocuronium, vecuronium, and pancuronium

- Eliminated by the liver.
- Not associated with histamine release.

Benzylisoquinolinium class of drugs: atracurium and cisatracurium

- Histamine release occurs with atracurium but not with cisatracurium.
- Metabolized by Hoffman degradation and ester hydrolysis in the plasma (elimination is independent of the liver and kidneys).

Factors that enhance the effect of NMBAs

- Acid–base imbalance (acidosis and alkalosis).
- Hypothermia.
- Electrolyte imbalance (↓K^+, ↓Na^+, ↓Ca^{2+}, ↑Mg^{2+}).
- Neuromuscular disease.
- Medications:
  - depolarizing—neostigmine, metoclopramide, esmolol, etomidate.
  - non-depolarizing—Ca^{2+}-channel blockers, aminoglycosides, erythromycin, clindamycin, metronidazole, immunosuppressants, lithium, H_2-receptor antagonists.

Table 3.21 Suxamethonium chloride (succinylcholine chloride)

Clinical information	Side effects	Contraindications
Onset: 30–60 s Duration: 4–6 min Intubation dosage: 1–1.5 mg/kg IV Elimination: plasma cholinesterase	Hyperkalaemia Bradycardia Ventricular arrhythmias Hypotension ↑ Intra-ocular pressure ↑ Intragastric pressure ↑ Intracranial pressure Malignant hyperthermia Myalgia	Hyperkalaemia Major trauma Severe burns Spinal cord injury Low plasma cholinesterase activity (e.g. severe liver disease) Muscular dystrophy

Table 3.22 Non-depolarizing NMBAs

Drug	Timing	Dosage
Atracurium	Onset: 2–3 min Duration: 25–35 min	Initial 300–600 mcg/kg IV injection 270–1770 mcg/kg/h IV infusion
Cisatracurium	Onset: 2–3 min Duration: 25–45 min	Initial 150 mcg/kg IV injection 30–600 mcg/kg/h IV infusion
Rocuronium	Onset: 30–60 s Duration: 30–40 min	Initial 600 mcg/kg IV injection 300–600 mcg/kg/h IV infusion
Vecuronium	Onset: 1–2 min Duration: 20–30 min	Initial 80–100 mcg/kg IV injection 0.8–1.4 mcg/kg/min infusion
Pancuronium	Onset: 2–3 min Duration: 90–100 min	Initial 100 mcg/kg IV injection 60 mcg/kg IV every 60–90 min

Further reading

Gupta A and Singh-Radcliff N (eds). *Pharmacology in Anesthesia Practice*. Oxford University Press: Oxford, 2013.

Smith S, Scarth E and Sasada M. *Drugs in Anaesthesia and Intensive Care*, 4th edn. Oxford University Press: Oxford, 2011.

Sleep

Critically ill patients have disrupted circadian rhythms due to the severity of the underlying illness or injury causing changes to adrenocorticotropic hormone and melatonin levels, the physical environment of the critical care setting, and alterations of the light–dark cycle. An altered sleep pattern can then result in the patient sleeping during the day instead of at night, sleep fragmentation (frequently waking), and reduced slow-wave sleep (SWS) and rapid eye movement (REM) stages of sleep. Critical care patients commonly suffer from sleep deprivation, and this is significant because sleep is needed for the growth and rejuvenation of the immune system.[30]

Table 3.23 outlines a structured approach to assessment of sleep.

Pharmacological sedation vs. physiological sleep

- Benzodiazepines increase level 2 sleep and total sleep time but decrease SWS and REM sleep.
- Non-benzodiazepine hypnotics increase SWS and REM sleep.
- Sedative medications may increase quantity of sleep, but sleep fragmentation where the patient is frequently woken up decreases quality of sleep.

Effects of sleep deprivation

- Increased risk of delirium.
- Increased risk of post-traumatic stress disorder.
- Increased sympathetic stimulation.
- Reduced immune function.
- Respiratory fatigue and increase in weaning time.
- Increased number of mechanical ventilation days.
- Increased number of ICU days.
- Increased mortality.

Causes of sleep deprivation

- Noise—patients report that staff conversations and alarms are the most disturbing sources of noise.[31]
- Lights.
- Pain and discomfort.
- Medications.
- Stress.

Table 3.23 Sleep assessment

Quantity*	How many hours the patient has slept in a 24-h period
Distribution over 24 h	Timing of the sleep in relation to day and night
Continuity	How long sleep continued without being interrupted

* Assessment of quality of sleep is difficult because it requires polysomnography, which is not readily available to critical care nurses.

Factors that promote sleep

- Patient comfort.
- Noise and light reduction.
- Clustering of patient care.
- Uninterrupted time to sleep (a full sleep cycle requires ≥ 90 min).
- Optimal mechanical ventilation settings.
- Only essential early-morning care.
- Avoiding or minimizing the use of drugs that influence sleep.
- Melatonin.[32,33]

References

30 Wenham T and Pittard A. Intensive care unit environment. *Continuing Education in Anaesthesia, Critical Care & Pain* 2009; **9**: 178–83.

31 Xie H, Kang J and Mills GH. Clinical review: the impact of noise on patients' sleep and the effectiveness of noise reduction strategies in intensive care units. *Critical Care* 2009; **13**: 208.

32 Bourne RS, Mills GH and Minelli C. Melatonin therapy to improve nocturnal sleep in critically ill patients: encouraging results from a small randomised controlled trial. *Critical Care* 2008; **12**: R52.

33 Riutta A, Ylitalo P and Kaukinen S. Diurnal variation of melatonin and cortisol is maintained in non-septic intensive care patients. *Intensive Care Medicine* 2009; **35**: 1720–27.

Further reading

Castro R, Angus DC and Rosengart MR. The effect of light on critical illness. *Critical Care* 2011; **15**: 218.

Chan MC et al. Circadian rhythms: from basic mechanisms to the intensive care unit. *Critical Care Medicine* 2012; **40**: 246–53.

Eliassen KM and Hopstock LA. Sleep promotion in the intensive care unit—a survey of nurses' interventions. *Intensive and Critical Care Nursing* 2011; **27**: 138–42.

Tembo AC and Parker V. Factors that impact on sleep in intensive care patients. *Intensive and Critical Care Nursing* 2009; **25**: 314–22.

Immobility

Critically ill patients can remain immobile due to a combination of factors, including physiological instability, weakness, sedation, NMBAs, traction, and multiple invasive devices. Ideally, the patient should be frequently repositioned, with early mobilization as soon as their condition permits.

Complications

- **Chest infection:** due to decreased sputum clearance, impaired functional residual capacity (FRC), and reduced cough.
- **Muscle atrophy:** due to disuse—occurs rapidly with lack of use, and requires long periods to rebuild.
- **Joint stiffness and contractures:** stronger flexor muscles increase flexion, commonly the plantar, shoulder, hand, and hip flexors.
- **Demineralization and loss of long bone density:** loss of weight-bearing pressure decreases osteoblastic activity within 1–2 days.
- **Pressure ulcers:** high risk due to immobility plus altered tissue perfusion, reduced sensory function, malnutrition, and chronic disease factors.
- **Venous thromboembolism (VTE) and peripheral oedema:** venous stasis and increased coagulability due to loss of muscle pumps.
- **Urinary tract infection:** urinary stasis in the supine position due to dependent bladder portion filling and increased infection risk associated with urinary catheter.
- **Nephrolithiasis:** increased urinary calcium excretion due to disuse bone density loss.
- **Decreased gut motility and constipation:** partly due to muscle atrophy, and compounded by sedation and loss of enteral stimuli if the patient is not enterally fed.
- **Peripheral nerve injury:** the ulnar nerve is at particular risk from pronation and elbow flexion when the patient is supine.

Interventions to reduce the risk of complications are summarized in Box 3.8.

Box 3.8 Interventions to reduce the risk of complications of immobility

- Regular repositioning:
  - Use right and left lateral as well as supine positions, but maintain the bed head elevated at 30–45°.
  - Correct alignment and positioning of limbs to prevent nerve damage and contractures.
  - Early mobilization to chair.
  - Use hoists and stretchers for highly dependent patients.
  - Passive limb movements.
  - Maintain normal range of movement (ROM) and stretch flexors.
  - Maintain muscle strength and joint mobility.
  - Active isotonic limb and ROM exercises at regular intervals.
  - Spread the pressure load.
  - Use special support mattresses and surfaces, and check dependent points over bony structures (high-risk areas) every shift.
- Active chest physiotherapy.
- Commence enteral feeding as soon as possible.
- Observe and document bowel function, intervening as necessary.
- Maintain scrupulous infection control.
- Give VTE prophylaxis.

Communicating with patients

Normal communication processes are disrupted in the critically ill patient by sedation, opiates, endotracheal and tracheal tubes, and fluctuating consciousness. This is complicated by pain, fear, and anxiety. Communication requires patience, motivation, the ability to see the patient as an individual, perseverance, a willingness to try new methods, and experience. Many patients are able to hear, understand, and respond emotionally to what is said to them, even when they are not thought to be aware by critical care staff.

Patients can feel isolated, alienated, and fearful. This should be recognized in any communication by showing empathy, giving information, and acknowledging these concerns. Box 3.9 provides a list of suggestions on how to communicate effectively with critically ill patients, Box 3.10 lists examples of communication assistance devices, and Box 3.11 lists specific nursing skills that can enhance communication.

Critical care survivors have given accounts of their experiences, which are a valuable source of information about what is important. Orientation to time, day, and situation is an important baseline, in addition to a clear introduction of self and others.

Box 3.9 Communicating effectively with critically ill patients

- Ensure that the patient can see and hear you by positioning yourself in their line of sight, making eye contact, and speaking clearly.
- Use touch to signal that the patient has your attention and empathy.
- Use positive feedback—smiling, nodding attentively, and focusing your full attention on the patient's face.
- Orientate the patient to time, day, place, and your own identity.
- Assess the patient's ability to respond (by means of speech, signs, mouthing, nodding and facial gestures, writing, etc.).
- Enhance the response using communication devices such as word or symbol boards or computers.
- Use appropriate levels of questioning:
  - open questions for patients who can speak or communicate fully
  - closed questions for patients who communicate with gestures and nodding.
- Where possible, agree appropriate gestures for communication, and ensure that these are documented or handed over.
- Where language difficulties exist, obtain phonetic translations of simple words, such as pain, or use symbol boards (available from speech and language therapists).
- Involve the patient's family in planning and using the right method of communication.

Box 3.10 Communication assistance devices for intubated patients

- Passy-Muir valve.
- Possum Portascan.
- Pen or pencil and paper.
- Alphabet or symbol boards.
- Laptop computer.
- Magic writer or magic slate.
- Electronic communicator (e.g. Lightwriter).

Box 3.11 Nursing skills to enhance communication

- Lip-reading.
- Knowledge of other languages.
- Use of mime, gestures, and facial expressions.
- Eye contact.
- Touch.

Family care

Family members of critically ill patients commonly report the need for:[34,35]

- support
- comfort
- information
- proximity
- assurance.

Families require a positive, supportive relationship with the critical care staff, and documentation about family care should be kept to ensure that the entire multi-professional team is aware of what has been communicated (see Box 3.12). Strategies for helping to support and communicate with large families include the following:

- Establish who is next of kin, and ensure that this is clearly documented in the patient record.
- Ask the family to appoint one spokesperson who will be responsible for receiving information and communicating it to the rest of the family.
- Limit concurrent visiting numbers, and organize relays of attendance at the bedside.
- Ensure that visitors are aware of rest periods.
- Specify a daily update time.
- Encourage mutual support within the family.

Box 3.12 Meeting family needs in critical care

Information

- Anticipate and supply information needs.
- Supplement information with printed booklets, online resources, and explanations.
- Ensure that information is not conflicting.

Communication and explanation

- Communication should be open and honest.
- Distressing communications should be delivered in a private environment.
- Ensure that explanations are delivered in appropriate language.
- A common record of all communication between the family and the multi-professional team should be maintained.

Involvement in care

- Support family time, both at the bedside and away from it.
- Involve families in non-technical patient care as appropriate.
- Involve families in patient diaries, in personalizing the environment, and in stimulating the patient when they are more awake.
- If English is the family's second language, be very active in involving the family in reassuring the patient.

Support of the family

- Access to the patient should be tailored both to be in the patient's best interests and to meet the family's needs.
- Staff should monitor the family carefully for stressors and offer advice, support, and links to alternative support mechanisms as necessary.
- Assign consistent nurses to maintain continuity of care.
- Use volunteers, pastoral care, and ancillary staff to give added support.

References

34 Al-Mutair AS et al. Family needs and involvement in the intensive care unit: a literature review. *Journal of Clinical Nursing* 2013; **22**: 1805–17.

35 Obringer K et al. Needs of adult family members of intensive care unit patients. *Journal of Clinical Nursing* 2012; **21**: 1651–8.

Further reading

Buckley P and Andrews T. Intensive care nurses' knowledge of critical care family needs. *Intensive and Critical Care Nursing* 2011; **27**: 263–72.

Davidson JE. Family-centered care: meeting the needs of patients' families and helping families adapt to critical illness. *Critical Care Nurse* 2009; **29**: 28–34.

HealthTalkOnline. ℅ www.healthtalkonline.org/Intensive_care

ICUSteps. ℅ www.icusteps.org

Intensive Care Society. *Patients and Relatives Committee.* ℅ www.ics.ac.uk/about-us/council-and-committee-pages/patients-and-relatives-committee

Khalaila R. Patients' family satisfaction with needs met at the medical intensive care unit. *Journal of Advanced Nursing* 2013; **69**: 1172–82.

Visiting

The British Association of Critical Care Nurses (BACCN) Position Statement Standards[36] on visiting in adult critical care units in the UK state that:

'Patients should expect:

- to have their privacy, dignity and cultural beliefs recognized
- confidentiality
- the choice of whether or not to have visitors
- the choice to decide who they want to visit, including children and other loved ones
- the choice of care assisted by their relatives
- a critical care team who recognize the importance and value of visiting.

Relatives should have:

- a comfortable and accessible waiting room with bathroom facilities nearby
- access to overnight accommodation in the vicinity of the ICU
- easy access to food and drink
- a telephone nearby
- access to relevant information regarding critical illness, the critical care environment and aftercare and support; this should be reinforced with written materials
- a separate area for private discussions with healthcare professionals
- involvement in patient care as the patient would wish
- written information regarding the unit procedures e.g. hand washing, time of ward rounds
- information concerning patient progress on at least a daily basis
- information when there are any significant changes to the patient's condition
- not have to wait for long periods of time in the waiting room without regular updates
- access to interpretation facilities if needed.' (Reproduced with permission of BACCN © 2012.)

Reference

36 Gibson V et al. *Position Statement on Visiting in Adult Critical Care Units in the United Kingdom.* British Association of Critical Care Nurses (BACCN)L: Newcastle Upon Tyne, 2012.

Non-technical skills

Communication with the multidisciplinary team

[illegible]

Teamwork

[illegible]

- patient care
- productivity
- staff satisfaction
- the working environment
- [illegible]

[illegible]

- [illegible]
- [illegible]
- [illegible]

[illegible]

[illegible]

Non-technical skills

Communication with the multidisciplinary team

Critical care nurses frequently interact with a variety of people within the multidisciplinary team, which requires them to have strong communication skills. Use of a handover structure, such as the nursing care plan or SBAR (Situation, Background, Assessment, Recommendation) tool,[37] will ensure that essential information is handed over in a systematic manner (see Table 3.24). Closed loop communication encourages checking back and verifying that information was received and understood by the person to whom it was being communicated.

Teamwork

Collaborative, team-based working is essential within the critical care unit, and helps to improve:

- patient care
- productivity
- staff satisfaction
- the working environment
- outcomes, including mortality.

Teamwork requires mutual respect among professionals, and recognition that all team members' contributions are necessary to give the patient the best outcome. Teams should have a recognized team leader, although there are often several different team groupings, such as:

- unit clinical team—team leader is a medical consultant.
- unit nursing team—team leader is a sister or charge nurse.
- bedside team—team leader is nurse at bedside.
- unit management team—team leader is general manager or clinical director.

Effective teamworking requires a key decision-making point, such as the traditional ward round, during which the patient's case can be discussed and a plan of care decided on. However, the key to effective and safe teams is the opportunity for all team members to raise concerns and question decisions.

Table 3.24 SBAR tool[37]

S	Situation	What is going on with the patient?
B	Background	What clinical information is pertinent to the situation?
A	Assessment	What are the key aspects of your assessment?
R	Recommendation	What actions are needed? What do you want to happen for this patient?

Markers of effective teamwork

- Common goals and values are shared by all team members, focus on patient-centred care, and foster staff empowerment, support, and development.
- Roles within the team are clearly defined, with all members of the team fully understanding and respecting the role of each of the other members.
- Team members monitor each other's performance and step in to help out and support each other—trust is implicit in this.
- Giving and receiving feedback is the norm for all team members and is seen as part of their role.
- Communication is made real (i.e. senders check that messages are received as they intended).
- Team members collectively learn from experiences, enable constructive feedback from critical incidents, and show a willingness to address and resolve causes of conflict.
- A range of qualities, skills, and knowledge is evident within the team, along with commitment from all team members.

Methods of improving team effectiveness

- Enhance multidisciplinary decision making by drawing from a broad spectrum of knowledge about the patient's condition. This could also include listening to the patient and their family.
- Reward the team as a whole.
- Encourage innovative solutions to problems.
- Promote a shared multidisciplinary team approach to clinical practice, education, research, and management activities.
- Establish clear roles and responsibilities for all members of the critical care team.
- Endorse a positive working culture with strong leadership, flexible service planning, successful communication systems, and effective resource use.
- Ensure that all members of the team are aware of clear procedures for:
  - daily routine practice
  - admissions and discharges
  - acting upon early warning signs of the deteriorating patient
  - outreach systems
  - unplanned events (e.g. resuscitation, evacuation, major incident).

Time management

It is important for critical nurses to demonstrate effective time management skills in order to provide safe, high-quality nursing care despite the pressures and demands placed on nurses in a busy critical care unit (see Table 3.25). Improving the productivity and efficiency of critical care nursing practice through effective time management also helps to reduce waste and thus the overall financial and environmental cost of critical care. These are significant considerations in view of current initiatives for the NHS to become a more sustainable healthcare service.[38,39]

Table 3.25 The implications of time management

Poor use of time	Good use of time
Unsafe practice	Safe practice
Poor quality of care	High-quality nursing care
Loss of productivity	Productivity and efficiency
Increase in cost	Increase in cost-effectiveness
Increase in stress levels of staff	Improved working culture

Strategies for improving time management skills

- Prioritize urgent care.
- Actively engage in early recognition of risk factors for patient deterioration in order to initiate preventive measures and trouble-shoot potential clinical problems.
- Collaborate with colleagues.
- At the beginning of a clinical shift, plan out nursing care so as to efficiently complete nursing care for the patient and their family and also ensure that breaks can be taken and arrange break coverage of other colleagues.
- Consider rationales for clinical decisions to help to justify and prioritize nursing care while making nursing practice more efficient (e.g. protocols, guidelines, care bundles, research, intuition, local culture, and past experience).

Situation awareness

Critical care nurses must not only be aware of and understand the clinical context of their patients, but also have an appreciation of what is happening within the surrounding environment in the critical care unit (see Box 3.13). In addition, they need to be able to consider the implications of acting or not acting upon specific events that occur within the current situation. The process of situation awareness has three elements:[40]

- **perception**—awareness of the environment and context of the current situation
- **comprehension**—understanding, interpreting, and evaluating the current situation
- **projection**—anticipation of future possibilities and ability to plan trouble-shooting measures.

Box 3.13 Situation awareness for critical care nurses

Are you aware of the following?

- The current clinical context, including physical and non-physical health needs of the patient and their family.
- The immediate bed-space environment of your patient, including monitoring, equipment, and therapies.
- Possible reasons for deterioration in your patient's health status.
- Effectiveness of current therapies and treatments.
- Staffing levels and skill mix for the shift.
- Acuity and nursing workload for other patients.
- Patients who are about to be admitted or discharged.
- Break coverage for yourself and nearby colleagues.
- Shift-leader support that you may be able to provide.

Notes and references

37 NHS Institute for Innovation and Improvement. SBAR: situation-background-assessment-recommendation, 2008. http://www.institute.nhs.uk/quality_and_service_improvement_tools/quality_and_service_improvement_tools/sbar_-_situation_-_background_-_assessment_-_recommendation.html.

38 National Audit Office. *Securing the Future Financial Sustainability of the NHS.* http://www.nao.org.uk/report/securing-the-future-financial-sustainability-of-the-nhs/

39 NHS Sustainable Development Unit. *Sustainability in the NHS: Health Check 2012.* www.sdu.nhs.uk/documents/publications/Sustainability_in_the_NHS_Health_Check_2012_On-Screen_Version.pdf

40 Schulz CM et al. Situation awareness in anaesthesia: concept and research. *Anesthesiology* 2013; **118**: 729–42.

Further reading

Coleman NE and Pon S. Quality: performance improvement, teamwork, information technology and protocols. *Critical Care Clinics* 2013; **29**: 129–51.

Manthous C, Nembhard IM and Hollingshead AB. Building effective critical care teams. *Critical Care* 2011; **15**: 307.

Reader TW et al. Developing a team performance framework for the intensive care unit. *Critical Care Medicine* 2009; **37**: 1787–93.

Rose L. Interprofessional collaboration in the ICU: how to define? *Nursing in Critical Care* 2011; **16**: 5–10.

Stubbings L, Chaboyer W and McMurray A. Nurses' use of situation awareness in decision-making: an integrative review. *Journal of Advanced Nursing* 2012; **68**: 1443–53.

Chapter 4

Respiratory assessment and monitoring

Respiratory assessment

If an actual or potential respiratory abnormality is identified during a general ABCDE assessment (see ➔ p. 18) or while monitoring the patient, a more detailed and focused respiratory assessment can provide further information to guide clinical management. Patients with dyspnoea or acute respiratory failure will often also manifest systemic signs and symptoms, including altered consciousness, cardiovascular compromise, and gastrointestinal dysfunction.

Focused health history

Subjective information about the respiratory history can be taken from the patient if they are awake, or from other sources (e.g. family, caregivers, or patient notes).

Respiratory symptom enquiry

Check whether the patient has recently experienced any of the following:

- cough (productive)
- haemoptysis
- dyspnoea (acute, progressive)
- wheeze
- chest pain
- fever/night sweats
- sleep apnoea.

Focused physical assessment

- Respiratory rate over 1 min (normal range, 10–20 breaths/min).
- Obvious signs of discomfort or distress.
- Inability to lie flat or cough due to respiratory distress.
- Inability to complete full sentences.
- Oxygen therapy.
- Fluid assessment (see ➔ p. 24).
- Respiratory-focused assessment (see Table 4.1).

Normal breath sounds

- **Tracheal**—heard over the trachea as very loud, harsh, and high-pitched. Inspiration duration < expiration duration.
- **Bronchial**—heard over the manubrium as loud, harsh, and high-pitched. Inspiration duration = expiration duration.
- **Bronchovesicular**—heard below the clavicles, between the scapulae as medium-pitched. Inspiration duration = expiration duration.
- **Vesicular**—heard over areas of lung tissue as soft and low-pitched. Inspiration duration > expiration duration.

If the trachea is not in the midline it may be deviated toward the site of injury, as in the case of lung collapse, or away from the site of injury, as in pneumothorax. *Note that tracheal deviation is a late sign of respiratory pathology.*

Respiratory landmarking

Any abnormal findings during the health history and physical assessment should be documented and reported according to the specific area of the chest where the abnormality was identified (see Figure 4.1).

Table 4.1 Respiratory-focused assessment

	Normal	Abnormal
Inspection	Pink, moist mucous membranes Mucoid sputum Symmetrical breathing pattern Midline trachea	Pallor or cyanosis Dry mucous membranes Mucopurulent, purulent, blood in sputum Respiratory asymmetry Dyspnoea/tachypnoea Accessory muscle use Chest wounds, drains, scarring Tracheal deviation
Palpation	Bilateral chest expansion Non-tender	Unilateral and/or reduced expansion Subcutaneous emphysema Fremitus Localized pain across chest
Percussion	Tympanic/resonant in all zones	Dull/hyper-resonant in all or some zones
Auscultation	Patent airway Normal breath sounds throughout chest	Stridor Abnormal breath sounds, wheeze, crackles, pleural rub, diminished breath sounds

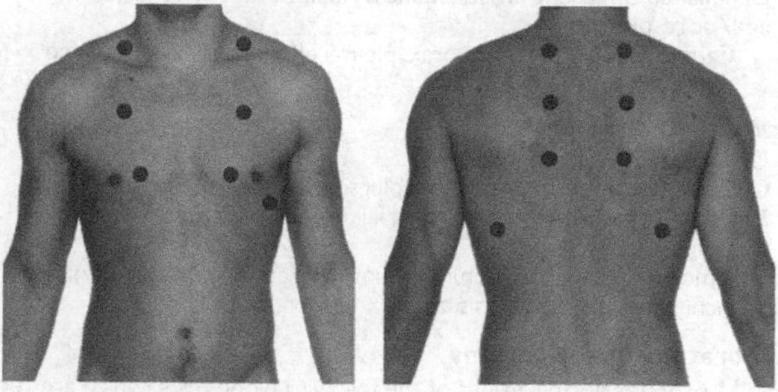

Figure 4.1 Posterior, anterior, and lateral landmarking of the thorax. (Reproduced from Thomas J & Monaghan T, *Oxford Handbook of Clinical Examination and Practical Skills*, 2014, with permission from Oxford University Press.)

Abnormal percussion sounds

- **Dullness**—indicates a solid structure, a consolidated or collapsed area of lung, or a fluid-filled area, which produces a dull note on percussion.
  - Causes include pleural effusion, infection, and lung collapse.
- **Hyper-resonance**—indicates a hollow structure, which produces a hyper-resonant note on percussion.
  - Causes include pneumothorax.

Abnormal breath sounds

- **Wheeze**—indicates airway restriction which is typically heard on expiration. An inspiratory wheeze indicates severe airway narrowing. High-pitched when produced in small bronchioles, and low-pitched when produced in larger bronchi. Monophonic (i.e. single pitch) when heard in an isolated area, and polyphonic (i.e. multi-pitched) when heard throughout the lung area.
  - Causes include bronchoconstriction, airway inflammation, secretions, and obstruction.
- **Crackles**—indicate instability of airways collapsing on expiration. Fine crackles can be heard in small airways, and coarse crackles can be heard in larger airways.
  - Causes include pulmonary oedema, secretions, atelectasis, and fibrosis.
- **Pleural rub**—indicates inflammation of the parietal and visceral layers of the pleura. Stiff creaking sound heard throughout inspiration and expiration.
  - Causes include pleurisy.
- **Diminished or absent breath sounds**—indicate lack of ventilation and/or respiration.
  - Causes include pneumothorax, pleural effusion, gas trapping, and collapse.

Causes of key abnormalities

- Consolidation—pneumonia.
- Collapse—post-operative, mucus plugs.
- Pleural effusion—transudate (heart failure), exudate (neoplasm), empyema.
- Pneumothorax—bullae rupture, trauma (penetrating chest injury).
- Bronchiectasis—tuberculosis, allergic reaction, cystic fibrosis.

Laboratory investigations

See ➔ p. 36 for normal values of the following blood tests, which are relevant to check for a respiratory review:

- full blood count (FBC)
- C-reactive protein (CRP)
- urea and electrolytes (U&E).

Further reading

Broad MA et al. *Cardiorespiratory Assessment of the Adult Patient: a clinician's guide*. Churchill Livingstone Elsevier: Edinburgh, 2012.

Heuer AJ and Scanlan CL (eds). *Wilkins' Clinical Assessment in Respiratory Care* 7th ed. Elsevier Mosby: Maryland Heights, Missouri, 2014.

Jarvis C. *Physical Examination and Health Assessment*, 6th edn. Saunders Elsevier: St Louis, MO, 2012.

Respiratory monitoring

Specific respiratory monitoring may be undertaken during the care of a critically ill patient, as part of the ongoing evaluation and assessment. Familiarity with these monitoring devices will enable accuracy of the results. In addition to the respiratory monitoring devices [illegible] this section, the following systems will provide further support for the respiratory assessment in care of the patient: chest X-ray, mechanical ventilation [illegible] and arterial blood gas analysis (see [illegible] p. 32).

- [illegible] [illegible] [illegible] [illegible] [illegible]
- [illegible] [illegible] [illegible] [illegible] [illegible] [illegible] [illegible] [illegible] [illegible] [illegible] [illegible] [illegible]
- [illegible] [illegible] [illegible] [illegible]

Respiratory monitoring

Specific respiratory monitoring may be indicated during the care of a critically ill patient. An understanding of the indications and practices associated with these monitoring devices will ensure accuracy of the results. In addition to the respiratory monitoring described in this section, the following systems will provide further support for the respiratory assessment and care of the patient: chest X-ray, mechanical ventilation waveform analysis and blood gas analysis (see ➲ p. 32).

Pulse oximetry

This provides continuous, non-invasive measurement of oxygen saturation in arterial blood (SpO_2). Pulse oximetry is used to assess for hypoxaemia, to detect variations from the patient's oxygenation baseline (e.g. due to procedures or activity level), and to support the use of oxygen therapy.

Method

A probe is placed over a digit, earlobe, cheek, or the bridge of the nose. It emits light at two specific wavelengths—red and infrared. Light passes through the tissue and is sensed by a photodetector at the base of the probe. Most of the emitted light is absorbed by skin (including pigment), bone, connective tissue, and venous vessels (baseline measurement). This amount is constant, so the only relevant fluctuations are caused by increases in blood flow during systole. The peaks and troughs of the pulsatile and baseline absorption for each wavelength are detected and the ratios of each are compared. This provides the ratio of oxyhaemoglobin to total haemoglobin (i.e. the saturation). Oxygen content dissolved in plasma is 3% and that bound to haemoglobin is 97%.

Pulse oximetry measures the oxygen content bound to haemoglobin, not the oxygen content dissolved in the blood. Consequently an anaemic patient may still have an oxygen saturation of 100%.

It also does not identify whether the patient is making any respiratory effort, oxygen consumption, or carbon dioxide retention.

Limitations

- Accuracy is within 2% *only* when the SpO_2 is ≥ 70%.
- Haemoglobin abnormality—for example, carboxyhaemoglobin (as a result of carbon monoxide poisoning or smoke inhalation) or methaemoglobinaemia (due to local anaesthetics, antibiotics, or radio-opaque dyes).
- Impaired peripheral perfusion—due to hypothermia, hypovolaemia, peripheral vascular disease, or vasoconstriction (distal to blood pressure cuff).
- Heart rate abnormality—weak, arrhythmia, absent.
- Impaired light absorption—due to nail polish, high bilirubin concentration, high levels of ambient light (e.g. sunlight, phototherapy, surgical lamp).
- Motion artefact—tremor, shivering, ill-fitting probe.

Ongoing care

- Attach the probe securely.
- Confirm that there is a clear pulsatile waveform.
- Set alarm limits—individualized to the patient.
- Observe the probe site 4-hourly for pressure ulceration.
- Confirm abnormal readings with other assessment findings, such as arterial blood gas (ABG).

Capnography

This provides a measurement of carbon dioxide (CO_2) with a continuous waveform at the end of expiration—that is, end-tidal CO_2 ($ETCO_2$). Capnography is used to assess the adequacy of ventilation, to detect oesophageal intubation (i.e. very little or no CO_2 is detected), to indicate disconnection from the ventilator, and to diagnose circulatory problems, such as pulmonary embolus (a sudden fall in $ETCO_2$).

Method

Most analysers utilize infrared absorption spectroscopy, whereby the infrared light is absorbed by CO_2 at a specific wavelength (4.3 millimicrons). Since the amount of light absorbed is proportional to the concentration of CO_2 gas molecules, the concentration of CO_2 can be determined by comparing the measured absorbance with the absorbance of a known standard. The CO_2 concentration is expressed as a partial pressure in kPa.

A large difference between $ETCO_2$ and $PaCO_2$ may represent an increase in the dead space to tidal volume ratio, poor pulmonary perfusion, auto-positive end expiratory pressure (auto-PEEP), or intra-pulmonary shunting.

A progressive rise in $ETCO_2$ may represent hypoventilation, airway obstruction, or increased CO_2 production due to an increase in metabolic rate.

Limitations

The $ETCO_2$ approximates to $PaCO_2$ only if the patient shows cardiorespiratory stability and is normothermic. It is not so reliable in patients with respiratory failure—for example, ventilation/perfusion mismatch or significant gas trapping (e.g. asthma).

Capnogram

There are four phases (see Figure 4.2).

Phase 1

Gas is sampled during the start of expiration from the anatomical and sampling device dead space. The concentration of CO_2 should be negligible. However, if the CO_2 level is significant this indicates re-breathing of exhaled gas. The commonest causes are failure of the expiratory valve to open during mechanical ventilation, or an inadequate amount of fresh gas in the reservoir of a non-rebreathing face mask.

Phase 2

Gas is sampled from the alveolar gas. The concentration of CO_2 rapidly rises.

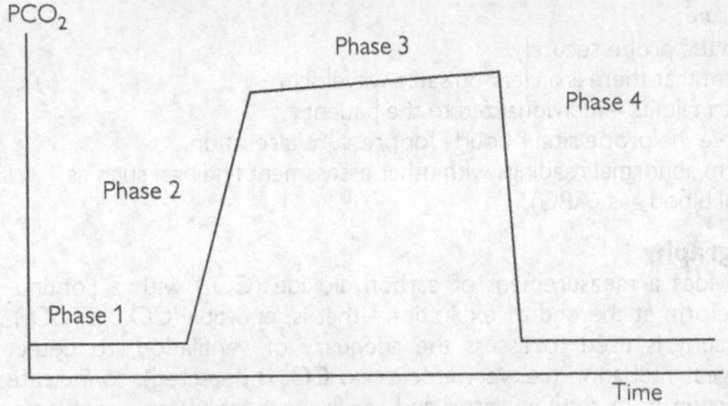

Figure 4.2 The normal capnogram. (Reproduced from Singer M and Webb A, *Oxford Handbook of Critical Care*, Third Edition, 2005, with permission from Oxford University Press.)

Phase 3

This is known as the alveolar plateau, and it represents the CO_2 concentration in mixed expired alveolar gas. There is normally a slight increase in CO_2 concentration as alveolar gas exchange continues during expiration. Airway obstruction or a high rate of CO_2 production will increase the slope. The gradient during Phase 3 depends on the rate of alveolar gas exchange. A steep gradient can indicate ventilation/perfusion mismatch.

Phase 4

As inspiration begins there is a rapid fall in the concentration of CO_2.

Peak flow meter

This provides a measurement of peak expiratory flow rate (PEFR). Peak flow is used to assess the trends in airway obstruction, but the accuracy of the results is dependent on patient effort. As it is a measure of airflow it cannot detect restrictive ventilatory defects, such as those caused by pulmonary fibrosis, as these reduce lung volume but do not affect airflow.

Method

The patient is required to take a full breath in and produce a rapid forced maximal expiratory puff into the single-use mouthpiece attached to the meter. The result is recorded in L/min and is interpreted according to the patient's age, gender, and height. Peak flows can be checked twice daily, preferably at the same time.

Pneumonia

Definition

[illegible]

Causes

[illegible]

Respiratory findings

[illegible]

Management

[illegible]

[illegible]

[illegible]

Pneumonia

Definition

Pneumonia is an inflammation of the lung, which is characterized by exudation into the alveoli. It can be classified anatomically as lobar or by aetiology (see Box 4.1).

Causes

Pneumonia can be caused by any of over 100 microorganisms. Therefore the treatment should be started before the causative organism has been identified. Box 4.2 lists some of the most common causative organisms.

Assessment findings

- The clinical findings are often referred to as consolidation.
- Expansion is reduced on the affected side.
- There is percussion dullness over the area of consolidation.
- Breath sounds are bronchial.
- Added sounds are crackles.
- Tachypnoea and central cyanosis.
- Fever, sweats, and rigors.
- Cough and sputum.

Management

- Chest X-ray.
- ABG and pulse oximetry.
- FBC, serum creatinine, U&E, and LFTs.
- Blood cultures prior to administering antimicrobial therapy.

Box 4.1 Types of pneumonia

- **Community acquired**—not hospitalized or residing in a long-term care facility for ≥ 14 days prior to onset of symptoms.
- **Hospital acquired**—more than 48 h between admission and onset of symptoms.
- **Ventilator associated**—more than 48–72 h between intubation and onset of symptoms. See ➲ p. 153.
- **Aspiration**—micro-aspiration of bacteria colonizing the upper respiratory tract, macro-aspiration of gastric contents, indirect transmission from staff, inhaled aerosols.
- **Atypical.**

Box 4.2 Microorganisms that can cause pneumonia

Streptococcus pneumoniae (90% of cases)
Haemophilus influenzae
Staphylococcus aureus
Pseudomonas species
Legionella species

- Sputum microscopy, culture, and sensitivity.
- Bronchoalveloar lavage may be used for patients who are immunocompromised, those who do not respond to antimicrobial therapy, or those from whom a sputum sample cannot be obtained.
- Urinary *Legionella* antigen.
- Antimicrobial therapy.
- Monitor haemodynamics (see ➲ p. 172).
- Monitor electrolytes and treat imbalances (see ➲ p. 36).
- Monitor fluid status and treat imbalances (see ➲ pp. 24 and 52).
- Oxygen therapy (see ➲ p. 138).
- Adherence to infection prevention and control.
- Ventilator-associated pneumonia care bundle (see Box 4.3 and p. 153).

Box 4.3 Measures to reduce ventilator-associated pneumonia

1 Elevation of the head of the bed to 30–45° unless contraindicated.
2 Sedation level assessment unless contraindicated or patient is awake.
3 Oral hygiene with chlorhexidine gluconate (≥ 1–2%) 6-hourly.
4 Subglottic aspiration of secretions 1- to 2-hourly.
5 Tracheal cuff pressure is maintained at 20–30 cmH_2O (or 2 cmH_2O above peak inspiratory pressure) 4-hourly.
6 Stress ulcer prophylaxis.

Further reading

BRITISH Thoracic Society (BTS). *BTS Guidelines for the Management of Community Acquired Pneumonia in Adults*. BTS: London, 2009.

Department of Health. *High Impact Intervention: care bundle to reduce ventilator-associated pneumonia*. Department of Health: London, 2010.

Melsen WG, Rovers MM and Bonten MJ. Ventilator-associated pneumonia and mortality: a systematic review of observational studies. *Critical Care Medicine* 2009; 39: 2709–18.

National Institute for Health and Care Excellence (NICE). *Technical Patient Safety Solutions for Ventilator-Associated Pneumonia in Adults*. PSG002. NICE: London, 2008. www.nice.org.uk/guidance/psg002

Pleural effusion

Definition

This is a collection of fluid in the pleural space. It is the result of excessive fluid accumulating between the thin layers of tissue that line the lungs and thorax. Pleural fluid is normally a clear pale yellow colour. A large amount of purulent drainage indicates an *empyema*.

Causes

Transudate may be caused by cardiac failure, kidney disease, hypoalbuminaemia due to chronic liver disease, or hypothyroidism. The fluid has similar protein levels to those found in normal pleural fluid, with no evidence of blood, inflammation, or infection.

Exudate may develop as a result of pneumonia, neoplasm, tuberculosis, or pulmonary infarction. The fluid contains increased levels of protein, blood, or evidence of inflammation or infection.

Empyema is pus in the pleural space, and it may develop as a result of pneumonia, lung abscess, bronchiectasis, or tuberculosis.

Assessment findings

- Trachea displaced *away* from a massive effusion.
- Expansion reduced on the affected side.
- Percussion dullness over the area of fluid.
- Breath sounds reduced or absent.
- Added sounds bronchial above the effusion due to compression of overlying lung.
- Tachypnoea and central cyanosis.
- Fever.
- Cough.
- Pleuritic pain.

Management

- Chest X-ray.
- Ultrasound examination.
- ABG and pulse oximetry.
- FBC, serum creatinine, U&E, and LFTs.
- Treatment for pleural effusions will require management of the underlying cause (e.g. antimicrobial therapy for pneumonia, diuretics for cardiac failure).
- Monitor haemodynamics (see ➲ p. 172).
- Monitor electrolytes and treat imbalances (see ➲ p. 36).
- Monitor fluid status and treat imbalances (see ➲ pp. 24 and 52).
- Oxygen therapy (see ➲ p. 138).
- Adherence to infection prevention and control.

Large, infected, or inflamed pleural effusions often require drainage to improve symptoms and prevent complications. Various procedures may be used to treat pleural effusions, including the following:

- **Thoracentesis**—to remove large amounts of pleural effusion or for diagnostic purposes.
- **Pleurodesis**—an irritant (e.g. talc, doxycycline) is injected through a chest tube into the pleural space. The irritant creates an inflammatory

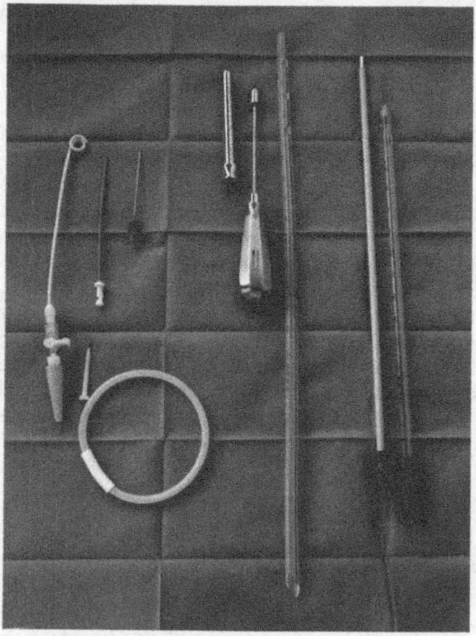

Figure 4.3 Chest drain. (Reproduced from Tubaro M et al. *The ESC Textbook of Intensive and Acute Cardiac Care* (2011), with permission from the European Society of Cardiology.)

response that causes the surfaces of the pleura and chest wall to adhere, sealing the space and thus preventing further fluid collection.
- **Tube thoracotomy (chest drain)**—a plastic tube is inserted into the pleural space via a small incision made in the chest wall. The tube is attached to suction and may remain *in situ* for several days (see Figure 4.3).

Nursing care of a chest drain

A chest drain has three functions:
- to drain fluid and/or air
- to prevent additional air from entering the chest
- to facilitate lung re-expansion using suction.

Monitor the appearance of drained fluid and record measurements hourly. If a chest drain was indicated for a pneumothorax, drainage of fluid is less likely.

Use of a water seal prevents air from entering the chest tube and the patient's lungs. Fluctuation of the water in the tubing on inspiration and expiration is normal, and if not present this could indicate kinked, blocked tubing or a fully reinflated lung. Bubbling of the water indicates that air is escaping from the pleural cavity (e.g. in the case of a pneumothorax). New bubbling could indicate a new undiagnosed pneumothorax or disconnection of the tubing. It is possible to distinguish between an air leak and a pneumothorax by clamping the tubing close to the chest wall, which will stop the bubbling if the air is caused by a pneumothorax, but the bubbling will continue if it is due to a loose connection or a disconnection.

Clamping of a chest tube should only be performed to identify the cause of an air leak and on medical orders.

Removal of a chest tube can be undertaken at the bedside with the patient in bed, using an aseptic non-touch technique. Two sutures are usually inserted—the first to assist later closure of the wound after drain removal, and the second (a stay suture) to secure the drain which needs to be removed. Care must be taken to avoid air entering the pleural cavity. Clamping prior to removal is not recommended on the basis of the latest evidence. The patient should be instructed to exhale while the tube is being removed. Once the tube has been removed the closure suture should be tied and an occlusive dressing applied. The patient should be monitored for signs of respiratory distress. Disposal of the chest drain must include safe disposal of the fluid (absorbent gels can be used to avoid spillage of the contents).

Further reading

Frazer C. Managing chest tubes. *MedSurg Matters!* 2012; **21**: 9–12.

Maslove DB et al. The diagnosis and management of pleural effusions in the ICU. *Journal of Intensive Care Medicine* 2013; **28**: 24–36.

Pneumothorax

Definition

A pneumothorax occurs when there is air in the pleural space surrounding the lung, and it requires a chest tube to allow the air to escape. [illegible] pneumothorax occurs when there is [illegible] between the lung and the pleural space [illegible] from [illegible]. As a result of the [illegible] of the pleural space [illegible] of blood vessels [illegible] will further [illegible].

Causes

The causes can be classified [illegible] (see Table [illegible]).

Assessment findings

- Trachea [illegible] from the affected side [illegible]
- Subcutaneous emphysema
- [illegible] on the affected side
- [illegible]
- Breath sounds reduced or absent [illegible]
- [illegible]

Management

- [illegible]
- [illegible]
- [illegible]
- [illegible] chest drain [illegible] the pleural space via a small incision made in the chest wall. The tube is attached [illegible]
- [illegible] (see p. [illegible])
- [illegible] (see p. [illegible])
- [illegible] (see p. [illegible])
- Oxygen therapy (see p. [illegible])
- [illegible]

Pneumothorax

Definition

A pneumothorax occurs when there is air in the pleural space surrounding the lungs, and it requires a chest tube to allow the air to escape. Similarly, a haemothorax occurs when blood collects within the pleural cavity. A tension pneumothorax occurs when there is communication between the lung and the pleural space. Air is able to enter during inspiration, but is prevented from exiting on expiration. As a result the accumulation of air in the pleural space will cause displacement of the mediastinum and obstruction of blood vessels, and will restrict ventilation.

Causes

The causes can be classified as spontaneous or traumatic (see Table 4.2).

Assessment findings

- Trachea displaced *away from* a massive pneumothorax.
- Subcutaneous emphysema.
- Expansion is reduced on the affected side.
- Percussion is hyper-resonant over the area of pneumothorax.
- Breath sounds reduced or absent.
- Tachypnoea and central cyanosis.

Management

- Chest X-ray.
- ABG and pulse oximetry.
- FBC, serum creatinine, U&E, and LFTs.
- *Tube thoracotomy (chest drain)*—a plastic tube is inserted into the pleural space via a small incision made in the chest wall. The tube is attached to suction and may remain *in situ* for several days.
- Monitor haemodynamics (see ➲ p. 172).
- Monitor electrolytes and treat imbalances (see ➲ p. 36).
- Monitor fluid status and treat imbalances (see ➲ pp. 24 and 52).
- Oxygen therapy (see ➲ p. 138).
- Adherence to infection prevention and control.

Table 4.2 Causes of pneumothorax

Spontaneous
Subpleural bullae rupture—usually in tall young males
Emphysema bullae rupture—usually in middle-aged or elderly patients with generalized emphysematous changes
Iatrogenic—central venous catheter insertion, high positive airway pressures with mechanical ventilation
Traumatic
Rib fracture
Penetrating chest wall injury
Pleural aspiration

Further reading

British Thoracic Society (BTS). *Pleural Disease Guideline*. BTS: London, 2010.

Haynes D and Baumann M. Management of pneumothorax. *Seminars in Respiratory and Critical Care Medicine* 2010; 31: 769–80.

Asthma

Definition

Asthma is a chronic respiratory condition with the following features:

- reversible airway obstruction (depending on the severity, this can be complete or partial) (see Table 4.3)
- airway inflammation
- airway hyper-responsiveness to various stimuli.

An exacerbation of asthma is an acute event characterized by a worsening of the patient's respiratory symptoms that exceeds normal day-to-day variations. It is typified by cough, wheeze, dyspnoea, chest tightness, and decreasing expiratory flow.

Status asthmaticus is a medical emergency that can be identified by failure to respond to nebulized bronchodilators (see Box 4.4).

A patient may have more than one cause of airway obstruction—for example, COPD and asthma often coexist.

Table 4.3 Levels of severity of acute asthma exacerbations

Moderate asthma	Increasing symptoms PEF > 50–75% of best or predicted No features of acute severe asthma	
Acute severe asthma	Any one of the following: • PEF 33–50% of best or predicted • respiratory rate ≥ 25 breaths/min • heart rate ≥ 110 beats /min • inability to complete sentences in one breath	
Life-threatening asthma	Any one of the following in a patient with severe asthma:	
	Clinical signs	Measurements
	Altered conscious level	PEF < 33% of best or predicted
	Exhaustion	SpO_2 < 92%
	Arrhythmia	PaO_2 < 8 kPa
	Hypotension	'Normal' $PaCO_2$ (4.6–6.0 kPa)
	Cyanosis	
	Silent chest	
	Poor respiratory effort	
Near-fatal asthma	Raised $PaCO_2$ and/or requiring mechanical ventilation with raised inflation pressures	

Reproduced from British Thoracic Society and Scottish Intercollegiate Guidelines Network, British guideline on the management of asthma, *Thorax* 2014; **69**: i1–192, with permission from the BMJ Publishing Group Ltd.

Box 4.4 Patients at risk of developing near-fatal or fatal asthma

A combination of **severe asthma**, recognized by one or more of the following:

- previous near-fatal asthma (e.g. previous ventilation or respiratory acidosis)
- previous admission for asthma, especially if in the last year
- requiring three or more classes of asthma medication
- heavy use of a β_2-agonist
- repeated attendances at Emergency Department for asthma, especially if in the last year

and adverse behaviour or psychosocial features, recognized by one or more of the following:

- non-compliance with treatment or monitoring (including few GP contacts, self-discharge from hospital)
- psychiatric illness, deliberate self-harm, alcohol or drug abuse
- current or recent use of major tranquillizers
- denial
- obesity
- learning impairment
- employment or financial problems
- social isolation
- high levels of domestic, relationship, or legal stress.

Reproduced from BTS British Guidelines on Management of Asthma, with permission from Publishing Company (BTS 2012).

Causes

Both genetic and environmental factors have been implicated in the aetiology of asthma. Immunoglobulin E (IgE) appears to be involved in the characteristic airway inflammation and hyper-responsiveness, with the allergens in the local environment determining the level of antibody response.

Triggers for asthma can be non-specific (e.g. exercise, air temperature, pollutants), specific allergens (e.g. animal dander, house mite, pollen), or an alteration in airway control (e.g. beta blockers, aspirin).

Assessment findings

- Accessory muscle use.
- Decreased PEFR.
- Expansion reduced bilaterally (hyperinflated chest).
- Breath sounds diminished or absent.
- Added sounds—expiratory/inspiratory wheeze.
- Tachypnoea and central cyanosis.
- Cough and sputum.

Management

- ABG and pulse oximetry.
- Peak flow.
- β_2-agonist bronchodilators—in most cases nebulized salbutamol or terbutaline given in high doses acts quickly to relieve bronchospasm, with few side effects. Repeat doses of β_2-agonists at 15- to 30-min intervals, or give continuous nebulization of salbutamol at 5–10 mg/h if there is an inadequate response to initial treatment. Reserve the intravenous route for patients in whom the inhaled route is unreliable.
- Steroid therapy—steroid tablets are as effective as injected steroids, provided that they can be swallowed and retained. Use prednisolone 40–50 mg daily or parenteral hydrocortisone 400 mg daily (100 mg 6-hourly).
- Anticholinergic therapy—nebulized ipratropium bromide with a β_2-agonist produces significantly greater bronchodilation than a β_2-agonist alone. Add nebulized ipratropium bromide (0.5 mg 4- to 6-hourly).
- Magnesium sulfate—use a single dose of IV magnesium sulfate for patients with life-threatening or near-fatal asthma who have not shown a good initial response to inhaled bronchodilator therapy (1.2–2 g IV infusion over 20 min).
- Some patients with life-threatening near-fatal asthma who show a poor response to initial therapy may gain additional benefit from IV aminophylline (5 mg/kg loading dose over 20 min unless on maintenance oral therapy, followed by an infusion of 0.5–0.7 mg/kg/h). If given to patients taking oral aminophylline or theophylline, blood levels should be checked on admission and daily.
- Monitor haemodynamics (see ➔ p. 172).
- Monitor electrolytes and treat imbalances (see ➔ p. 36).
- Monitor fluid status and treat imbalances (see ➔ pp. 24 and 52).
- Oxygen therapy (see ➔ p. 138).
- Adherence to infection prevention and control.
- Mechanical ventilation strategies for asthma:
  - limit airway pressures (i.e. low tidal volumes)
  - extend expiratory time
  - low respiratory rate
  - minimize intrinsic PEEP
  - permissive hypercapnia (higher risk of hypoxia and barotrauma).

Further reading

British Thoracic Society (BTS). *British Guideline on the Management of Asthma: a national clinical guideline*. BTS: London, 2014.

Chronic obstructive pulmonary disease (COPD)

Definition

Around 900 000 people in the UK are known to have COPD, with a further 2 million people remaining undiagnosed. The Global Initiative for Chronic Obstructive Lung Disease (GOLD) has established an internationally recognized definition of COPD as 'a common preventable and treatable disease, characterized by persistent airflow limitation that is usually progressive and associated with an enhanced chronic inflammatory response in the airways and the lung to noxious particles or gases. Exacerbations and comorbidities contribute to the overall severity in individual patients.'

An exacerbation of COPD is an acute event characterized by a worsening of the patient's respiratory symptoms that is beyond normal day-to-day variations. Exacerbations are often precipitated by [illegible] respiratory tract infection. Less [illegible], or [illegible].

Causes

The chronic airflow limitation that is characteristic of COPD is caused by a mixture of small airways disease (obstructive bronchiolitis) and parenchymal destruction (emphysema). Chronic inflammation causes structural changes and narrowing of the small airways. Destruction of the lung parenchyma, also by inflammatory processes, leads to the loss of alveolar attachments to the small airways and decreases lung elastic recoil; in turn, these changes diminish the ability of the airways to remain open during expiration.

Assessment findings

- Accessory muscles [illegible]
- Barrel-shaped chest
- Expansion reduced bilaterally (hyperinflated chest)
- [illegible] diminished/wheezes
- [illegible] expiratory [illegible]
- Dyspnoea, [illegible]
- Cough and sputum

Management

- [illegible]
- ABG (or pulse oximetry)
- CXR
- FBC, [illegible]
- [illegible] and sensitivity
- [illegible]

[illegible]

Chronic obstructive pulmonary disease (COPD)

Definition

Around 900 000 people in the UK are known to have COPD, with a further 2 million people remaining undiagnosed.[1] The Global Initiative for Chronic Obstructive Lung Disease (GOLD)[2] has established an internationally recognized definition of COPD as a common but preventable disease, characterized by persistent airflow limitation that is usually progressive and associated with an enhanced chronic inflammatory response in the airways and the lung to noxious particles or gases. Exacerbations and comorbidities contribute to the overall severity in individual patients.

An exacerbation of COPD is an acute event characterized by a worsening of the patient's respiratory symptoms that exceeds normal day-to-day variations. Exacerbations are often precipitated by a viral upper respiratory tract infection, heart failure, or retained secretions.

Causes

The chronic airflow limitation that is characteristic of COPD is caused by a mixture of small airways disease (obstructive bronchiolitis) and parenchymal destruction (emphysema). Chronic inflammation causes structural changes and narrowing of the small airways. Destruction of the lung parenchyma, also by inflammatory processes, leads to the loss of alveolar attachments to the small airways and decreases lung elastic recoil. In turn these changes reduce the ability of the airways to remain open during expiration.

Assessment findings

- Accessory muscle use.
- Barrel-shaped chest.
- Expansion reduced bilaterally (hyperinflated chest).
- Breath sounds diminished or absent.
- Added sounds—expiratory wheeze.
- Tachypnoea and central cyanosis.
- Cough and sputum.

Management

- Chest X-ray.
- ABG and pulse oximetry.
- Peak flow.
- FBC, serum creatinine, U&E, and LFTs.
- Sputum microscopy, culture, and sensitivity.
- **β_2-agonist bronchodilators**—in most cases, nebulized salbutamol or terbutaline given in high doses acts quickly to relieve bronchospasm, with few side effects. Repeat doses of β_2-agonists at 15- to 30-min intervals or give continuous nebulization of salbutamol at 5–10 mg/h if there is an inadequate response to initial treatment. Reserve the intravenous route for patients in whom the inhaled route is unreliable.

- **Steroid therapy**—steroid tablets are as effective as injected steroids, provided that they can be swallowed and retained. Use a dose of 30–40 mg prednisolone per day for 10–14 days.
- **Anticholinergic therapy**—nebulized ipratropium bromide with a β_2-agonist produces significantly greater bronchodilation than a β_2-agonist alone. Add nebulized ipratropium bromide (0.5 mg 4- to 6-hourly).
- **Antibiotic therapy.**
- Monitor haemodynamics (see ➲ p. 172).
- Monitor electrolytes and treat imbalances (see ➲ p. 36).
- Monitor fluid status and treat imbalances (see ➲ pp. 24 and 52).
- Oxygen therapy, taking into consideration the patient's normal PCO_2 and PO_2 (see ➲ p. 138).
- Chest physiotherapy.
- Adherence to infection prevention and control.
- Mechanical ventilation strategies for COPD:
  - limit airway pressures (i.e. low tidal volumes)
  - extend expiratory time
  - low respiratory rate
  - minimize intrinsic PEEP
  - permissive hypercapnia (higher risk of hypoxia and barotrauma).

The decision to ventilate a patient with an exacerbation of COPD must take into consideration the stage of lung disease, the aggressive treatment, and the weaning process, together with the wishes of the patient.

References

1 Health Care Commission. *Cleaning the Air: a national study of chronic obstructive pulmonary disease.* Commission for Health Care Audit and Inspection: London, 2006.

2 Global Initiative for Chronic Obstructive Lung Disease (GOLD). *Global Strategy for Diagnosis, Management, and Prevention of COPD.* GOLD: 2015.

Further reading

Ward NS and Dushay KM. Clinical concise review: mechanical ventilation of patients with chronic obstructive pulmonary disease. *Critical Care Medicine* 2008; **36**: 1614–19.

Wildman MJ et al. Implications of prognostic pessimism in patients with chronic obstructive pulmonary disease (COPD) or asthma admitted to intensive care in the UK within the COPD and asthma outcome study (CAOS): multicentre observational cohort study. *British Medical Journal* 2007; **335**: 1132.

Pulmonary oedema

Definition

Pulmonary oedema is an accumulation of fluid in the interstitial space of the lung tissue. This excess fluid will impair gas exchange at the alveolar–capillary membrane.

Causes

Fluid accumulation within the lung itself has either a *cardiogenic cause* (failure of the heart to remove fluid from the lung circulation) or a *non-cardiogenic cause* (direct injury to the lung parenchyma) (see Table 4.4).

Assessment findings

- Added sounds—crackles.
- Tachypnoea and central cyanosis.
- Cough and sputum.

Management

- Chest X-ray.
- ABG and pulse oximetry.
- FBC, serum creatinine, U&E, and LFTs.
- Nitrate—sublingually or by infusion.
- Diuretic—furosemide IV 0.5–1.0 mg/kg.
- Morphine—IV 5 mg.
- Monitor haemodynamics (see ➔ p. 172).
- Monitor electrolytes and treat imbalances (see ➔ p. 36).
- Monitor fluid status and restrict fluids (see ➔ pp. 24 and 52).
- Oxygen therapy (see ➔ p. 138).
- Adherence to infection prevention and control.
- Non-invasive ventilation strategies for pulmonary oedema:
  - continuous positive airway pressure (CPAP) with high-level PEEP.

Table 4.4 Cardiogenic and non-cardiogenic causes of pulmonary oedema

Cardiogenic causes	Non-cardiogenic causes
Cardiogenic shock	Chest trauma (smoke inhalation)
Cardiac failure (left ventricle)	Oxygen toxicity
Myocardial infarction	Sepsis
Post-cardiac arrest	Multiple transfusions
	Pancreatitis
	Liver disease

Further reading

Salman A, Milbrandt E and Pinksy M. The role of noninvasive ventilation in acute cardiogenic pulmonary oedema. *Critical Care* 2010; 14: 303.

Pulmonary embolism (PE)

Definition

Embolization of a venous thrombosis to the lungs will lead to pulmonary artery occlusion, obstruction of the pulmonary circulation, and sudden death. The effect of the obstruction will cause inflammatory changes, which will lead to pulmonary hypertension and subsequent coronary oedema. In addition, the obstruction will cause a ventilation/perfusion mismatch, leading to hypoxaemia.

Causes

Most pulmonary embolisms result from lower limb, pelvic, or inferior vena cava thrombus. Patients are at higher risk if they manifest any or all three of Virchow's triad—venous stasis, hypercoagulability, or vein wall injury. Immobility is the main cause.

Assessment findings

- Pulmonary embolism can often occur without any symptoms.
- Sudden dyspnoea.
- Pleuritic chest pain.
- Haemoptysis.
- Tachypnoea and central cyanosis.
- Signs of venous thromboembolism (VTE).
- Signs of right ventricle dysfunction (e.g. jugular venous distension).

Management

- Chest X-ray.
- ABG and pulse oximetry.
- D-dimer.
- FBC, serum creatinine, U&E, and LFTs.
- ECG.
- Anticoagulation.
- Inferior vena cava filter if anticoagulation is contraindicated.
- Thrombolysis.
- Embolectomy if thrombolysis is contraindicated.
- Monitor haemodynamics (see ➔ p. 172).
- Oxygen therapy (see ➔ p. 138).
- Adherence to infection prevention and control.
- VTE assessment and prophylaxis.

Further reading

British Thoracic Society Standards of Care Committee, Pulmonary Embolism Guideline Development Group. *D-Dimer in Suspected Pulmonary Embolism: a statement from the British Thoracic Society Standards of Care Committee*. British Thoracic Society: London, 2006.

Miller A and Boldy D. Pulmonary embolism guidelines: will they work? *Thorax* 2003; 58: 463.

Tuberculosis (TB)

Definition

TB is a contagious bacterial infection that mainly affects the lungs, although the pathogen *Mycobacterium tuberculosis* can infect other parts of the body, such as the gastrointestinal tract, cerebrospinal fluid, and other organs.

Exposure is through aerosol droplets from coughing, sneezing, or speaking. Duration and intimacy of contact determine the likelihood of transmission. Four outcomes are possible following exposure—immediate clearance of bacteria, primary disease, latent infection, and reactivation disease. Latent infection refers to the presence of TB without the disease.

Causes

Medical conditions that predispose to TB include HIV, diabetes, chronic renal failure, and chronic pulmonary disease. Social factors such as homeless shelters, prisons, population density, and poverty are associated with an increased risk of TB.

Assessment findings

- Productive and prolonged cough.
- Chest pain.
- Haemoptysis.
- Fever, chills, and night sweats.
- Weight loss and appetite loss.
- Fatigue.

Management

- Chest X-ray.
- ABG and pulse oximetry.
- FBC, serum creatinine, U&E, and LFTs.
- Sputum microscopy, culture, and sensitivity for acid-fast bacilli (AFB).
- Antiviral therapy (e.g. isoniazid, rifampicin, pyrazinamide, ethambutol).
- Corticosteroid therapy.
- Monitor haemodynamics (see ➔ p. 172).
- Monitor electrolytes and treat imbalances (see ➔ p. 36).
- Monitor fluid status and treat imbalances (see ➔ pp. 24 and 52).
- Oxygen therapy (see ➔ p. 138).
- Adherence to infection prevention and control.

Generally, patients with confirmed or suspected TB are cared for in isolation. If available, the ventilation for the room should be set to *negative pressure*, and the doors must be kept closed to achieve this.

If the patient is intubated or ventilated and a closed suction system is in use, masks do not need to be worn. However, high-filtration masks (e.g. FFP3) must be worn whenever the closed system is disconnected (e.g. when changing filters, catheter mounts, tubing, or suction apparatus, or for chest physiotherapy). Masks can be removed 30 min after the procedure has been completed. If the patient is not fully ventilated and a closed circuit cannot be maintained (e.g. on CPAP or T-piece), carers must wear high-filtration masks in the room at all times unless the patient is considered no longer infectious.

Further reading

World Health Organization. *Policy on TB Infection Control in Health-Care Facilities, Congregate Settings and Households*. World Health Organization: Geneva, 2009.

National Institute for Health and Care Excellence (NICE). *Tuberculosis: clinical diagnosis and management of tuberculosis, and measures for its prevention and control*. NICE: London, 2011. ➚ https://www.nice.org.uk/guidance/cg117

Interstitial lung disease

Definition

There are a number of similar diseases that affect the lung tissue, and these are grouped under the umbrella term *interstitial lung disease*. This group of diseases is classified in this way to distinguish them from obstructive airway diseases.

- *Pulmonary fibrosis*—injury to the epithelial surface that causes inflammation if prolonged, leading to fibrosis.
- *Granulomatous lung disease*—accumulation of T lymphocytes, macrophages, and epithelioid cells organized into discrete structures known as granulomas.

The lung tissue involved includes alveoli, alveolar epithelium, capillary endothelium, and the spaces between these structures.

Interstitial lung disease can be considered a comorbidity, which will have acute and chronic phases as well as exacerbating any new lung pathologies.

Causes

Interstitial lung disease may be caused by inhaled substances (e.g. asbestosis), medications (e.g. amiodarone, chemotherapy), connective tissue disease (e.g. sarcoidosis), or infection (pneumonia), or it may be idiopathic.

Assessment findings

- Finger clubbing.
- Expansion reduced.
- Added sounds—fine inspiratory crackles.
- Tachypnoea and central cyanosis.
- Fatigue.

Management

Management will not reverse fibrosis, but rather the goals are to remove the agents that are causing injury and to suppress the inflammatory process.

- Chest X-ray.
- ABG and pulse oximetry.
- FBC, serum creatinine, U&E, and LFTs.
- Sputum microscopy, culture, and sensitivity.
- Glucocorticoids to suppress inflammation, 0.5–1 mg/kg daily.
- Monitor haemodynamics (see ➲ p. 172).
- Monitor electrolytes and treat imbalances (see ➲ p. 36).
- Monitor fluid status and treat imbalances (see ➲ pp. 24 and 52).
- Oxygen therapy (see ➲ p. 138).
- Adherence to infection prevention and control.

Further reading

King T. Interstitial lung diseases. In: A Fauci et al. (eds) *Harrison's Principles of Internal Medicine*, 17th edn. McGraw-Hill Companies, Inc.: London, 2008. pp. 1643–50.

Acute respiratory distress syndrome (ARDS)

Definition

The 2012 Berlin definition of ARDS changed the terminology and slightly modified criteria that had previously been used (see Table 8.5). For example, the phrase 'acute lung injury' is no longer used; instead, ARDS is now categorized as mild, moderate, or severe.

ARDS is defined as a type of acute, diffuse, inflammatory lung injury that leads to increased pulmonary vascular permeability and loss of aerated lung tissue.

The clinical presentation consists of hypoxaemia, bilateral lung opacities, [illegible] decreased lung compliance. The acute phase is characterized by diffuse alveolar damage, [illegible] proliferation, or fibrotic repair.

Causes

Risk factors for ARDS or conditions associated with these include:

- pneumonia
- aspiration of gastric contents
- non-pulmonary sepsis
- inhalation injury
- pulmonary contusion
- multiple trauma
- [illegible]
- pancreatitis.

Sepsis [illegible] up to 40% of [illegible] increases [illegible] organ dysfunction [illegible] inflammatory response [illegible] ARDS [illegible] preventive measures.

Assessment findings

See the Berlin definition of ARDS in Table 8.5.

Management

- Chest radiograph
- ABG and pulse oximetry
- [illegible]
- [illegible]
- [illegible] (see [illegible] p. [illegible])
- [illegible] (see [illegible] p. [illegible])
- [illegible] therapy (see [illegible] p. [illegible])
- [illegible]
- [illegible]
- [illegible]
- [illegible] (see [illegible] p. [illegible])
- [illegible] airway pressure [illegible] ventilation [illegible] (see [illegible]

Acute respiratory distress syndrome (ARDS)

Definition

The 2012 Berlin definition of ARDS[3] changed the terminology and diagnostic criteria that had previously been used (see Table 4.5). For example, the phrase 'acute lung injury' is no longer to be used, and ARDS is now categorized as mild, moderate, or severe.

ARDS is defined as a type of acute, diffuse, inflammatory lung injury that leads to increased pulmonary vascular permeability and loss of aerated lung tissue.

The clinical presentation consists of hypoxaemia, bilateral lung opacities, increased physiological dead space, and decreased lung compliance. The acute phase is characterized by diffuse alveolar damage (i.e. oedema, inflammation, or haemorrhage).

Causes

Patients at clinical risk of developing ARDS include those with:

- pneumonia
- aspiration of gastric contents
- lung contusion
- inhalational injury
- non-pulmonary sepsis
- multiple trauma
- massive transfusion
- pancreatitis.

Sepsis precipitates ARDS in up to 40% of cases, and the risk increases if shock, organ dysfunction, or systemic inflammatory response is present. Early detection of patients with sepsis who are at risk of developing ARDS is an important preventive strategy.

Assessment findings

See the Berlin definition of ARDS in Table 4.5.

Management

- Chest X-ray.
- ABG and pulse oximetry.
- FBC, serum creatinine, U&E, and LFTs.
- Monitor haemodynamics (see ➲ p. 172).
- Monitor electrolytes and treat imbalances (see ➲ p. 36).
- Monitor fluid status and treat imbalances (see ➲ pp. 24 and 52).
- Oxygen therapy (see ➲ p. 138).
- Adherence to infection prevention and control.
- Ventilator-associated pneumonia care bundle (see Box 4.3).
  - consider I:E ratio change with prolonged inspiratory time
  - consider prone positioning (see ➲ p. 158)
- Consider airway pressure release ventilation (APRV) (see ➲ p. 155).

Table 4.5 The Berlin definition of acute respiratory distress syndrome (ARDS)[3]

	Acute respiratory distress syndrome
Timing	Within 1 week of known clinical insult or new or worsening respiratory symptoms
Chest imaging	Bilateral opacities that are not fully explained by effusions, lobar or lung collapse, or nodules
Origins of oedema	Respiratory failure that is not fully explained by cardiac failure, fluid overload, or hydrostatic oedema
Oxygenation	
Mild	PaO_2/FiO_2 < 200 mmHg or < 300 mmHg with PEEP or CPAP > 5 cmH_2O
Moderate	PaO_2/FiO_2 < 100 mmHg or < 200 mmHg with PEEP > 5 cmH_2O
Severe	PaO_2/FiO_2 < 100 mmHg PEEP > 5 cmH_2O

- Consider extracorporeal membrane oxygneation (ECMO) (see ➲ p. 161).
- Mechanical ventilation strategies for ARDS:
  - pressure control mode (in volume-controlled ventilation, gas is delivered preferentially to more compliant areas of lung with a risk of overstretch)
  - protective lung ventilation (see ➲ p. 157)
  - tidal volumes 6–8 ml/kg
  - maintain plateau pressure < 30 cm H_2O
  - high amounts of PEEP

Lung-protective strategies are the only supportive therapy that has been shown to improve survival in ARDS patients. Therefore they should be used for patients who have or are at risk of developing ARDS. It can be combined with an open lung approach in patients with moderate to severe ARDS (i.e. higher PEEP and recruitment manoeuvres). The ventilation strategy chosen should be modified in patients with obstructive lung disease in order to prevent dynamic hyperinflation (e.g. patients with COPD or asthma).

- Severe ARDS: early administration of neuromuscular blocking agent (see ➲ p. 82)
- Steroids—research inconclusive

Reference

3 The ARDS Definition Task Force. Acute respiratory distress syndrome: the Berlin definition. *Journal of the American Medical Association* 2012; **307**: 2526–33.

Further reading

deHaro C et al. Acute respiratory distress syndrome: prevention and early recognition. *Annals of Intensive Care* 2013; 3: 11.

National Heart, Lung, and Blood Institute (NHLBI) ARDS Network. www.ardsnet.org

Chapter 5

Respiratory support

Respiratory physiology

Lung volumes

- **Tidal volume (V_T)**—volume of gas that moves in and out of the lungs in one breath. Normal range is 5–9 mL/kg.
- **Minute volume (MV)**—volume of gas that moves in and out of the lungs in 1 minute. Normal range is V_T × respiratory rate = 5–9 mL/kg × 12 = 5–6 L.
- **Vital capacity (VC)**—volume of gas exhaled after maximum inspiration. Normal range is 3–4.8 L.
- **Functional residual capacity (FRC)**—volume of gas remaining in the lungs after normal exhalation. Normal range is 1.8–2.4 L.
- **Anatomical dead space**—volume of gas that fills the conducting airways (from nose to lower airways, but not including the bronchioles), which is not available for gas exchange. Alveoli that are ventilated but not perfused can also be included as dead space. Normal value is 2 mL/kg.

Gas exchange in the lungs

An area of approximately $70m^2$ is provided for gas exchange in the adult lung.

Diffusion of gases across the alveolar–capillary membrane is dependent on the difference in the concentration of the gas (i.e. its partial pressure) in the alveolus and in the capillary. Movement of the gases is explained by Dalton's law.

Dalton's law

The pressure exerted by a mixture of gases in a space is equal to the sum of the pressure that each gas exerts if occupying the space alone.

Air is a mixture of predominantly three gases—79% nitrogen, 21% oxygen, and 0.03% carbon dioxide. Air at atmospheric pressure = 101 kPa. Therefore each gas exerts a proportional (i.e. partial) pressure:

$$79 \text{ kPa N} + 21 \text{ kPa } O_2 + 0.03 \text{ kPa } CO_2 = 101 \text{ kPa.}$$

Boyle's law

For a fixed amount of gas kept at a fixed temperature, the pressure and volume are inversely proportional—that is, if the volume of a gas increases, the pressure that it exerts decreases, or if the volume of a gas decreases, the pressure that it exerts increases.

Partial pressure of alveolar oxygen (P_AO_2)

This is the oxygen level in the alveoli calculated using the alveolar gas equation. The normal range is 2.6–5.3 kPa.

$$P_AO_2 = F_iO_2 \times 94.8 - P_aCO_2/RQ$$

where RQ is the respiratory quotient, estimated to be 0.8.

The partial pressure of alveolar oxygen is less than that of arterial oxygen because the partial pressure of oxygen is reduced by the addition of water vapour from the humidification of the air in the upper airways and the ongoing exchange of oxygen and carbon dioxide in the pulmonary capillaries and the alveoli.

A–a gradient

This is the alveolar (A)–arterial (a) oxygen gradient. The normal range is 2–3.3 kPa (the value increases with age).

$$\text{A–a gradient} = F_iO_2 \times 94.8 - P_aCO_2/RQ - P_aO_2$$

P_aO_2/F_iO_2 ratio

This is the ratio of deoxygenated blood to oxygenated blood. The normal range is > 40 kPa (a ratio of < 26 kPa reflects intra-pulmonary shunting).

F_iO_2 is a fraction, not a percentage (i.e. 50% oxygen = 0.50 F_iO_2).

Work of breathing

This is the effort involved in moving air in and out of the lungs. Accessory muscles are used to assist breathing during exercise or when the work of breathing is increased.

It is affected by:

- elasticity of the lung tissue
- chest wall compliance
- resistance to gas flow in the airways
- obstruction to gas flow in the airways.

Elasticity of lung tissue

This is dependent on two factors:

- **Alveolar surface tension**—surfactant is secreted to reduce surface tension and reduce resistance to expansion. Surfactant secretion can be impaired by acidosis, hypoxia, hyperoxia, atelectasis, pulmonary oedema, and acute respiratory distress syndrome (ARDS).
- **Elastic fibres of the lung**—these contract and help to force air out of the lung.

Chest wall compliance

This is the change in volume of the lung divided by the amount of pressure required to produce the volume change.

Large volume changes produced by small pressure changes indicate a compliant lung. Table 5.1 lists the factors that affect lung compliance.

Lung compliance has two components—static and dynamic compliance.

Table 5.1 Factors that affect lung compliance

Factors that decrease lung compliance	Factors that increase lung compliance
Pulmonary congestion	Pulmonary oligaemia (decreased blood volume)
Increased pulmonary smooth muscle tone	Decreased pulmonary smooth muscle tone
Increased alveolar surface tension	Augmented surfactant secretion
Pulmonary fibrosis, infiltration, or atelectasis	Destruction of lung tissue (e.g. emphysema)

Static compliance

This is the compliance of the lung excluding resistance to gas flow. It is measured at the end of a known volume inspiration with the airway occluded for 2 s to achieve a plateau pressure.

Dynamic compliance

This is the compliance of the lung including resistance to gas flow. It refers to the change in pressure from end inspiration to end expiration.

In healthy lungs there is little difference between static and dynamic compliance. In patients with airway obstruction, dynamic compliance will decrease rapidly due to resistance to gas flow, without a significant change in static compliance.

Ventilation/perfusion match

Efficient gas exchange within the lung depends on the relationship between alveolar ventilation (V) and pulmonary capillary perfusion (Q).

- When V/Q = 1, there is good ventilation and good perfusion.
- When V/Q is > 1, there is good ventilation but poor perfusion (increased dead space).
- When V/Q is < 1, there is poor ventilation but good perfusion (increased venous admixture or shunt).

In the normal lung there is a certain degree of variation in ventilation and perfusion, with up to 15% mismatch. The pathological causes of V/Q mismatch are summarized in Table 5.2.

The body has two homeostatic responses to allow it to adjust to variations in ventilation and perfusion:

Table 5.2 Causes of V/Q mismatch

V/Q > 1 (dead space)	V/Q < 1 (shunt)
Pulmonary embolus	Atelectasis
Decreased cardiac output	Consolidation
Extrinsic pressure on pulmonary arteries (tumour, pneumothorax) Pulmonary oedema	Obstructive lung disease (emphysema, bronchitis, asthma)
Destruction of pulmonary vessels	Restrictive lung disease (ARDS, pulmonary and alveolar fibrosis, pneumonia)
Decreased cardiac output	
Obstruction of the pulmonary microcirculation (ARDS)	

Hypoxic pulmonary vasoconstriction

Capillaries in areas with low alveolar PO_2 will vasoconstrict to reduce perfusion to the affected areas.

Hypocapnic bronchoconstriction

Bronchioles in areas with low capillary PCO_2 will constrict to reduce ventilation to the affected areas.

Respiratory failure

The majority of patients who require ventilator support will have some degree of respiratory failure.

Type I respiratory failure

The patient is hypoxaemic, but has normal levels of carbon dioxide—that is, PO_2 is < 11 kPa on F_iO_2 0.4, with PCO_2 in the range 4.5–6.0 kPa.

Type II respiratory failure

The patient is both hypoxaemic and hypercapnic—that is, PO_2 is < 11 kPa on F_iO_2 0.4, or < 8.0 kPa on air, with PCO_2 > 6.5 kPa without a primary metabolic acidosis.

Patient indicators of respiratory failure

- Respiratory rate > 25 breaths/min or < 8 breaths/min.
- Deteriorating vital capacity.

Oxygen therapy

Oxygen is transported dissolved in plasma (3%) and bound to haemoglobin in the red blood cells (97%). The affinity of haemoglobin for oxygen is governed by the partial pressure of oxygen. At higher partial pressures (i.e. at the lungs) more oxygen binds to haemoglobin and it is 98–100% saturated. At lower partial pressures (i.e. at the tissues) only 75% of the haemoglobin remains saturated, to allow utilization of oxygen by the cells. In extreme circumstances more oxygen can be unbound, reducing saturation even further, to 20–30%.

When the partial pressure of oxygen is plotted against the haemoglobin saturation, an 'S'-shaped curve is produced. This is known as the oxyhaemoglobin dissociation curve (see Figure 5.1).

Specific factors affect oxyhaemoglobin dissociation by shifting the position of the curve to the right or left, making more or less oxygen dissociate from haemoglobin (see Box 5.1).

Carbon dioxide is transported dissolved in plasma (7%), bound to haemoglobin in the red blood cells (23%), or converted to bicarbonate in the red blood cells (70%).

In the presence of *deoxygenated blood* more carbon dioxide will bind to the red blood cells.

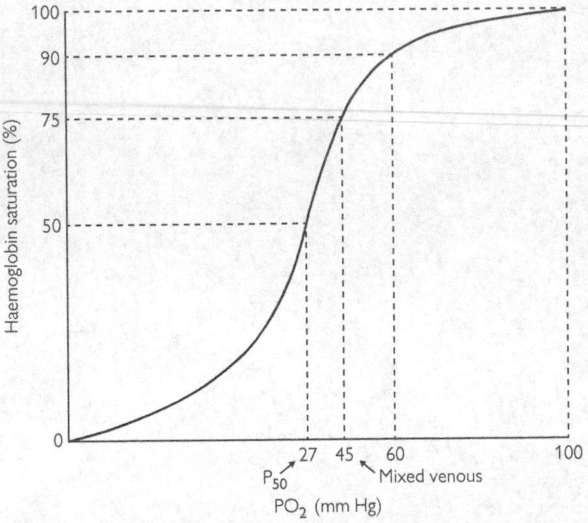

Figure 5.1 The oxyhaemoglobin dissociation curve. (Reproduced with permission from James Munis, *Just Enough Physiology* (Oxford University Press, 2011) © Mayo Foundation for Medical Education and Research.)

Box 5.1 Factors that cause a shift on the oxyhaemoglobin dissociation curve

Right shift = reduced affinity, so more oxygen is available to the tissues:
- ↓pH
- ↑ body temperature
- ↑ PCO_2
- ↑ 2,3-DPG.

Left shift = increased affinity, so less oxygen is available to the tissues:
- ↑ pH
- ↓ body temperature
- ↓ PCO_2
- ↓ 2,3-DPG.

2,3-DPG is 2,3-diphosphoglycerate, a chemical compound produced in the cell during anaerobic respiration (glycolysis).

Indications for administration of oxygen

- Respiratory distress (respiratory rate > 25 or < 8 breaths/min).
- Hypoxaemia (PO_2 < 8 kPa on air).
- Acute events, including:
  - acute coronary syndrome
  - major haemorrhage
  - pulmonary oedema
  - pulmonary embolus
  - seizures
  - low cardiac output
  - metabolic acidosis.

Oxygen is a drug, and should only be administered without a prescription in an emergency (see Table 5.3).

Target oxygen saturation should be > 92%.

Risks of oxygen therapy

A small proportion (approximately 12%) of patients with acute or chronic pulmonary disease, in type II respiratory failure, are dependent on the hypoxic drive. They may require lower target oxygen saturation in order to maintain adequate respiration. These patients should be closely monitored during oxygen delivery for signs of increasing drowsiness and decreased respiratory effort (respiratory rate < 10 breaths/min and shallow depth).

Oxygen is a dry gas, so will adversely affect cilia function and sputum clearance. This risk increases with duration of use and high flow rates. In any patient who requires oxygen for more than 24 h, humidification is required.

Use of high percentage oxygen (> 80%) is associated with nitrogen washout and alveolar collapse, as diffusion of most of the gas through to the capillary can occur and little nitrogen is left to maintain intra-alveolar pressure. When it is appropriate to do so, oxygen delivery should be at the lowest level possible to maintain normal PO_2.

Further reading

British Thoracic Society (BTS). *Emergency Oxygen Use in Adults*. BTS: London, 2008.

Table 5.3 Modes of oxygen delivery

Delivery mode	O_2 (%)	Associated problems	Safety priorities	Indication
Nasal cannulae	2 L/min 23–28% 3 L/min 28–30% 4 L/min 32–36%	Limited O_2 (%) Inaccurate O_2 delivery with high minute volumes Requires patent nasal passages Avoid if patient is a mouth breather Drying and discomfort of nasal passages	Regular monitoring of respiratory rate and pattern Pulse oximetry Check O_2 flow rate Position cannulae inside nares	Low-level O_2 supplementation Short to long term Disposable delivery system
Variable-performance face mask	5 L/min ~35% 6 L/min ~50% 8 L/min ~55% 10 L/min ~60% 15 L/min ~80%	Inaccurate O_2 delivery with high minute volumes Limits patient activities (e.g. eating and drinking) Drying and discomfort of upper respiratory tract Rebreathing	Regular monitoring of respiratory rate and pattern Pulse oximetry Check O_2 flow rate Check mask position	Low- to medium-level O_2 supplementation Short to medium term Disposable delivery system
Fixed-performance face mask (Venturi)	2 L/min 24% 4 L/min 28% 8 L/min 35% 10 L/min 40 15 L/min 60%	O_2 percentage may still not be achieved with high flow Limits patient activities (e.g. eating and drinking) Drying and discomfort of upper respiratory tract	Regular monitoring of respiratory rate and pattern Pulse oximetry Check O_2 flow rate Check mask position	Medium- to high-level O_2 supplementation Short to medium term Disposable delivery system

Humidified oxygen using nebulizer system	Varying rates of flow to deliver 28–60% O_2	Inaccurate O_2 delivery with high minute volumes Limits patient activities (e.g. eating and drinking)	Regular monitoring of respiratory rate and pattern Pulse oximetry Check O_2 flow rate, including on nebulizer circuit Check mask position	Low- to medium-level O_2 supplementation Medium to long term Disposable delivery system
Non-rebreathing mask with reservoir bag	80–85%, depending on respiratory rate and flow rate 15 L/min O_2	Reservoir bag should be partially inflated at all times	Ensure that reservoir bag is fully inflated before placing on patient	Emergency situations and short-term use only

Non-invasive ventilation (NIV)

Non-invasive ventilation (NIV) allows support of respiratory function without the requirement for intubation. Therefore the patient must be spontaneously breathing and have a level of consciousness to comply with the treatment. NIV can be delivered via a tight-fitting face mask, a nasal cannula, or a helmet. This is to ensure that there is no gas leak in order to maintain the positive pressure. There are two forms of NIV:

- continuous positive airway pressure (CPAP)
- bi-level positive airway pressure (BPAP).

Continuous positive airway pressure (CPAP)

CPAP maintains a positive pressure throughout inspiration and expiration; this is equivalent to positive end expiratory pressure (PEEP). The pressure level is set and adjusted according to patient response. It is used to increase or maintain functional residual capacity (FRC) (see ➲ p. 134). An increased FRC is associated with reduced work of breathing, improved oxygenation, and improved lung compliance.

Bi-level positive airway pressure (BPAP)

BPAP cycles between two positive pressure settings—inspiratory positive airway pressure (IPAP) and expiratory positive airway pressure (EPAP). The pressure levels are set and adjusted according to patient response. Respiratory rate is usually determined by the patient's spontaneous rate, but may be time cycled (i.e. the machine will cycle between IPAP and EPAP at set intervals). It is used to augment tidal volume (V_T) (see ➲ p. 134). An increased V_T is associated with a reduction in $PaCO_2$, reduced work of breathing, and improved oxygenation.

Indications

- Acute exacerbation of COPD.
- Acute pulmonary oedema.
- Specific groups of patients with acute respiratory failure in whom intubation is associated with poor outcomes (e.g. immunocompromised patients, and those with neuromuscular disease or end-stage COPD).
- Facilitation of weaning.
- Post-operative respiratory failure.
- Obstructive sleep apnoea.

Contraindications

- Inability to protect the airway and/or high risk of aspiration.
- Facial surgery or trauma.
- Poor patient tolerance or compliance.
- Claustrophobia.

Before starting NIV, establish a clear management plan and document the settings. Agreement on the escalation and/or discontinuation of treatment should be reached with the patient. A successful outcome should be evident within 4 h, and evidence shows that it is dependent on nursing care. NIV is supportive, and therefore the cause of the respiratory difficulty should be managed and treated. Often the key to successful NIV is developing the patient's trust and confidence. It is worth spending time explaining, reassuring, and trialling different set-ups so that the patient will tolerate the equipment, overcome their initial anxiety, and allow continuation of NIV. Nurse the patient in a highly visible area and ensure that the call bell is within easy reach of the patient. The use of NIV is highly dependent on patient monitoring and nursing support. In addition, effective NIV is improved by correct positioning of the patient to optimize respiratory expansion. Table 5.4 provides further information on nursing care.

Table 5.4 Nursing support for patients with NIV

Setting up
Provide patient explanation
Set up machine and/or attach correct PEEP valve for agreed level of support (usually 5–10 cmH_2O)
Choose the correct size of mask (use sizing guide)
Connect the mask to the machine
Allow the patient to try the mask without fixing the straps. Once the patient is confident, attach the straps and continue to offer support and reassurance until the patient can tolerate the secured mask
Monitoring: • Gas flow, PEEP valve, and O_2 levels • Ongoing respiratory assessment—ABG, saturations, and respiratory rate • Vital signs—haemodynamic changes due to reduced venous return resulting from raised intra-thoracic pressure may decrease blood pressure and cardiac filling pressures
Patient problems
Pressure damage: • Check fitting of mask and straps • Protect bridge of nose, ears, and chin with hydrocolloid dressing
Drying of eyes: • Check mask fitting for leaks
Gastric distension: • Insert nasogastric tube on free drainage
Difficulty eating or drinking: • Support fluid and nutrition delivery by alternative routes
Feelings of claustrophobia: • Offer a supportive presence • Allow the patient opportunities to remove the mask • Consider use of earplugs to reduce the noise of high-flow gas

Further reading

Esquinas Rodriguez AM et al. Clinical review: helmet and non-invasive mechanical ventilation in critically ill patients. *Critical Care* 2013; **17**: 223–35.
Nava S and Hill N. Noninvasive ventilation in acute respiratory failure. *Lancet* 2009; **374**: 250–59.

Intubation and extubation

A secure airway is the primary goal of airway management. There are a number of different airway adjuncts that can be used for this purpose, including a nasal or oral endotracheal tube or a tracheostomy tube. The tubes are most often made of polyvinyl chloride with an inflatable cuff to seal the trachea to prevent air leakage and aspiration of oropharyngeal and gastric secretions. The cuff pressure should be in the range 20–30 cmH_2O in order to maintain a seal and reduce the risk of capillary occlusion in the mucosa of the trachea, which could lead to tracheal erosion. Endotracheal tubes may also have a subglottic port for suctioning above the cuff to remove secretions (see Figure 5.2), and to aid extubation. An 'armoured' tube will be wire-reinforced and can be used for long-term intubation or for patients with compressible tracheas (e.g. flexed neck position in surgery). Tracheostomy tubes can have a single or double lumen with a replaceable inner tube to maintain tube patency, and can be fenestrated to allow the patient to vocalize and communicate. The tube must be secured in order to avoid unintended extubation.

Process of endotracheal intubation

Intubation requires the following equipment:

- laryngoscope
- stylet (guidewire)
- Magill's forceps
- endotracheal tube (internal diameter, range 6.0–10.5 mm), cut to length and lubricated (if indicated)
- 10-mL syringe
- suctioning equipment
- oxygen and bag-valve mask
- tapes to secure tube

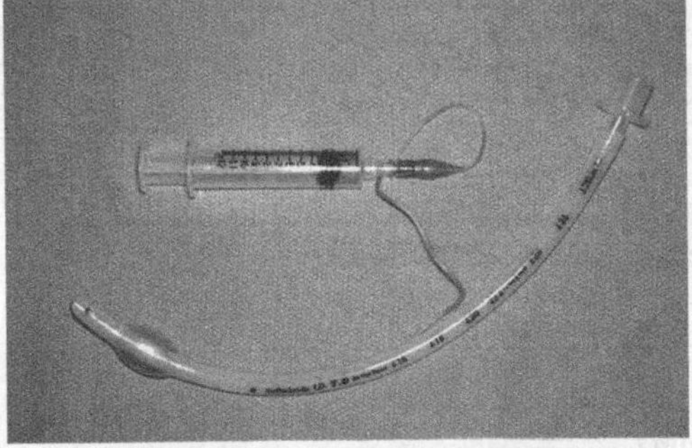

Figure 5.2 Endotracheal tube with subglottic port. (Reproduced with permission from Eelco Wijdicks, *The Practice of Emergency and Critical Care Neurology* (Oxford University Press, 2010). © Mayo Foundation for Medical Education and Research.)

- scissors
- stethoscope
- intravenous cannula
- capnography
- monitoring equipment (e.g. heart rate, saturations, blood pressure)
- nasogastric tube (this can be inserted at the same time, or if already present can be aspirated to empty the stomach contents; ensure that feed is stopped)
- catheter mount, ventilation tubing, and mechanical ventilator.

The patient should be prepared for the procedure by informing them of what will be happening, positioned supine with their neck slightly flexed and their head extended 'sniffing the air', and then pre-oxygenated for 3 min. Intubation should take no longer than 30 s (i.e. from loss of airway protection to secured airway and ventilation).

Rapid sequence induction (RSI) is indicated in patients who are at risk of aspiration of gastric contents into the lungs (e.g. in emergencies when the patient will not have been starved in advance of anaesthesia). Cricoid pressure is applied, to prevent gastric reflux, by compressing the cricoid cartilage against the cervical vertebrae. Once applied it should only be removed once, when indicated by the person intubating (i.e. once the trachea is intubated, the cuff is inflated, and both of the lungs are ventilating) (see Figure 5.3).

The nurse's role is to inform the person intubating of the vital signs and observe for complications. Once the tube is inserted, the cuff should be inflated and the patient's chest observed and auscultated for bilateral expansion. The tube must then be secured and the patient attached to the ventilator and a check X-ray performed. Arterial blood gas sampling should also be performed to confirm the initial ventilation settings and inform any changes that are required.

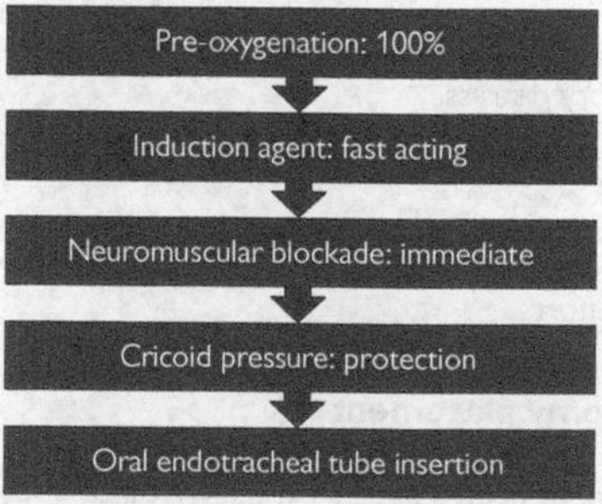

Figure 5.3 Process of intubation.

Drugs used during intubation

Safe intubation of a patient outside of a cardiac arrest situation will require the administration of drugs to enable insertion of the tube. The drugs used are subdivided into sedatives, neuromuscular blocking agents (NMBAs), and sympathomimetics (pp. 80 and 82):

- sedatives (e.g. propofol, etomidate, midazolam, ketamine)
- NMBAs (e.g. suxamethonium, which is a depolarizing muscle relaxant, or atracurium, pancuronium, and vecuronium, which are non-depolarizing muscle relaxants)
- sympathomimetics (e.g. metaraminol, ephedrine, adrenaline).

Process of endotracheal extubation

Extubation requires the following equipment and two individuals:

- 10-mL syringe
- suctioning equipment
- oxygen and oxygen mask/non-invasive ventilation
- scissors
- stethoscope
- monitoring equipment (e.g. heart rate, saturations, blood pressure)
- emergency reintubation equipment.

The decision to extubate the patient should be multidisciplinary and follow a period of weaning from mechanical ventilatory support. For further details on weaning, see ➲ p. 164. The reason for the intubation must be resolved and the patient must be able to maintain adequate gas exchange.

Reassess the patient's spontaneous respiratory rate, tidal volume, oxygen saturations, and arterial blood gas. Ensure that they are able to cough and clear secretions, that they have cardiovascular stability, and that they are able to obey commands. Aspirate the nasogastric tube.

The patient should be prepared for the procedure by informing them of what will be happening. Then position the patient upright in a seated position in the bed, suction the oropharynx and down the tube, and then cut the tapes. Simultaneously applying suctioning, deflate the cuff and withdraw the tube in a single rapid movement. Encourage the patient to cough, and suction secretions in the oropharynx. Apply the face mask to the patient and provide reassurance. Once the tube has been removed continue to monitor the patient for signs of respiratory distress.

Factors that can result in failed extubation

- Obstruction of airway.
- Inability to clear secretions, or the presence of copious secretions.
- Aspiration of gastric contents.
- Fatigue or poor respiratory effort.
- Poor gas exchange.

The process of tracheostomy placement

A tracheostomy can be sited surgically or percutaneously. The percutaneous method is generally used for intubated patients in the critical care setting (i.e. as a bedside intervention).

The following equipment is required for percutaneous insertion:

- sterile field and cleaning fluid
- lubricant

- local anaesthetic
- bronchoscope with catheter mount
- percutaneous tracheostomy kit (with tracheostomy, dilators and 10-mL syringe)
- suctioning equipment
- oxygen and bag-valve mask
- tapes to secure the tube
- stethoscope
- intravenous cannula
- monitoring equipment (e.g. heart rate, saturations, blood pressure)
- catheter mount, ventilation tubing, and mechanical ventilator.

The procedure is ideally performed under bronchoscopy guidance.

Local anaesthetic is infiltrated subcutaneously and a 1 cm incision is made in the skin midline above the trachea. The introducer needle and syringe are advanced at 45° until air is aspirated from the trachea. The guidewire is passed through the needle, and dilators of increasing diameter are used to extend the hole for insertion of the tracheostomy tube.

The nurse's role is to inform the person performing the tracheostomy of the vital signs and observe for complications. Once the tube has been inserted, the cuff should be inflated and the patient's chest observed and auscultated for bilateral expansion. The endotracheal tube can be removed. The tube must then be secured and the patient attached to the ventilator, and a check X-ray may be performed. Arterial blood gas sampling is also necessary, to confirm the initial ventilation settings and inform any changes that may be required.

Process of tracheostomy decannulation

The following equipment is required for decannulation:

- suctioning equipment
- gauze
- clear semi-permeable dressing
- stethoscope
- monitoring equipment (e.g. heart rate, saturations, blood pressure)
- emergency reintubation equipment.

The decision to decannulate the patient should be multidisciplinary and follow a period of weaning from mechanical ventilatory support (for further details about weaning, see ➔ p. 164). The reason for the tracheostomy insertion must be resolved, and the patient must be able to maintain adequate gas exchange.

Reassess the patient's spontaneous respiratory rate, tidal volume, oxygen saturations, and arterial blood gas. Ensure that they are able to cough and clear secretions, that they have cardiovascular stability, and that they are able to obey commands. Aspirate the nasogastric tube.

The patient should be prepared for the procedure by informing them of what will be happening. Position the patient upright in a seated position in the bed. Generally the patient will have had the cuff deflated for a period of time before the decannulation. Suction the oropharynx and down the tube, and then loosen the tapes. Withdraw the tube in a single rapid movement. Encourage the patient to cough, and suction secretions in the oropharynx. Apply the gauze dressing over the stoma and provide reassurance. Once the tube has been removed, continue to monitor the patient for signs of respiratory distress. Advise the patient to support the stoma when speaking or coughing. Inspect the stoma site daily. Once skin closure has occurred the site can remain exposed for ongoing healing.

Factors that can result in failed decannulation

- Obstruction of the airway.
- Inability to clear secretions, or the presence of copious secretions.
- Aspiration of gastric contents.
- Fatigue or poor respiratory effort.
- Poor gas exchange.

Management of the patient with an endotracheal tube or tracheostomy

The nurse is responsible for the ongoing management of patients with an endotracheal tube or a tracheostomy. Considerations with regard to the care of the patient include infection prevention and control, suctioning, humidification, analgesia and/or sedation, and communication.

Checks to be completed at the start of a shift

- Tube patency.
- Tube position—lip level.
- Cuff pressure (20–30 cmH_2O).
- Tube security (change the tapes only if they are soiled or loose, observe for ulceration, and ensure that venous drainage is unimpeded).
- Emergency ventilation equipment (bag-valve-mask, suction equipment and catheters, oxygen).
- Tracheostomy emergency equipment (one tube of the same size and one tube of a smaller size, obturator, disposable inner cannulas, 10-mL syringe, tracheostomy ties, tracheostomy dressing, dilator forceps, disconnection wedge).

Checks to be completed routinely during a shift

- Inner cannula patency (inspect and replace).

Infection prevention and control

The intubated patient is at high risk of infection, particularly ventilator-associated pneumonia (see ➔ p. 153). Measures to minimize contamination, colonization, and infection must be adhered to at all times and with each patient (e.g. hand hygiene, patient hygiene, single-use or sterilized equipment and fluid, patient screening, and environmental cleaning). Tubes should remain *in situ* for as long as indicated in the manufacturer's guidance (which ranges from 7 days up to 60 days).

The tracheostomy stoma should be assessed 4- to 8-hourly and the stoma cleaned and dressed as required.

Suctioning

- Use closed suction to minimize cross-contamination.
- Suction catheter size—multiply inner diameter by 3, and divide by 2.
- Suction catheter length—caution is needed when suctioning via tracheostomy.
- Suction only as needed—presence of secretions, flow loop changes, hypoxaemia.

- Consider pre-oxygenation prior to suctioning.
- Limit suction pressure to < 120 mmHg.
- Ensure that non-fenestrated inner tube is *in situ* in tracheostomy.
- Apply suction for a maximum of 10 s with each pass of the catheter.
- Undertake a maximum of three passes in a single episode.
- Note the colour, consistency, and quantity of the secretions.

Hypoxaemia may result from suctioning due to entrainment of alveolar air rather than air around the catheter. This can be minimized by using the correct catheter diameter, pre-oxygenation, minimal negative pressure, minimal time suctioning, and minimal number of catheter passes.

Mucosal irritation can be minimized by minimal negative pressure, rotation of the catheter, and withdrawal of the catheter from the carina before applying negative pressure.

Humidification

All patients with an artificial airway should receive continuous humidification. As the upper airway is bypassed during mechanical ventilation, humidification is necessary in order to avoid damage to the airway mucosa, atelectasis, thickened secretions, and airway obstruction. Humidification can be active, via a heated humidifier, or passive, via a heat and moisture exchanger (HME). Heated humidifiers increase the heat and water content (water vapour) of inspired gas. Set temperatures are in the range 37–41°C. Excess fluid will condense and should be collected in a water trap. HMEs trap exhaled heat and water vapour in order to warm and moisten the subsequently inspired gas. HMEs will increase dead space and should be used with caution in lung-protective ventilation strategies with low tidal volumes. Both forms of humidification can increase work of breathing, aerosol contaminants if disconnected, and may not adequately humidify inspired gas.

Communication

Communication with the patient while they are intubated is vital irrespective of the patient's level of sedation. The patient will be unable to vocalize, so the nurse must continue to observe and assess non-verbal signs of pain, anxiety, delirium, and discomfort (➔ p. 20). The inability to communicate can in itself contribute to the patient's anxiety. The patient's family will need to be educated about the care and communication of their relative, with ongoing explanations and reassurance.

Key considerations include the following:

- Introduce yourself to the patient.
- Orientate the patient.
- Explain the interventions to the patient.
- Allow the patient time to respond.
- Provide reassurance to the patient.

With a tracheostomy it is possible to trial cuff deflation to allow air to pass through the vocal cords. This can be achieved using a one-way valve once the patient is able to clear secretions and is spontaneously breathing.

In the conscious patient, alternative means of communication include devices such as tablets and alphabet, picture, or writing boards. Support from a speech and language therapist is also recommended.

Further reading

Restrepo R and Walsh B. Humidification during invasive and non-invasive mechanical ventilation. *Respiratory Care* 2012; **57**: 782–8.

Dawson D. Essential principles: tracheostomy care in the adult patient. *Nursing in Critical Care* 2014; **19**: 63–72.

Khalaila R et al. Communication difficulties and psychoemotional distress in patients receiving mechanical ventilation. *American Journal of Critical Care* 2011; **20**: 470–79.

Morris L et al. Tracheostomy care and complications in the Intensive Care Unit. *Critical Care Nurse* 2013; **33**: 18–30.

Ortega R et al. Endotracheal extubation. *New England Journal of Medicine* 2014; **370**: e4(1)–(4).

Stollings J et al. Rapid-sequence intubation: a review of the process and considerations when choosing medications. *Annals of Pharmacotherapy* 2014; **48**: 62–75.

Mechanical ventilation

[illegible]

Indications for mechanical ventilation

- [illegible]
- [illegible] hypoxaemia
- [illegible] the work of breathing

[illegible]

- Respiratory [illegible]
- [illegible]
- [illegible]
- [illegible]
- [illegible]

[illegible] hypoxaemia

- [illegible]
- [illegible]
- [illegible]

[illegible] work of breathing

- [illegible]
- [illegible]
- [illegible]

Physiological effects of mechanical ventilation

[illegible]

[illegible] cardiac output and venous return

[illegible]

Mechanical ventilation

Although it is a life-saving intervention, mechanical ventilation or intermittent positive pressure ventilation (IPPV) exposes the patient to a large number of potential risks and complications. These include the effects of positive intra-thoracic and intra-pulmonary pressure (barotrauma, decreased venous return) and the increased risks associated with endotracheal intubation. Nurses must be fully aware of these risks and understand how to reduce them in order to protect the patient.

Indications for mechanical ventilation

- To support acute ventilatory failure.
- To reverse life-threatening hypoxaemia.
- To decrease the work of breathing.

Causes of acute ventilatory failure

- **Respiratory centre depression**—decreased conscious level, intra-cerebral events, sedative or opiate drugs.
- **Mechanical disruption**—flail chest (multiple rib fractures resulting in a free segment of chest wall), diaphragmatic trauma, pneumothorax, pleural effusion.
- **Neuromuscular disorders**—acute polyneuropathy, myasthenia gravis, spinal cord trauma or pathology, Guillain-Barré syndrome, critical illness.
- **Reduced alveolar ventilation**—airway obstruction (foreign body, bronchoconstriction, inflammation, tumour), atelectasis, pneumonia, pulmonary oedema (cardiac failure and ARDS), obesity, fibrotic lung disease.
- **Pulmonary vascular disruption**—pulmonary embolus, ARDS, cardiac failure.

Causes of hypoxaemia

- **V/Q mismatch**—pulmonary embolus, obstruction of the pulmonary microcirculation, ARDS.
- **Shunt**—pulmonary oedema, pneumonia, atelectasis, consolidation.
- **Diffusion (gas exchange) limitation**—pulmonary fibrosis, ARDS, pulmonary oedema.

Causes of increased work of breathing

- Airway obstruction.
- Reduced respiratory compliance.
- High CO_2 production (e.g. due to burns, sepsis, overfeeding).
- Obesity.

Physiological effects of mechanical ventilation

IPPV has significant effects on the respiratory, cardiac, and renal systems. These are principally related to increased intra-thoracic pressure and its effect on normal physiological responses.

Decreased cardiac output and venous return

Increased intra-thoracic pressure reduces venous return (the passive flow of blood from central veins to the right atrium) and increases right ventricular afterload (the resistance to blood flow out of the ventricle by the pulmonary circulation). This reduces right ventricular output and consequently left ventricular filling and ultimately output. The use of PEEP means that this occurs throughout the respiratory cycle.

- **Effects**—hypotension, tachycardia, hypovolaemia, decreased urine output.
- **Management**—fluid loading to optimize stroke volume and cardiac output. Inotropes may be necessary if cardiac function is compromised.

Increased incidence of barotrauma

The pressure required to deliver gas to the alveoli through airways which may be resistant to gas flow can cause damage to more compliant areas through over-distension. Greater damage is caused at higher tidal volumes, causing gas to escape into the pleura and interstitial tissues. Up to 15% of patients develop barotrauma. The risk is particularly high in conditions with increased airway resistance due to bronchoconstriction, such as asthma.

- **Effects**—pneumothorax, pneumomediastinum, subcutaneous emphysema.
- **Management**—tidal volumes that are close to physiological values (e.g. 6–8 mL/kg). Avoid high airway pressures, if necessary by manipulating the inspiratory:expiratory (I:E) ratio. Chest drain management of pneumothorax is required.

Decreased urine output

The response to reduced cardiac output includes release of antidiuretic hormone, activation of the renin–angiotensin–aldosterone (RAA) response, and increased salt and water retention.

- **Effects**—oliguria, increased interstitial fluid, and generalized peripheral oedema.
- **Management**—fluid filling to optimize stroke volume and cardiac output, and careful fluid monitoring.

Ventilator-associated pneumonia

Ventilator-associated pneumonia (VAP) develops 48 h or later after commencement of mechanical ventilation via endotracheal tube or tracheostomy. It develops as a result of colonization of the lower respiratory tract and lung tissue by pathogens. Intubation compromises the integrity of the oropharynx and trachea, allowing oral and gastric secretions to enter the airways.

VAP is the most frequent post-admission infection in critical care patients, and significantly increases the number of mechanical ventilation days, the length of critical care stay, and the length of hospital stay overall.[1] Patients at increased risk include those who are immunocompromised, the elderly, and those with chronic illnesses (e.g. lung disease, malnutrition, obesity).

Diagnosis of VAP is difficult due to the number of differential diagnoses that present with the same signs and symptoms (e.g. sepsis, ARDS, cardiac failure, lung atelectasis). Radiological changes include consolidation and new or progressive infiltrates. Clinical signs include pyrexia > 38°C, raised or reduced white blood cell (WBC) count, new-onset purulent sputum, increased respiratory secretions/suctioning requirements, and worsening gas exchange. Microbiology criteria include a positive blood culture growth not related to any other source, and positive cultures from bronchoalveolar lavage.

Use of a care bundle approach has been demonstrated to be an effective preventive strategy. The Department of Health has established a care bundle[1] with six elements for the prevention of ventilator-associated pneumonia, which should be reviewed daily:

1. **Elevation of the head of the bed**—the head of the bed is elevated to 30–45° (unless contraindicated).
2. **Sedation level assessment**—unless the patient is awake and comfortable, sedation is reduced or held for assessment at least daily (unless contraindicated).
3. **Oral hygiene**—the mouth is cleaned with chlorhexidine gluconate (≥ 1–2% gel or liquid) 6-hourly. Teeth are brushed 12-hourly with standard toothpaste.
4. **Subglottic aspiration**—a tracheal tube (endotracheal or tracheostomy) that has a subglottic secretion drainage port is used if the patient is expected to be intubated for > 72 h. Secretions are aspirated via the subglottic secretion port 1- to 2-hourly.
5. **Tube cuff pressure**—cuff pressure is measured 4-hourly, and maintained in the range 20–30 cmH_2O (or 2 cmH_2O above peak inspiratory pressure).
6. **Stress ulcer prophylaxis**—stress ulcer prophylaxis is prescribed only for high-risk patients, according to locally developed guidelines.

Modes of mechanical ventilation

There are no generic terms for modes of ventilation and therefore the principles of mechanical ventilation and common terminology/abbreviations are discussed here. Refer to individual ventilator specifications for comprehensive information on the modes and settings available.

Controlled mechanical ventilation (CMV)

There is a set frequency of patient breaths delivered as either pressure controlled (with a set inspiratory pressure) or volume controlled (with a set tidal volume).

Synchronized intermittent mandatory ventilation (SIMV)

There is a set frequency of patient breaths, but this mode of ventilation allows spontaneous breaths to be taken in between. Ventilator breaths are synchronized to these spontaneous breaths, and can be pressure controlled (SIMV-PC) or volume controlled (SIMV-VC). The current trend is for pressure-controlled ventilation in order to control pressure and limit potential barotrauma.

Volume-controlled ventilation

The set tidal volume is delivered at a constant flow rate, resulting in changes to airway pressure through inspiration. The set tidal volume remains constant as lung compliance and resistance change. A high inspiratory flow rate delivers the set tidal volume more quickly. Therefore if ventilation is time cycled and the set tidal volume has been reached before the end of inspiration, there will be a pause before expiration and the airway pressure will drop. High inspiratory flow rates will also elevate the peak airway pressure. Therefore low inspiratory flow rates are recommended to keep the peak airway pressure as low as possible. Pressure-limited, volume-controlled ventilation ensures that the tidal volume delivered is as close as possible to the set tidal volume for the set pressure limit (e.g. 30–35 cmH_2O).

Pressure-controlled ventilation

Set pressures throughout the inspiratory and expiratory cycle are delivered at a decelerating flow rate, resulting in a tidal volume that varies with lung compliance and resistance. For example, an increase in resistance or a reduction in lung compliance will decrease the tidal volume delivered, resulting in hypoventilation. Common pressure controlled modes which also allow for pressure supported spontaneous breaths (see ➲ p. 155) include BIPAP, PCV+, DuoPAP, BiLevel and Bi-vent (terms and abbreviations depend on the Trademark name of the specific ventilator being used).

Airway pressure release ventilation (APRV)

This is a pressure-regulated mode of ventilation, with set inspiratory pressure and PEEP. The settings produce an inverse ratio in ventilation, with the time at the higher pressure exceeding the time at the lower pressure. A combination of patient spontaneous and mandatory set breaths is allowed.

Pressure support ventilation/assist (PSV/assist)

A set level of inspiratory pressure support or tidal volume is delivered when the patient triggers a breath. The tidal volume of each breath is dependent on lung compliance and respiratory rate. In addition, a back-up rate of breaths will occur if the patient does not initiate (trigger) breaths at the required rate. PSV is used to provide ventilator support (e.g. when the patient's own respiratory efforts are diminished). This mode reduces the requirement for sedation, allows ongoing use of respiratory muscles, and provides the opportunity to gradually reduce the level of support to facilitate weaning. Pressure supported breaths can also be added into other modes which allow for spontaneous breaths over and above the set mandatory controlled breaths (e.g. SIMV, BIPAP).

Mechanical ventilator settings

Respiratory rate (f) (breaths/min)

Typically the respiratory rate is 10–15 breaths/min, but it may be altered in order to optimize minute volume and/or PCO_2.

Tidal volume (V_T) (mL/kg)

Typically this is in the range 6–8 mL/kg, but it may be altered to optimize minute volume and/or PCO_2.

Minute volume (MV or V_E) (L/min)

Typically this is in the range 3–10 L/min. It is derived from tidal volume and respiratory rate

Flow rate (V) (L/min)

Typically this is in the range 40–80 L/min, and adjusted to ensure that tidal volume is achieved within inspiratory time. A decelerating flow pattern is always seen in pressure support modes.

Positive end expiratory pressure (PEEP) (cmH_2O)

Typically this is in the range 5–10 cmH_2O.

Airway pressure (cmH2O)

Typically plateau pressure is limited to < 30 cmH_2O in order to reduce barotrauma.

Pressure support/assist (cmH_2O)

Typically this is in the range 5–20 cmH_2O, set according to patient requirements for assistance.

Inspiratory:expiratory (I:E) ratio

Typically this is 1:2 (i.e. expiratory time is twice as long as inspiratory time). It may vary with extended or inverted ratios in order to increase time for inspiration in patients with severe airflow limitation (e.g. due to asthma), or to assist expiration by lengthening expiratory time and avoid air trapping.

Trigger

This can be flow based, pressure based, volume based, or time based, and is vital for reducing the delay between the initiation of a breath and the ventilator response and thus the patient's work of breathing.

- Flow-based triggers require the patient to produce a minimum flow rate of 1 L/min to initiate a breath.
- Pressure-based triggers require the patient to generate a negative pressure of –1 to –10 cmH_2O to initiate a breath.
- Volume-based triggers require the patient to inhale a certain volume of gas to initiate a breath.
- Time-based triggers are independent of the patient effort, with preset frequency and delivered at regular intervals of time.

The ventilator settings are summarized in Table 5.5.

Pressure–volume relationships

Pressure–volume loops can be viewed graphically on most modern ventilators, and the information obtained can be used to inform ventilator settings, such as PEEP and upper airway pressure limits.

Table 5.5 Ventilator settings

Parameter	Initial setting for ventilator
Respiratory rate	10–15 breaths/min
Tidal volume	6–8 mL/kg
Positive end expiratory pressure	3–10 cmH_2O
Peak airway pressure	≤ 35 cmH_2O
Inspiratory: expiratory ratio	1:2
Oxygen (adjusted to blood gas results)	0.4–0.6 F_iO_2

The pressure–volume relationship in a ventilator breath consists of three stages:

- initial increase in pressure with little change in volume
- linear increase in volume as pressure increases
- pressure increase with no further volume increase.

The inflection points represent the change between the different stages of the ventilator breath (see Figure 5.4).

Lower inflection point

This occurs between stages 1 and 2, and is the point at which airway resistance is overcome, allowing alveolar opening. In a patient who is fully ventilated and making little or no respiratory effort, the lower inflection point is the point at which lower airways would close on expiration. PEEP should therefore be set at this level to avoid gas trapping.

Upper inflection point

This occurs between stages 2 and 3, and is the point at which lung capacity for the breath has been reached. It can be used to adjust settings for maximum inspiratory pressure.

Protective lung ventilation

Protective lung ventilation is the current standard of care for mechanical ventilation for both ARDS and non-ARDS patients. Features include permissive hypercapnia, lower plateau pressures, and low tidal volume ventilation (4–8 mL/kg) (ideal body weight, not actual body weight).

Ideal body weight

Male patients: 50 kg + 2.3 kg for each inch over 5 feet.
Female patients: 45.5 kg + 2.3 kg for each inch over 5 feet.

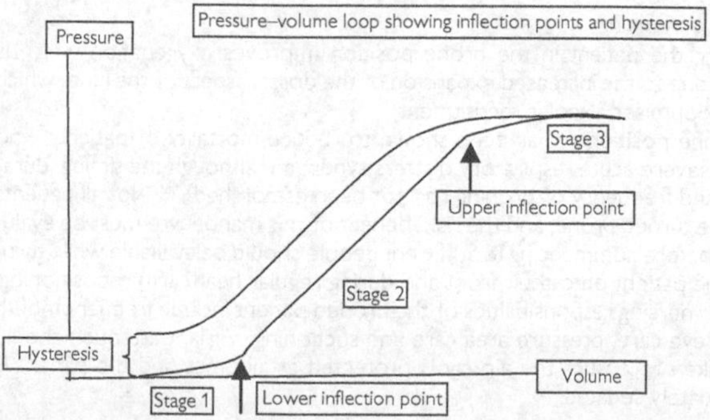

Figure 5.4 Pressure–volume loop showing inflection points and hysteresis.

Mechanical ventilation: troubleshooting

The patient is highly vulnerable to a number of problems while dependent on a mechanical ventilator. The critical care nurse is responsible for the patient's safety, and it is his or her responsibility to ensure that any problems are recognized as soon as possible and dealt with in an effective and timely manner.

A guide to recognition and management of the more common problems is provided in Table 5.6. If there is any doubt about the functioning of the ventilator, and the patient is deteriorating, the nurse should immediately:

- call for help
- manually ventilate the patient using a manual ventilation bag with high-flow oxygen
- review the patient for indicators of what is causing the problem.

Improving oxygenation in the ventilated patient

In patients with severe acute lung pathology (e.g. ARDS), simply increasing the FiO_2 may not be sufficient to support the patient's oxygen requirements. Alternative interventions may also be needed, including the following.

Positive end expiratory pressure

- PEEP will increase FRC by improving V/Q match and will prevent collapse of recruited alveoli.
- Increase by increments of 1–2 cmH_2O.
- Response to any alteration in PEEP should be monitored using blood gas analysis.
- Pressure–volume loops can be used to identify the lower inflexion point to determine the optimal PEEP setting.
- ARDS.net suggests higher PEEP to lower F_iO_2 ratios. For example:
  - PEEP 8–14 cmH_2O with 0.3 F_iO_2
  - PEEP 14–16 cmH_2O with 0.4 F_iO_2
  - PEEP 16–20 cmH_2O with 0.5 F_iO_2
  - PEEP 22–24 cmH_2O with 0.5–1.0 F_iO_2.

Prone positioning

Placing the patient in the prone position improves oxygenation which is likely due to the increased expansion of the dorsal aspect of the lungs which then optimises alveolar recruitment[2].

Prone positioning has been shown to reduce mortality of patients who have severe acute respiratory distress syndrome although the timing, duration and frequency of proning has not been established[3,4,5]. Not all patients can be turned prone, and the risk–benefit of this manoeuvre must be evaluated before commencing it. Sufficient people should be available while turning the patient onto their front and during regular head/arm repositioning. Other nursing responsibilities of the proned patient include frequent mouth care, eye care, pressure area care and suctioning. Vigilant attention should be taken to ensure the airway is protected at all times and the patient is adequately sedated.

Nitric oxide (NO)

Inhaled NO crosses the alveolar membrane, acting locally on the pulmonary vasculature by dilating vessels and increasing blood flow. This improves

Table 5.6 Troubleshooting problems in the ventilated patient

High airway pressure: airway pressure alarm sounds, persistent rise in peak airway pressure, evidence of patient distress, haemodynamic instability

Life-threatening causes

- Endotracheal tube (ETT) and/or ventilator tubing obstruction
- Pneumothorax
- Severe bronchospasm

Other causes

- Build-up of airway secretions
- Asynchrony with mechanical ventilation (tidal volume too high)
- Patient coughing
- ETT displacement

Interventions

- Ascertain cause of high airway pressure and treat accordingly
- Consider manual ventilation if patient is in respiratory distress
- Emergency re-intubation
- Review ventilator settings
- Check tubing and filter integrity
- Auscultate lungs for abnormal breath sounds
- Perform suction
- Check arterial blood gas and treat accordingly
- Review sedation if an increase with or without paralysis is indicated

Low airway pressure: airway pressure alarm sounds, audible air leak, decreased minute volume, evidence of patient distress, haemodynamic instability

Life-threatening causes

- ETT and/or ventilator tubing disconnection or leak

Interventions

- Ascertain cause of low airway pressure and treat accordingly
- Consider manual ventilation if patient is in respiratory distress
- Emergency re-intubation
- Check connections
- Check tubing integrity
- Check cuff pressure
- Review ventilator settings
- Auscultate lungs for abnormal breath sounds
- Perform suction
- Check arterial blood gas and treat accordingly
- Review sedation if an increase with or without paralysis is indicated

Low minute volume: low MV alarm sounds, audible air leak, evidence of patient distress, haemodynamic instability

Life-threatening causes

- Disconnection from the ventilator,
- Asynchrony with mechanical ventilation (i.e. flow rate may be too low to allow set volume in time allocated by set respiratory rate)
- Air leak via chest drain

(*continued*)

Table 5.6 (*Contd.*)

Interventions

- Ascertain cause of low minute volume and treat accordingly
- Consider manual ventilation if patient is in respiratory distress
- Emergency re-intubation
- Check connections and tubing integrity
- Check cuff pressure
- Review ventilator settings (increase to compensate for chest drain)
- Auscultate lungs for abnormal breath sounds
- Check arterial blood gas and treat accordingly
- Review sedation if an increase with or without paralysis is indicated

High minute volume: high MV alarm sounds, evidence of patient making respiratory effort

Effects

- Ventilator malfunction
- Asynchrony with mechanical ventilation (patient making respiratory effort)

Interventions

- Check causes of patient's tachypnoea (e.g. pain, hypoxia, hypercapnia)
- Review ventilator settings

Auto-PEEP (intrinsic PEEP, air-trapping): failure of alveolar pressure to return to zero at the end of exhalation, causing increased resistance to airflow and increased work of breathing

Causes

- Incomplete or impeded exhalation, as a result of either high MV (> 10 L/min) or airway resistance (due to chronic pulmonary disease)

Interventions

- Ensure low-compressible-volume ventilator tubing is used
- Review ventilator settings to reduce MV by decreasing respiratory rate or altering inspiratory flow rate to decrease inspiratory time and increase expiratory time
- Reduce metabolic workload to reduce respiratory demand

V/Q match and therefore gas exchange. As soon as it enters the blood, NO is bound to haemoglobin and has no further systemic (i.e. hypotensive) effect.

NO gas is added to the gas delivery of the ventilator or in the inspiratory limb of the ventilation circuit. Optimal delivery is titrated according to PO_2 at least once a shift. Withdrawal of NO should be slow, as there may be rebound pulmonary hypertension and hypoxaemia. Significant increases in oxygenation are seen in up to 60% of patients. However, this has not been associated with an improvement in overall mortality.

The safe use of nitric oxide is summarized in Box 5.2.

Box 5.2 Safe use of nitric oxide

- Monitoring of exhaled levels of nitrogen dioxide (a toxic substance produced when NO combines with O_2) is required. Levels of > 0.005 ppm are rare, and only levels of > 5 ppm are considered dangerous.
- Avoid high levels of condensation or water pooling in ventilator circuits by using HME filters, as nitrogen dioxide in solution produces nitric acid.
- Monitor levels of methaemoglobin (> 5% total haemoglobin is significant), which is formed when NO combines with haemoglobin.

Extracorporeal membrane oxygenation (ECMO)

ECMO uses an artificial lung (the membrane) to oxygenate the blood outside the body (hence 'extracorporeal') in a similar way to heart and lung bypass. By providing oxygenation outside the body the lungs can be rested (i.e. not exposed to high ventilator pressures or high oxygen levels), and the use of a blood pump can provide support for reversible heart disorders. ECMO can be either veno-venous or veno-arterial.

The main risk associated with ECMO is bleeding due to anticoagulant use.

There are ECMO centres throughout the UK for adult and paediatric patients, with referral and acceptance criteria. Specialist retrieval teams from these centres will transfer the patient, and in extreme circumstances ECMO may be started prior to transfer of the patient.

Managing hypercapnia in severe pulmonary disease

In patients with severe pulmonary disease, such as ARDS, where there is a risk of further lung damage being caused by the high airway pressures necessary to reduce PCO_2, it may be *preferable* to tolerate high levels of CO_2 provided that acidosis is adequately compensated for. This is termed 'permissive hypercapnia.' Rather than increasing the likelihood of barotrauma by increasing the volume of the breath, the patient's PCO_2 is allowed to rise to 10 kPa or more, provided that the pH can be maintained at ≥ 7.2. As a high CO_2 level is a very strong respiratory stimulant, permissive hypercapnia can only be tolerated if the patient is well sedated.

High-frequency ventilation (HFV)

This incorporates techniques using ventilation frequencies greater than 60–2000 breaths/min and tidal volumes of 1–5 mL/kg. This is useful when the lungs are non-compliant or there is a bronchopleural fistula causing large leaks of gas (and subsequent loss of tidal volume) during normal mechanical ventilation.

High-frequency oscillation

A rapidly oscillating gas flow is created by a device that acts like a woofer on a loudspeaker, producing a high-frequency rapid change in direction of gas flow. Most of the experience that has been gained with this approach has been in the paediatric population, but recent research in adults with severe ARDS suggests that it may be beneficial. Oscillation can be applied externally or via the endotracheal tube.

High-frequency jet ventilation

High-pressure air and oxygen are blended and then supplied through a non-compliant injection (jet) system to the patient via an open (uncuffed) circuit. The driving pressure of this gas can be adjusted to alter the rate of flow from the maximum (2.5 atm) down to zero. Added (warmed and humidified) gas is entrained from an additional circuit via a T-piece attached to the endotracheal tube. The entrainment circuit should provide at least 30 L/min of flow. Highly efficient humidification (usually via a hot-plate vaporizer humidifier) is necessary due to the high flows of otherwise dry gas. The usual frequency set is 100–200 breaths/min delivering tidal volumes of 2–5 mL/kg.

In an entrainment system, the tidal volume delivered by the ventilator increases with driving pressure and decreases with respiratory frequency. It remains the same with alterations in I:E ratio.

References

1 Department of Health. *High Impact Intervention No.5: care bundle to reduce ventilation-associated pneumonia*. Department of Health: London, 2010.

2 Gattinoni L et al. Prone position in acute respiratory distress syndrome: rationale, indications, and limits. *American Journal of Respiratory and Critical Care Medicine* 2013; **188**: 1286–1293.

3 Guérin C et al. (PROSEVA Study Group). Prone positioning in severe acute respiratory distress syndrome. *New England Journal of Medicine* 2013; **368**: 2159–2168.

4 Lee JM et al. The efficacy and safety of prone positional ventilation in acute respiratory distress syndrome: updated study-level meta-analysis of 11 randomized control trials. *Critical Care Medicine* 2014; **14**: 1252–1262.

5 Sud S et al. Effect of prone positioning during mechanical ventilation on mortality among patients with acute respiratory distress syndrome: a systematic review and meta-analysis. *Canadian Medical Association Journal* 2014; **186**: E381–E390.

Further reading

de Beer J and Gould T. Principles of artificial ventilation. *Anaesthesia and Intensive Care Medicine* 2013; **14**: 83–93.

Grossbach I et al. Overview of mechanical ventilatory support and management of patient- and ventilator-related responses. *Critical Care Nurse* 2011; **31**: 30–44.

Henzler D. What on earth is APRV? *Critical Care* 2011; **15**: 115.

Lambert M-L et al. Prevention of VAP: an international online survey. *Antimicrobial Resistance and Infection Control* 2013; **2**: 1–8.

Mireles-Cabodevila E et al. A rational framework for selecting modes of ventilation. *Respiratory Care* 2013; **58**: 348–66.

National Heart, Lung, and Blood Institute (NHLBI) ARDS Network. www.ardsnet.org

National Institute for Health and Care Excellence (NICE). *Technical Patient Safety Solutions for Ventilator-Associated Pneumonia in Adults*. PSG002. NICE: London, 2008. www.nice.org.uk/guidance/psg002.

Singer M and Webb AR. *Oxford Handbook of Critical Care*, 3rd edn. Oxford University Press: Oxford, 2009.

Tobin M. *Principles and Practice of Mechanical Ventilation*, 3rd edn. McGraw-Hill: London, 2013.

Weaning

With the growing awareness of the hazards of prolonging the period of ventilation, there is an increasing emphasis on effective weaning strategies. Weaning can be defined as a gradual reduction in ventilatory support so that the patient no longer requires [illegible] support is [illegible] positive [illegible] of mechanical ventilation [illegible] a critical [illegible] study [illegible] evaluation of the patient's ability [illegible] protocol [illegible] is [illegible] to wean.

[illegible] concepts of [illegible] ventilation [illegible] support [illegible] progress [illegible] to achieve [illegible].

[illegible] evidence [illegible] protocol [illegible].

The decision to wean

The decision to wean can be informed by the RSBI [illegible] (RSBI). The use of an RSBI [illegible] the ratio of respiratory frequency to tidal volume (f/VT) [illegible] measured as follows:

- [illegible] the patient [illegible] breathing spontaneously [illegible]
- [illegible] respiratory rate and [illegible] with a spirometer.
- [illegible] to calculate the f/VT.

For example, [illegible] breaths [illegible] tidal volume [illegible]

= [illegible] breaths/min/L

An RSBI of ≤ 100 breaths/min/L [illegible] weaning [illegible].

Other typical parameters include the following:

- [illegible]
- [illegible]

[illegible] weaning [illegible] assessment [illegible] patient [illegible] the cause of respiratory failure [illegible] mechanical ventilation [illegible].

Weaning methods

The [illegible] process of weaning involves [illegible] the mode of ventilation [illegible] to assess the patient's ability to maintain their own work of breathing. [illegible] spontaneous breathing trial (SBT) [illegible] The SBT may [illegible] (see [illegible]) [illegible] CPAP [illegible] pressure support [illegible].

Weaning

With the growing awareness of the hazards of prolonged mechanical ventilation there is an increasing emphasis on effective weaning strategies. Weaning can be defined as a gradual reduction in ventilatory support so that the patient either requires no assistance with their breathing or no further reduction in support is possible. Protocol-directed weaning has shown positive outcomes, with shorter duration of mechanical ventilation and decreased critical care stay. It also counters the under-estimation by physicians of the patient's ability to be successfully weaned. A current trend in protocol use is nurse-led weaning.

Weaning often consists of a succession of stages rather than a single transition from full ventilatory support to independent breathing. The implication is that in order for progress to be made the patient only has to be fit enough to achieve each stage.

Weaning must take place alongside other care activities, and therefore consideration should be given to time of day, nursing interventions, medical treatments, and patient response.

The decision to wean

The decision to wean can be informed by the Rapid Shallow Breathing Index (RSBI). The use of the RSBI as a weaning predictor was first reported in the early 1990s.[6] It is the ratio of respiratory rate to tidal volume (f/V_T), and is measured as follows:

- Perform a 1-min trial of unassisted breathing with a T-piece.
- Measure the respiratory rate and tidal volume with a spirometer.
- Divide the respiratory rate by the tidal volume to calculate the RSBI.

For example, 25 (breaths/min)/450 (mL/breath) → 25/0.45 L = 55 (breaths/min/L).

An RSBI of ≤ 105 breaths/min/L, indicating a relatively low respiratory rate to tidal volume, is used as an indication of readiness to wean or extubate. RSBI is most accurate when used to predict failure to wean, rather than readiness to wean.

Additional parameters include the following:

- $PaO_2/F_iO_2 < 200$ mmHg
- PEEP < 5 cmH_2O.

The decision to wean will also be based on an assessment of patient improvement—that is, whether the cause of respiratory failure requiring mechanical ventilation has been resolved, and whether the patient is stable (see Box 5.3).

Weaning methods

The initial process of weaning involves changing the mode of ventilation or support to assess the patient's ability to maintain their own work of breathing. A spontaneous breathing trial (SBT) for 30 min is used. The SBT may be coupled with a sedation hold (See ➲ p. 77). SBT can be achieved by using a T-piece, pressure support plus PEEP, CPAP or flow-by. If the patient shows no signs of fatigue (i.e. they display no cardiovascular or respiratory distress) this can then be followed by a pressure support or external

Box 5.3 Prerequisites for weaning[7]

- Able to cough and clear secretions (minimal amount).
- $F_iO_2 < 0.5$.
- Adequate minute ventilation.
- Alert and able to follow commands.
- Reason for mechanical ventilation resolved or resolving.
- No significant acid–base abnormalities.
- No evidence of severe sepsis, septic shock, or systemic inflammatory response syndrome (SIRS).
- Vasopressor support minimal.
- No electrolyte imbalances.
- No fluid shifts or fluid resuscitation required.

Box 5.4 Signs of respiratory distress

- Respiratory rate > 35 breaths/min or < 8 breaths/min
- Saturations < 90%
- Heart rate > 140 beats/min
- Systolic blood pressure > 180 mmHg or < 90 mmHg
- Signs of increased work of breathing

CPAP trial prior to extubation. If respiratory distress is identified, no further attempt to wean should be undertaken until the following day (see Box 5.4). The exception to this practice is in patients ventilated on APRV, as this is a spontaneous breathing mode. The aim of weaning from this mode is to adjust gas flow to the level of CPAP, with progressively fewer releases occurring per minute.

Non-invasive ventilation has been utilized in the weaning process in the following ways:

- as an alternative weaning method for patients who are unsuccessful in initial weaning trials
- for patients who are extubated but develop acute respiratory failure within 48 h
- as prophylaxis after extubation for patients who are at high risk for reintubation.

Weaning classification[8]

- Simple weaning—patients who proceed from initiation of weaning to successful extubation on the first attempt without difficulty.
- Difficult weaning—patients who fail initial weaning and require up to three SBTs or as long as 7 days from the first SBT to achieve successful weaning.
- Prolonged weaning—patients who fail at least three weaning attempts or require > 7 days weaning after the first SBT.

Prolonged weaning

Prolonged weaning is often a direct consequence of the complexities of critical illness. Patients who survive the acute phase of their admission will experience a range of physical and psychological disturbances (including neuromyopathy, weakness, sleep deprivation, and delirium). These can all have a negative impact both on the patient's readiness to wean and on the weaning process itself.

Measures to support the patient with prolonged weaning include rehabilitation, tracheostomy insertion, and specialized weaning units.

References

6 Crocker C. Weaning from ventilation—current state of the science and art. *Nursing in Critical Care* 2009; 14: 185–90.

7 Kaplan L and Toevs C. Weaning from mechanical ventilation. *Current Problems in Surgery* 2013; 50: 489–94.

8 Boles J-M et al. Weaning from mechanical ventilation. *European Respiratory Journal* 2007; 29: 1033–56.

Further reading

Blackwood B et al. Protocolized versus non-protocolized weaning for reducing the duration of mechanical ventilation in critically ill adult patients. *Cochrane Database of Systematic Reviews* 2010; Issue 5: CD006904.

Burns K et al. Non-invasive positive-pressure ventilation as a weaning strategy for intubated adults with respiratory failure. *Cochrane Database of Systematic Reviews* 2013; Issue 12: CD004127.

Intensive Care Society. *Weaning Guidelines*. Intensive Care Society: London, 2007.

Chapter 6

Cardiovascular assessment and monitoring

Cardiovascular assessment

If an actual or potential cardiovascular abnormality has been identified during a general ABCDE assessment (see ➲ p. 18) or while monitoring the patient, a more detailed and focused cardiovascular assessment can provide further information to guide clinical management.

Focused health history

Subjective information about the cardiovascular history can be taken from the patient if they are awake, or from other sources (e.g. family, caregivers, or patient notes). For an overview of history taking, see ➲ p. 16.

Cardiovascular symptom enquiry

- Chest pain, indigestion, and arm or jaw numbness.
- Palpitations.
- Shortness of breath—in the daytime and/or at night.
- Syncope.
- Fatigue.
- Oedema.
- Leg cramps.
- Cough—if productive, note the type, amount, and colour of sputum.
- Previous hypertension, angina, or myocardial infarction.

Focused physical assessment

- Supporting therapies—oxygen, inotropes, intra-aortic balloon pump, pacing, oxygen, non-invasive or invasive mechanical ventilation.
- Obvious signs of discomfort or distress.
- Fluid assessment (see ➲ p. 24).
- Cardiovascular-focused assessment of the face, neck, thorax, and peripheries (see Table 6.1).

Precordial landmarking

The following landmarking areas (see Figure 6.1) are used for precordial palpation to rule out thrills, heaves, and thrusts and for auscultation of heart sounds:

- aortic area—second intercostal space, right sternal border
- pulmonary area—second intercostal space, left sternal border
- Erb's point—third intercostal space, left sternal border
- tricuspid area—fourth intercostal space, left sternal border
- mitral area—fifth intercostal space, left mid-clavicular line.

Causes of key abnormalities

- Chest pain—angina, acute coronary syndromes, non-cardiac cause.
- Irregular pulse—arrhythmia, ectopics.
- Bounding pulse—sepsis.
- Weak pulse—hypovolaemia, hypotension, left ventricular failure.
- Peripheral oedema—right ventricular failure, sepsis.
- Cool, diaphoretic skin.
- Peripheral cyanosis—hypoxia, poor tissue perfusion.
- Absent or weak pedal pulses—left ventricular failure, oedema, vascular insufficiency.
- Prolonged capillary refill—poor tissue perfusion.

Table 6.1 Cardiovascular-focused assessment

	Normal	Abnormal
Inspection	Pink, moist mucous membranes Symmetrical precordium Pink peripheries	Central cyanosis Dry mucous membranes Raised JVP Precordial wounds, drains, scarring, or bruising Oedema Signs of VTE Peripheries pale, cyanotic, or mottled
Palpation	Point of maximal impulse fifth intercostal space, mid-clavicular line Bilateral, strong, regular pulses Capillary refill < 2 s Warm peripheries	Thrills, heaves, and thrusts Displaced point of maximal impulse Pulses—weak, absent, bounding, or irregular Capillary refill > 2 s Peripheries cool, cold, hot, or diaphoretic
Auscultation	Clear S1 and S2 heart sounds No bruits Clear breath sounds	Heart sounds—murmur, S3, S4, split, rub, or muffled Bruits—carotid, aortic, renal, or iliac Breath sounds—crackles, wheeze, or diminished

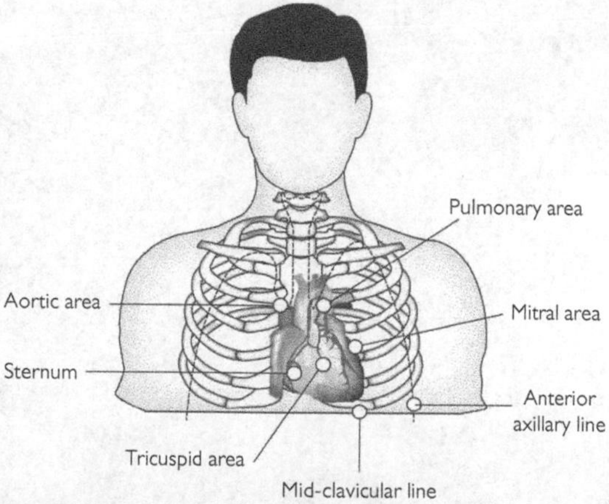

Figure 6.1 Precordial landmarking. (Adapted with permission from Spiers C (2011) Cardiac auscultation. *British Journal of Cardiac Nursing* 6(10), 482–6. © MA Healthcare.)

Laboratory investigations

See ➲ p. 36 for normal values and further explanation of the following blood tests which are relevant to check for a cardiovascular review:

- FBC
- U&E
- LFTs
- clotting
- troponin T
- arterial blood gas analysis, including lactate
- glucose.

Cardiovascular monitoring: a brief introduction

There is [illegible] need for effective and accurate [illegible] monitoring of all critically ill patients. [illegible] Standard cardiovascular [illegible] include:

- continuous electrocardiography [illegible]
- arterial blood pressure monitoring
- central venous pressure [illegible]
- cardiac output measurement [illegible]
- fluid balance assessment
- [illegible]

Cardiovascular monitoring: a brief introduction

There is clearly a need for effective and accurate cardiovascular monitoring of all critically ill patients. There are a number of monitoring tools available for this, and these will be described in more detail in Chapter 7.

Standardized cardiovascular monitoring tools include:

- continuous electrocardiogram (either a 3- or 5-lead system)
- arterial blood pressure recording
- central venous pressure measurement
- cardiac output measurement (several tools are available)
- fluid balance assessment
- central temperature recording.

Hypotension

Definition

Hypotension is normally defined as a low blood pressure. The [illegible] [illegible] [illegible] there is considerable [illegible] normal blood pressure as being within a range of values. The normal systolic blood pressure is in the range 100–139 mmHg, and normal diastolic blood pressure is in the range [illegible] mmHg.

In critical care it may be more useful to define hypotension as a systolic blood pressure below 90 mmHg or a mean arterial pressure below [illegible] mmHg. Hypotension results in reduced organ and tissue perfusion, and if the underlying cause is not rectified [illegible] [illegible] [illegible] [illegible] organ dysfunction, and organ failure.

Assessment/monitoring

[illegible] assessment of patients with hypotension [illegible] [illegible] [illegible] useful to review patients' trends, as these changes may indicate deterioration earlier [illegible]. This includes monitoring of:

- heart rate
- respiratory rate (oxygen saturation)
- [illegible]
- [illegible]
- urine output
- level of consciousness (if not sedated)
- blood lactate

It is suggested that monitoring [illegible] more beneficial for the [illegible] [illegible] [illegible] and [illegible] cardiac output are [illegible] [illegible] assessment and [illegible] [illegible] [illegible] [illegible] [illegible] [illegible] of adequate [illegible] [illegible]. [illegible] [illegible] (Table 6.[illegible]):

- warm, well-perfused peripheries (normal skin colour, capillary refill [illegible])
- [illegible]
- blood pressure within acceptable limits
- [illegible]
- evidence [illegible] (e.g. urine output [illegible])
- absence of [illegible] (normal lactate)

Low cardiac output can occur in a critically ill patient for a number of reasons. However, hypotension predominantly [illegible] [illegible] [illegible] [illegible] [illegible] including:

- hypovolaemic shock
- cardiogenic shock
- septic shock/systemic inflammatory response syndrome (SIRS)
- anaphylactic shock
- neurogenic shock
- obstructive shock
- mixed shock

The cardiovascular assessment findings for each type of shock are summarized in Table 6.2.

Hypotension

Definition

Hypotension is normally defined as a low blood pressure. The National Institute for Health and Care Excellence (NICE)[1] defines normal blood pressure as being within a range of values. Normal systolic blood pressure is in the range 100–139 mmHg, and normal diastolic blood pressure is in the range 60–89 mmHg.

In critical care it may be more useful to define hypotension as a systolic blood pressure below 90 mmHg or a mean arterial pressure below 60 mmHg. Hypotension needs to be recognized and treated quickly, as all of the body's organs require sufficient arterial pressure to maintain perfusion. Inadequate blood pressure will lead to reduced organ perfusion, organ dysfunction, and organ failure.

Assessment findings

When assessing for signs of hypotension in the critically ill patient it is essential to review other vital signs, as other changes may indicate cardiovascular deterioration. This includes changes in:

- heart rate
- respiratory rate (if self-ventilating)
- peripheral perfusion
- vascular resistance
- urine output
- level of consciousness (if not sedated)
- blood pH.

It is suggested that it may be more beneficial for the critically ill patient if parameters of effective cardiac output are managed, rather than basing assessment and management on one parameter alone. To that end, Soni and Watson[2] have highlighted a number of criteria that might suggest cardiac output is effective. These include:

- warm, well-perfused peripheries (normal skin colour, cap refill < 3 seconds, palpable peripheral pulses)
- blood pressure within acceptable limits
- heart rate within acceptable range
- evidence of functioning organs (e.g. urine output > 0.5 ml/kg/hr)
- absence or improvement of acidosis.

Ineffective cardiac output can occur in the critically ill patient for a number of reasons. However, hypotension is commonly linked to various forms of shocks, including:

- hypovolaemic shock
- cardiogenic shock
- septic shock or systemic inflammatory response syndrome (SIRS)
- anaphylactic shock
- neurogenic shock
- obstructive shock
- trauma shock.

Key cardiovascular assessment findings for each type of shock are summarized in Table 6.2.

Table 6.2 Key cardiovascular changes for each type of shock

Type of shock	Heart rate	Cardiac output	Systemic vascular resistance	Central venous pressure
Hypovolaemic	↑	↓	↑	↓
Cardiogenic	↑	↓	↑	↑
Septic or SIRS	↑	↑*	↓	↓
Anaphylactic	↑	↓	↓	↓
Neurogenic	↓	↓	↓	↓
Obstructive	↑	↓	↓	↓
Trauma	↑	↓	↓	↓

* Cardiac output may be low with late sepsis.

Hypovolaemic shock

Definition

Hypovolaemia is an ineffective cardiac output status related to low volume within the vascular compartment. There are many causes of hypovolaemia, including:

- excessive blood loss
- haemorrhage
- excessive vomiting and/or diarrhoea
- excessive diuresis
- plasma loss (e.g. severe burns)
- third spacing
- excessive dialysis.

Assessment findings

The hypovolaemic patient may present with some or all of the following findings on assessment:

- tachycardia
- decreased blood pressure (narrowing of pulse pressure)
- pallor and diaphoresis
- increased systemic vascular resistance (SVR)
- extended capillary refill time
- low central venous pressure
- decreased urine output.

Management

This should relate to establishing and treating the cause of hypovolaemia (e.g. a patient who is haemorrhaging may require surgical intervention). Common aspects of management include:

- appropriate fluid replacement (see ➔ p. 52)
- electrolyte replacement
- continuous monitoring (blood pressure, heart rate, CVP, and JVP)
- careful assessment of renal function (see ➔ p. 282)
- prevention of organ damage related to low perfusion.

Cardiogenic shock

Definition

Cardiogenic shock is a low cardiac output status related to reduced cardiac function. The heart does not pump effectively because of damage to the muscle. Poor cardiac output is then worsened by increased peripheral resistance resulting from normal compensatory mechanisms. The main causes of cardiogenic shock are:

- myocardial infarction
- cardiac tamponade
- cardiac valve disease (particularly mitral valve disease)
- cardiac arrhythmias.

Assessment findings

The patient with cardiogenic shock will present with all or some of the following symptoms:

- hypotension
- tachycardia
- arrhythmias
- increased SVR
- signs of heart failure (increased CVP, pulmonary oedema, shortness of breath, hypoxia increased JVP).

Management

Treatment will focus on supporting the failing cardiovascular system to ensure adequate but not excessive fluid balance, and includes:

- ensuring accurate fluid assessment to prevent both fluid overload and dehydration
- careful and appropriate use of inotropic support
- reduction in peripheral resistance
- cautious use of glyceryl trinitrate (GTN)
- intra-aortic balloon pump
- left ventricular assist devices.

Septic shock and systemic inflammatory response syndrome (SIRS)

Definition

An acute inflammatory response as a result of either severe infection or another inflammatory injury. This is a distributive form of shock, resulting in profound vasodilatation and increased microvascular permeability.

Assessment findings

The patient with septic shock or SIRS will present with some or all of the following symptoms:

- tachycardia
- initial widening of pulse pressure, followed by hypotension in the later stages
- initially increased and then decreased cardiac output
- increased or decreased temperature
- decreased SVR
- relative hypovolaemia.

Management

For details of the management of sepsis and SIRS, see ➲ p. 328.

Anaphylactic shock

Definition

This is a distributive form of shock related to severe allergic reaction following exposure to an antigen. Anaphylaxis triggers profound vasodilatation, misdistribution of fluid, and capillary leakage. It is treated as a medical emergency, as deterioration may be rapid, and prompt effective treatment is required (see ➲ p. 412). It may be caused by exposure to a number of antigens that may be infused, inhaled, or ingested. Examples include:

- infusion or drug reactions
- blood transfusion
- latex
- immunoglobulins
- ingested food substances.

Assessment findings

The patient with anaphylactic shock will present with all or some of the following symptoms:

- hypotension
- tachycardia
- increased respiration
- decreased SVR
- bronchospasm, laryngeal oedema, and/or stridor
- pulmonary oedema
- nausea and vomiting
- urticaria
- angio-oedema.

Management

Treatment should follow the Resuscitation Council guidelines[3] (see ➲ pp. 413 and p. 381 for further details).

Neurogenic shock

Definition

This is another distributive form of shock, in which severe vasodilatation is caused by disruption of sympathetic nerve activity that normally regulates and maintains vasomotor tone. It may occur within hours, and can persist for 1–3 weeks after spinal cord injury above T1 level, or more rarely after severe head injury affecting the medulla.

Assessment findings

The patient with neurogenic shock will present with all or some of the following symptoms:

- hypotension
- bradycardia
- decreased SVR
- loss of reflexes
- warm dry skin
- poikilothermia.

Management

This relates to protection of the spine, management of hypotension, and supportive measures until the period of neurogenic shock has passed. It includes:

- stabilization of the spinal cord
- assessment and management of other injuries
- protection of the airway and supportive ventilation if needed
- fluid replacement
- inotropic support (increased SVR is the goal of support)
- atropine or pacing for bradycardia
- careful temperature regulation.

Obstructive shock

Definition

This is a form of shock caused by an inherent problem within the thoracic cavity that prevents effective cardiac contraction and the forward flow of blood through the cardiovascular system. It may be caused by:

- pulmonary embolism
- pericardial tamponade
- tension pneumothorax.

Assessment findings

The patient with obstructive shock will present with all or some of the following symptoms:

- tachycardia
- cardiac arrhythmias
- paradoxical pulse
- hypotension
- increased CVP
- increased JVP
- cardiac or respiratory arrest.

Treatment

Treatment focuses on removal of the obstructive mechanism. Therefore treat the cause as follows:

- pneumothorax—chest drain insertion
- pulmonary embolism—thrombolysis if appropriate
- pericardial tamponade—drain tamponade.

Traumatic shock

Definition

Although trauma patients may present with any of the other forms of shock discussed previously, trauma practitioners have observed a specific form of shock following blunt trauma. Traumatic shock represents a unique pathological condition that appears to follow severe trauma and may lead to multi-organ dysfunction syndrome. This form of shock is characterized by an overwhelming inflammatory response, and supportive care is required for multi-organ dysfunction syndrome. See ➔ p. 460 for more details of trauma assessment and management.

Assessment findings

Rapid deterioration may be seen in this form of shock, and the patient may appear to be presenting with other forms of shock, including hypovolaemic shock and distributive shock (e.g. hypovolaemic shock without any other clinical signs of haemorrhage, or marked vasodilatation without other clinical signs of sepsis). See Chapter 18 (➔ p. 460) for further details about trauma assessment and management.

The patient with trauma shock may present with very sudden deterioration and some or all of the following symptoms:

- severe hypotension
- vasodilatation
- tachycardia
- tachypnoea
- symptoms of SIRS (see ➔ p. 328).

Treatment

Treatment focuses on:

- surgery or other interventions addressing the specific cause of the trauma
- effective management of blood pressure
- effective fluid resuscitation (see ➔ p. 470)
- treatment of the symptoms of SIRS (see ➔ p. 339)
- possible use of corticosteroids.

Other causes of hypotension

Hypotension in the critically ill patient may be unrelated to shock status, and other mechanisms may be responsible for a fall in blood pressure and the associated effects on effective cardiac output status.

In these cases it is important to isolate and treat the causative factor. This may include:

- side effects of medications such as sedatives or muscle relaxants
- hypoadrenalism
- hypopituitarism
- poisoning.

References

1 National Institute for Health and Care Excellence (NICE). *Hypertension: clinical management of primary hypertension in adults.* CG127. NICE: London, 2011. www.nice.org.uk/guidance/cg127

2 Soni N and Watson D. Cardiovascular support. In: GR Nimmo and M Singer (eds) *ABC of Intensive Care*, 2nd edn. Wiley-Blackwell: Chichester, 2011.

3 Resuscitation Council (UK). *Emergency Treatment of Anaphylactic Reaction: guidelines for health care workers.* Resuscitation Council (UK): London, 2008.

Hypertension

Definition

Hypertension is currently classified by NICE according to the level of the blood pressure above recognized normal limits.[4] NICE defines normal blood pressure as being within a range of values. Normal systolic blood pressure is in the range 100–139 mmHg, and normal diastolic blood pressure is in the range 60–89 mmHg.

NICE[4] classifies hypertension as follows:

- Stage 1 hypertension—systolic pressure above 140 mmHg and diastolic pressure above 90 mmHg.
- Stage 2 hypertension—systolic pressure above 160 mmHg and diastolic pressure above 100 mmHg.
- Stage 3 hypertension—systolic pressure above 180 mmHg and diastolic pressure above 110 mmHg.

A combination of medication in the form of angiotensin-converting enzyme (ACE) inhibitors, calcium-channel blockers, and thiazide diuretics is recommended to reduce elevated blood pressure. The combination depends on the level of elevation and the type of hypertension. There are many causes of chronic elevation of blood pressure, and these are treated in accordance with the NICE guidelines.

The critically ill patient may also present with a hypertensive crisis. This is clinically defined as an acute elevation of blood pressure (greater than 180/120 mmHg).

Causes

There are many causes of a hypertensive crisis, including:

- exacerbation of chronic hypertension
- sudden withdrawal of antihypertensive medication
- phenochromocytoma
- pre-eclampsia and eclampsia
- raised intracranial pressure
- idiopathic causes
- autonomic dysreflexia.

Assessment findings

In an acute hypertensive crisis the patient may present with various signs and symptoms, including:

- cardiovascular changes—elevated blood pressure, chest pain, palpitations
- neurological changes—headaches, visual disturbances, acute confusion, papilloedema, nausea and vomiting, seizures
- renal changes—acute kidney injury, proteinurea.

Treatment

Patients who present with a hypertensive crisis require immediate medical intervention, but care should be taken to ensure that the blood pressure is not reduced dramatically. Recommendations are as follows:

- Reduce the mean arterial pressure by no more than 25% in the initial hour.
- Gradually reduce the blood pressure once that goal has been achieved using appropriate antihypertensive therapy.
- Ensure that the patient receives adequate haemodynamic monitoring to facilitate continuous arterial pressure recordings to prevent sudden falls in blood pressure.
- Monitor for side effects of hypertensive crisis, such as neurological and/or other organ damage.

Reference

4 National Institute for Health and Care Excellence (NICE). *Hypertension: clinical management of primary hypertension in adults.* CG127. NICE London, 2011. www.nice.org.uk/guidance/cg127

Acute coronary syndrome

Definition

Acute coronary syndrome (ACS) refers to a number of clinical conditions, including:

- ST-segment elevation myocardial infarction (STEMI)
- non-ST-segment elevation myocardial infarction (NSTEMI)
- unstable angina (no changes to biological markers of ischaemia).

It is important that patients with ACS receive timely care to prevent further deterioration, potential irreversible damage to the myocardial wall, and potential heart failure. ACS has a high mortality rate, and approximately one-third of patients will die within 24 h of onset of symptoms. Risk factors for ACS include:

- smoking
- hypertension
- diabetes
- hyperlipidaemia.

Assessment findings

Chest pain is the main symptom associated with ACS, and a careful assessment of the pain is essential. It may be helpful to use the SOCRATES mnemonic (see Table 6.3).

In addition to pain, patients may also present with:

- anxiety
- increased parasympathetic activation (nausea and vomiting)
- increased sympathetic activity (sweating, tachycardia, increased respiratory rate, pallor, and a slight increase in blood pressure).[5]

It is important to remember that atypical presentation may occur, and that some groups of patients may present with no symptoms or atypically. This is common in:

- elderly patients
- female patients
- patients with diabetes.

NICE[6] emphasizes the importance of careful history taking, which should include:

- the type of pain
- associated symptoms, including nausea, vomiting, sweating, and shortness of breath
- family history of cardiovascular disease
- risk factors for the development of cardiovascular disease
- previous investigations and treatments.

Clinical diagnosis of STEMI is made on the basis of:

- presentation and patient history
- 12-lead ECG changes
- cardiac markers.

Table 6.3 SOCRATES mnemonic

Site	Where is the pain?
Onset	When did it start?
Characteristics	What is the pain like? (stabbing, aching, tight, crushing)
Radiation	Does it spread or radiate anywhere?
Associated symptoms	Are there any other symptoms associated with the pain?
Timing	What is the timing of the pain, and how long does it last?
Exacerbating factors	Does anything relieve the pain symptoms?
Severity	How severe is the pain (perhaps using a numerical scale of 1 to 5)?

Acute coronary syndrome: ECG findings

12-lead ECG changes

Diagnosis of STEMI is based on the following criteria:[7]

- new ST-segment elevation at the J point in two contiguous leads with the cut-points: ≥0.1 mV in all leads other than leads V2–V3 where the following cut points apply: ≥0.2 mV in men ≥40 years; ≥0.25 mV in men <40 years, or ≥0.15 mV in women[7]
- new left bundle branch block.

A 12-lead ECG showing STEMI is illustrated in Figure 6.2.

Diagnosis of NSTEMI is more complicated and requires further investigations, but in summary the patient may experience acute chest pain without the presence of persistent ST-segment elevation. Subtle ECG changes may be seen, including[7]:

- new horizontal or down-sloping ST-segment depression ≥ 0.05 mV in 2 continguous leads *and/or*
- T-wave inversion ≥ 0.1 mV in two contiguous leads with prominent R wave or R/S ratio >1.

However, the ECG may be normal. Cardiac markers (troponins) will be elevated. If cardiac markers are unchanged the patient may be diagnosed with unstable angina.

Acute coronary syndrome: treatment for STEMI

The goals of treatment of STEMI include:

- alleviating the patient's pain
- monitoring their CVS status
- restoring patency to the occluded artery or arteries
- reducing the patient's anxiety
- monitoring for complications of STEMI.

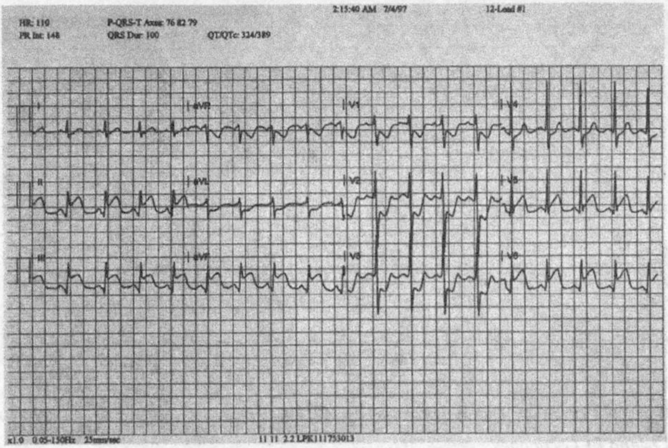

Figure 6.2 12-lead ECG showing STEMI. (Reproduced from Creed F and Spiers C, *Care of the Acutely Ill Adult: an essential guide for nurses*, 2010, with permission from Oxford University Press.)

Pain alleviation strategies

- Assessment using an appropriate tool.
- Opiate-based analgesia (usually morphine or diamorphine). Caution should be exercised if the patient is hypotensive or if they have underlying respiratory pathophysiology. Care should be taken to observe for signs of respiratory depression. Anti-emetics should be administered alongside analgesia to prevent further nausea and vomiting.
- Nitrates may be given either sublingually or intravenously, taking care to monitor the effect on blood pressure. Nitrates will reduce preload and afterload as well as dilating the coronary arteries, so they act to reduce myocardial oxygen demand and enhance myocardial perfusion.
- Intravenous beta blockers may also be given to reduce oxygen demand and thus help to alleviate pain.
- Oxygen may be administered to keep oxygen saturation ≥ 94%, but there is no clinical evidence that routine use of oxygen reduces pain or improves myocardial oxygenation.[8,9]

Monitoring of CVS status

- Careful monitoring is required to enable observation both of the effects of STEMI on the cardiovascular system, and of the side effects of treatment.
- Careful assessment should include monitoring of blood pressure, heart rate, heart rhythm, and fluid balance.
- The patient should be monitored using a continuous ECG and automated blood pressure recordings.

Restoring patency to the occluded artery or arteries

- The most important aspect of treatment is the reperfusion of the myocardium.
- Low-dose aspirin should be administered as soon as possible.
- The gold-standard treatment for STEMI is considered to be primary percutaneous coronary intervention (P-PCI). This should be undertaken as quickly as possible, and within 1 h of the initial presenting symptoms.
- If P-PCI is not available or is not suitable for the patient, thrombolysis medication (second or third generation) may be given to break down the fibrin thrombus. This should only be administered if it is not contraindicated (see Box 6.1 for contraindications to thrombolysis).
- The patient should be closely monitored for reperfusion arrhythmias and potential haemorrhage.

Reduction of anxiety

- Anxiety may exacerbate the sympathetic response, and the patient will require reassurance.
- Opiate-based analgesia will help to reduce anxiety, as will reassurance, effective communication, and a confident professional approach to care delivery.

Monitoring for complications of STEMI

- Some STEMI patients may be at higher risk of developing complications.
- Patients in whom STEMI affects the anterior left ventricle and patients with left bundle branch block (LBBB) are at increased risk.
- Complications to monitor for include:
  - left ventricular failure (LVF)
  - right ventricular failure (RVF)
  - cardiogenic shock
  - arrhythmias and cardiac arrest.

Box 6.1 Contraindications to thrombolysis

- Bleeding disorders
- Active bleeding
- Surgery
- Stroke
- Intracranial neoplasm or aneurysm
- Serious trauma
- Aortic dissection or aneurysm
- Prolonged CPR
- Recent gastrointestinal bleed

Acute coronary syndrome: treatment for NSTEMI

Treatment focuses on assessment and management of pain, and managing the patient's NSTEMI with medication. It is currently recommended that the following groups of medication are administered[10]:

- antiplatelet therapy
- antithrombin therapy
- nitrates
- beta blockers.

References

5 Spiers C. Cardiovascular assessment and care. In: F Creed and C Spiers (eds) *Care of the Acutely Ill Adult: an essential guide for nurses*. Oxford University Press: Oxford, 2010. pp. 59–104.

6 National Institute for Health and Care Excellence (NICE). *Myocardial Infarction with ST-Segment Elevation: the acute management of myocardial infarction with ST-segment elevation*. CG167. NICE: London, 2013. www.nice.org.uk/guidance/cg167

7 Thygesen K et al. Universal definition of myocardial infarction. *Circulation* 2007; **116**: 2634–53.

8 British Thoracic Society. BTS guideline for emergency oxygen use in adult patients. *Thorax* 2008; **63** (Suppl. 6): vi1–68.

9 Cabello JB et al. Oxygen therapy for acute myocardial infarction. *Cochrane Database of Systematic Reviews* 2013; Issue 8. Art. No.: CD007160.

10 National Institute for Health and Care Excellence (NICE). *Unstable angina and NSTEMI: the early management of unstable angina and non-ST-segment-elevation myocardial infarction*. CG94. NICE: London, 2013. https://www.nice.org.uk/guidance/cg94.

Acute heart failure

Definition

[illegible]

A number of factors may cause heart failure. These include:

- acute coronary syndrome
- [illegible]
- cardiac valve disorders
- cardiomyopathy
- pulmonary embolism
- cardiac tamponade
- sepsis.

Assessment findings

[illegible]

- [illegible]
- [illegible]
- [illegible]
- [illegible]
- altered level of consciousness
- increased anxiety.

[illegible]

- pleural effusion
- [illegible]
- cardiogenic shock

Investigations may include:

- chest X-ray
- echocardiogram
- [illegible]
- [illegible]
- 12-lead ECG
- [illegible]

Acute heart failure

Definition

Heart failure is defined by NICE as 'a complex clinical syndrome that suggests impairment of the heart as a pump supporting physiological circulation. It is caused by structural or functional abnormalities of the heart.'[11]

Acute heart failure represents a potential life-threatening emergency that requires immediate assessment and treatment, and is usually characterized by rapid onset of symptoms. The heart may fail in several ways:

- left-sided heart failure (left ventricular failure)
- right-sided heart failure (cor pulmonale or right ventricular failure)
- both sides (biventricular failure).

A number of factors may cause heart failure. These include:

- acute coronary syndrome
- arrhythmias
- cardiac valve disorders
- cardiomyopathy
- pulmonary embolism
- cardiac tamponade
- sepsis.

Assessment findings

The patient may present with:

- acute breathlessness, dyspnoea, hypoxaemia, and reduced oxygen saturations
- hypotension and tachycardia
- pallor, sweating, capillary refill > 3 seconds and cyanosis
- cool peripheries
- metabolic acidosis (raised lactate levels)
- altered level of consciousness
- increased anxiety.

In right-sided failure the patient may present with:

- peripheral oedema
- raised CVP
- raised JVP
- clear breath sounds.

In left-sided heart failure the patient may present with:

- evidence of pulmonary oedema (pink frothy sputum, and fine crackles on auscultation)
- pleural effusion
- cardiomegaly
- cardiogenic shock (see ➲ p. 176).

Investigations may include:

- chest X-ray
- echocardiogram
- biochemical markers of heart failure
- assessment of fluid status and fluid balance
- 12-lead ECG
- cardiac output studies.

Treatment

If possible the cause of the heart failure should be identified, as this will facilitate treatment.

Left-sided heart failure treatment

- Position the patient upright and support them with pillows (this reduces venous return and facilitates gas exchange).
- Give oxygen therapy to maintain oxygen saturations ≥ 94%.
- CPAP may be useful for the treatment of pulmonary oedema (this improves oxygenation and prevents further formation of pulmonary oedema).
- Mechanical ventilation may be required in cases of severe respiratory failure.
- Careful monitoring of cardiovascular status, fluid balance, and urine output is required.
- Give diamorphine or morphine (this has anxiolytic properties and facilitates venous dilation) and anti-emetic cover.
- Give a loop diuretic if there is evidence of hypervolaemia (this reduces blood volume and preload).
- Administer IV nitrates with caution to prevent severe hypotension.
- Give inotropic support with caution. See ➲ p. 232.
- Use an intra-aortic balloon pump if there is no improvement in response to medication. See ➲ p. 236.
- Use a left ventricular assist device if there is no improvement in response to medication.

Right-sided heart failure treatment

- Position the patient upright and support them with pillows.
- Give oxygen therapy to maintain oxygen saturations ≥ 94%.
- Careful monitoring of cardiovascular status, fluid balance, and urine output is required.
- Give anti-arrhythmic therapy if arrhythmias are present.
- Volume loading should be undertaken with caution (100–200 mL) to try to improve ventricular contractility.
- Provide inotropic support with an appropriate inotropic agent. See ➲ p. 232.
- Use an intra-aortic balloon pump (see ➲ p. 236).

Treatment for cardiogenic shock is described on ➲ p. 178.

Reference

11 National Institute for Health and Care Excellence (NICE). *Chronic Heart Failure: management of chronic heart failure in adults in primary and secondary care*. CG108. NICE: London, 2010. ✆ www.nice.org.uk/guidance/cg108

Pericarditis

Definition

The pericardium is a double-walled fibrous inelastic sac that surrounds the heart. Its purpose is to:

- fix the heart to the mediastinum
- prevent dilatation of the heart
- function as a barrier to infection.

Pericarditis is inflammation of the layers of the pericardium, which may be caused by:

- viral infection
- malignancy
- tuberculosis
- connective tissue disorders
- hypothyroidism
- idiopathic causes
- cardiac surgery
- myocardial infarction (late-onset pericarditis after MI is referred to as Dressler's syndrome, and is thought to be an autoimmune response).

Assessment findings

The patient with pericarditis may present with all or some of the following symptoms:

- chest pain (usually localized to the retrosternal area and left precordium); the pain may lessen if the patient sits forward, and it may worsen if the patient lies flat
- pericardial rub on cardiac auscultation
- 12-lead ECG changes (ECGs are abnormal in 90% of patients with acute pericarditis, and generally show diffuse ST-segment elevation in almost all of the 12-lead ECG).

Treatment

- Treat the cause where possible.
- Give non-steroidal anti-inflammatory medication.
- Observe for complications of pericarditis, which may include:
  - pericardial effusion
  - pericardial tamponade.

Pericardial effusion

Definition

A pericardial effusion is the abnormal accumulation of fluid (usually more than 50 mL) in the pericardial sac. Effusions may be non-compressive or compressive. Non-compressive effusions do not interfere with normal cardiac functioning, and may present with fewer symptoms. Compressive effusions may cause sudden increases in pericardial pressure which may lead to cardiac tamponade. The factors that affect the impact of the effusion include:

- the volume of fluid
- the rate of fluid accumulation
- the compliance of the pericardium.

Assessment findings

The patient may be asymptomatic (if non-compressive), or may have any of the following:

- dull chest pain
- signs of cardiac compression
- 12-lead ECG changes, especially a dampening effect (reduced voltage) because of the insulation effect of the accumulated fluid; the QRS height may also fluctuate between beats because of the fluid accumulation
- pericardial rub may be reduced because of the insulating effect of the fluid
- reduced percussion (dull) over the left lung (Ewart's sign), due to compression atelectasis.

The ECG should be considered to aid diagnosis.

Treatment

This involves pericardial drainage using pericardiocentesis.

Pericardial tamponade

Definition

Pericardial tamponade is a life-threatening condition that requires emergency medical intervention. It is caused by the accumulation of fluid that results in compression of the heart muscle and prevents normal cardiac contraction. The high pressure changes within the pericardium prevent ventricular filling, which leads to significantly reduced cardiac output, haemodynamic compromise, and potential circulatory collapse. Pericardial tamponade may be caused by:

- infection
- cardiac surgery
- aortic dissection
- trauma
- malignancy
- myocardial infarction
- central line insertion
- biopsy.

Assessment findings

Pericardial tamponade should be suspected if a patient with pericarditis or pericardial effusion shows signs of significant haemodynamic instability or compromise. Key findings may include:

- systemic hypotension
- tachycardia
- dyspnoea
- tachypnoea
- cool peripheries, pallor and capillary refill > 3 seconds
- raised JVP
- increased CVP
- quiet heart sounds on auscultation
- paradoxical pulse.

The patient may suffer cardiac arrest if the tamponade is not quickly identified and treated.

Treatment

- Pericardial drainage using pericardiocentesis. This may be performed either by open surgery, or percutaneously using echocardiography.
- Cardiac resuscitation may be required if the patient has suffered cardiac arrest (see ➔ p. 406).

Infective endocarditis

Definition

[illegible]

[illegible]

[illegible]

[illegible]

Infective endocarditis

Definition

The endocardium is the innermost lining of the heart, and its cells are biologically similar to the endothelial cells that line blood vessels. It has an important role in ensuring smooth blood flow through the heart.

Infective endocarditis is an infection that affects the endocardium, usually caused by a bacterial translocation from another area of the body. During the infection organisms are able to adhere to the surface of the valve and destroy the valvular leaflets. Vegetations may develop and these may break off, causing emboli distal to the heart (e.g. in the brain, gut, or limbs). Infective endocarditis may lead to heart failure. It may be divided into:

- acute endocarditis, in which symptoms progress rapidly
- subacute endocarditis, in which symptoms may develop over several months.

Endocarditis may be caused by:

- invasive procedures that may allow bacterial infiltration (e.g. pacing wires, CVP lines)
- cancer
- dental manipulation
- poor dental care
- IV drug abuse.

Assessment findings

Patients with infective endocarditis may present with:

- fever
- breathlessness
- signs of cardiac failure
- effects of thromboemboli (e.g. stroke)
- vascular changes (haemorrhagic lesions on the palms and soles, and splinter haemorrhages underneath the nail beds)
- cardiac murmurs
- arrhythmias
- signs of chronic illness.

Treatment

- High-dose intravenous antibiotics (often for several weeks).
- Treatment of specific disorders (e.g. heart failure, arrhythmias).
- Surgery to replace the affected valve.

Cardiac arrhythmias

Introduction

A common cardiac problem for critically ill patients is the development of cardiac arrhythmias. In health, normal cardiac electrical activity is stimulated by the sinoatrial node, and the normal cardiac rhythm is one that originates from the sinoatrial node and causes a normal sinus rhythm (see Figure 6.3).

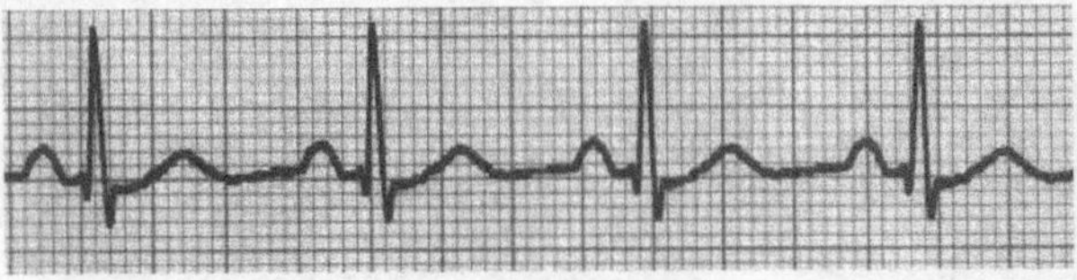

Figure 6.3 ECG showing sinus rhythm. (Reproduced from Creed F and Spiers C, *Care of the Acutely Ill Adult: an essential guide for nurses*, 2010, with permission from Oxford University Press.)

However, critically ill patients may develop:

- disorders of impulse formation—this may lead to the cardiac rhythm being stimulated by another pacemaker cell within the heart
- disorders of impulse conduction—this may lead to electrical impulses being slowed , blocked, or using an alternative pathway.

There are many factors that may contribute to arrhythmia and conduction disturbances in the critically ill, including:

- cardiac disease
- acute coronary syndrome
- factors that affect autonomic control (e.g. neurological damage)
- electrolyte disturbances
- acid–base imbalances
- endocrine influences
- side effects of medication
- invasive monitoring.

Brief diagnosis and management of common arrhythmias seen in critical care is discussed in the remainder of this chapter.

Analysing the ECG rhythm strip

It is important to adopt a systematic approach to ECG rhythm interpretation, as advocated by Spiers.[12] Each part of the ECG requires attention. The normal ECG complex is shown in Figure 6.4.

- Rate—the rate may be calculated by counting the number of small squares between two R waves and dividing into 1500.
- Rhythm—the rhythm should be inspected to see if it is regular or irregular. Even a normal sinus rhythm may be irregular in some individuals (sinus arrhythmia).
- P:QRS ratio—there should be one P wave for each QRS complex.

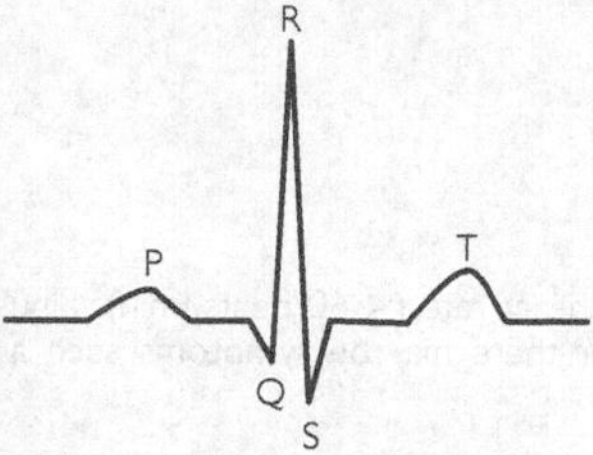

Figure 6.4 The normal ECG complex.

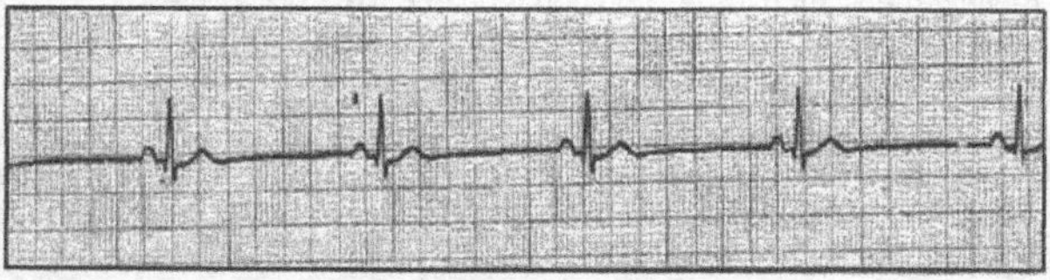

Figure 6.5 Sinus bradycardia. (Reproduced from Creed F and Spiers C, *Care of the Acutely Ill Adult: an essential guide for nurses*, 2010, with permission from Oxford University Press.)

- PR interval—this should be counted from the beginning of the P wave to the beginning of the R wave, and should be between 120–200 ms (milliseconds). A long PR interval may indicate first-degree heart block. A short PR interval may indicate ventricular pre-excitation syndromes.
- QRS complex—this should be narrow and less than 120 ms in width. A widened QRS complex may indicate conduction problems or ventricular hypertrophy.
- ST segment—this should be flat and on the isoelectric line at the J point which is the end of the QRS complex. Any deviation may indicate ischaemia or infarction, but a 12-lead ECG is required to determine this.
- T waves—the T wave should always be in the same direction as the QRS complex.

Sinus bradycardia

Definition

In sinus bradycardia the rhythm originates from the sinoatrial node, and so presents with a normal P wave and normal QRS complex. However, the rate is slower than normal (usually < 60 beats/min) (see Figure 6.5).

Causes

Sinus bradycardia may be normal for patients who are physically fit or in patients who are monitored while they are asleep. Pathophysiological causes of sinus bradycardia include:
- hypothermia
- inferior myocardial infarction
- raised intracranial pressure

- hypothyroidism
- medication—for example :
  - beta blockers
  - calcium-channel blockers
  - digoxin.

Assessment findings

The patient will present with a slow heart rate (< 60 beats/min). Sinus bradycardia may be asymptomatic, or there may be symptoms such as hypotension or syncope.

Treatment

This is rarely needed, but if required because of haemodynamic consequences it is best to treat the underlying cause. For example:

- Review medication if the condition is related to cardiac drugs.
- Slowly increase the body temperature if the patient is hypothermic.
- Correct hypothyroidism.

In some instances where the patient is adversely affected by bradycardia they may receive IV atropine and if this is ineffective, adrenaline may be given as an IV infusion. Pacing may also be considered if bradycardia is related to cardiac problems.

Sinus tachycardia

Definition

In sinus tachycardia the rhythm originates from the sinoatrial node and so presents with a normal P wave and normal QRS complex. However, the rate is faster than normal (usually > 100 beats/min) (see Figure 6.6).

Causes

Sinus tachycardia is a normal physiological response to stress and exercise. Pathophysiological causes of sinus tachycardia include:

- high temperature
- most forms of shock (except neurogenic shock)
- low cardiac output states
- heart disease
- respiratory disease
- hyperthyroidism
- pain
- stimulants
- some medications (e.g. salbutamol).

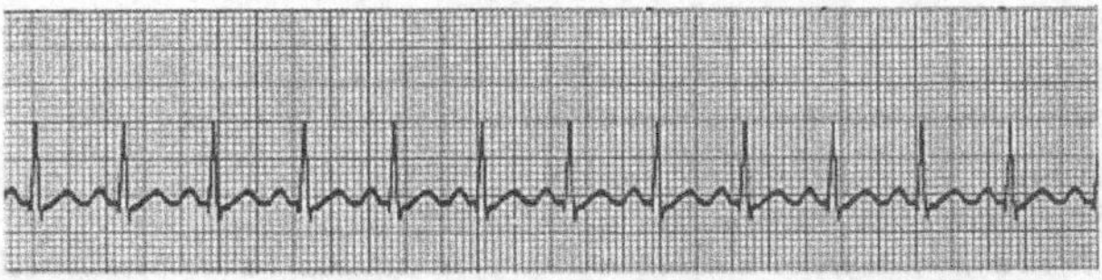

Figure 6.6 Sinus tachycardia. (Reproduced from Creed F and Spiers C, *Care of the Acutely Ill Adult: an essential guide for nurses*, 2010, with permission from Oxford University Press.)

Assessment findings

The patient will present with a heart rate of > 100 beats/min. They may be asymptomatic or there may be haemodynamic consequences. Diastolic filling will be reduced, so blood pressure may be affected and the patient may present with hypotension. Coronary artery filling is also reduced, so the patient may present with chest pain if they have cardiac disease.

Treatment

Treatment necessitates establishing the cause. For example:

- If the patient is hypovolaemic, fluid should be administered to correct hypovolaemia.
- If the patient is pyrexial, the cause of the high temperature should be addressed.
- Pain should be managed with appropriate assessment and treatment.
- On some occasions, medications may be required to slow the heart rate (e.g. beta blockers or digoxin).

Extrasystoles

Definition

Extrasystoles are premature beats that arise from an ectopic focus in the atria, the junctional area, or the ventricles. The beat is earlier than anticipated, and is followed by a compensatory pause. The normal heart rhythm may follow the compensatory pause, or further arrhythmias may be precipitated. The shape of the waveform of the ectopic beat will be determined by the focus. Therefore atrial and junctional extrasystoles are usually narrow complexes with an abnormal or absent preceding P wave. Ventricular extrasystoles have wide, often bizarre waveforms, and the T wave is normally in the opposite direction to the QRS complex (see Figure 6.7).

Causes

Occasional extrasystoles are common, even in healthy individuals. However, they may be caused by:

- stimulants
- cardiac disease
- hypoxaemia
- electrolyte disturbances
- acid–base disturbances.

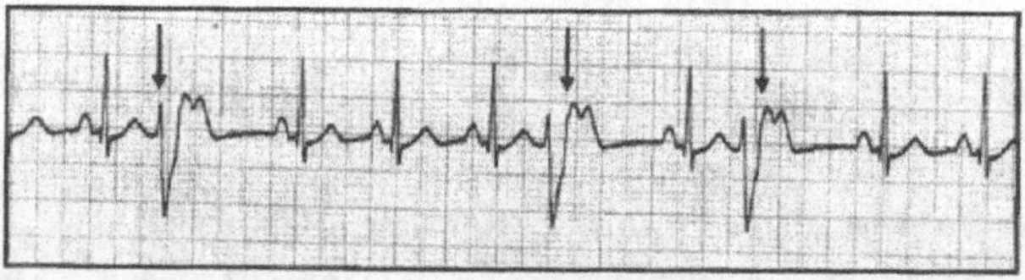

Figure 6.7 Ventricular extrasystole. (Reproduced from Creed F and Spiers C, *Care of the Acutely Ill Adult: an essential guide for nurses*, 2010, with permission from Oxford University Press.)

Assessment findings

ECG changes will be noted by the nurse, but occasional extrasystoles that do not precipitate arrhythmias will be unlikely to have any haemodynamic consequences for the patient. If the patient is having frequent extrasystoles and they are awake, they may be aware of 'palpitations.' Care should be taken if the extrasystoles are frequent or if they are multifocal (different shaped), as this may precipitate the development of arrhythmias.

Treatment

There is usually no need to treat atrial or junctional extrasystoles. However, treatment may be required for frequent or multifocal ventricular extrasystoles. This may include:

- checking serum electrolyte levels (especially potassium) and correcting any deficiencies
- increasing supplemental oxygen if the patient is hypoxic
- correcting the acid–base balance
- checking digoxin levels if the patient is receiving digoxin, as frequent extrasystoles may be a sign of digoxin toxicity.

Atrial fibrillation

Definition

Atrial fibrillation is the commonest arrhythmia seen in critically ill patients. It is generally a fast arrhythmia and usually caused by a re-entry circuit within the atria. In atrial fibrillation there is no coordinated conduction, and atrial contraction is ineffective. Ventricular conduction is normally faster than 100 beats/min. Atrial fibrillation may be classified as paroxysmal, persistent, or permanent, and is illustrated in Figure 6.8.

Causes

There are many causes of atrial fibrillation, including:

- underlying cardiac disease
- cardiac ischaemia
- congenital defects
- trauma
- hypoxia
- age over 50 years.

Assessment findings

The impact of atrial fibrillation is rate dependent. Atrial fibrillation will cause loss of atrial kick, which accounts for about 20% of stroke volume, so blood

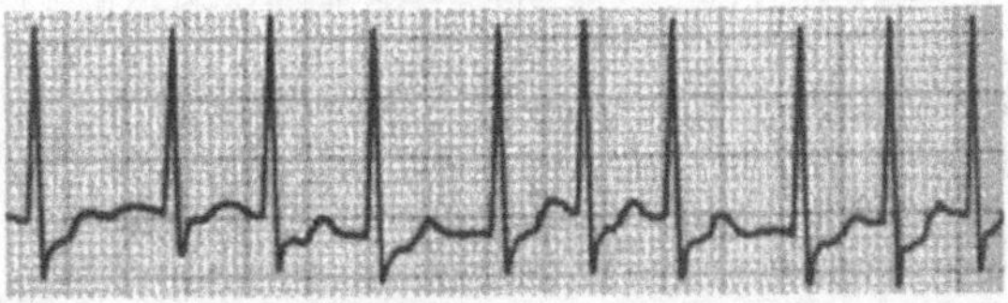

Figure 6.8 Atrial fibrillation. (Reproduced from Creed F and Spiers C, *Care of the Acutely Ill Adult: an essential guide for nurses*, 2010, with permission from Oxford University Press.)

pressure may quickly become affected. There is an associated risk of blood clot development. Patients may present with:

- hypotension
- palpitations
- chest pain
- breathlessness
- syncope.

Treatment

Treatment options are complex, and depend on the cause, nature, and duration of the arrhythmia.[12] Sudden onset should be reported immediately to the doctors, and NICE has provided guidelines on treatment.[13]

Supraventricular tachycardia

Definition

Supraventricular tachycardia (SVT) is a narrow complex tachycardia with a very fast rate, normally in the range 140–250 beats/min. In this arrhythmia, P waves are normally absent or obscured by the QRS complex, and the QRS remains narrow. SVT is illustrated in Figure 6.9.

Causes

SVT may be seen in healthy patients, and in this group may be caused by alcohol or stimulants.

In patients who are ill it may be caused by ischaemic heart disease or Wolff–Parkinson–White syndrome.

Assessment findings

Symptoms are likely to be rate related, but patients may experience:

- hypotension
- palpitations
- breathlessness
- syncope.

It may be necessary to slow the rate to facilitate diagnosis, and this can be done using:

- carotid sinus massage
- adenosine administration.

Treatment

Persistent SVT may require:

- administration of anti-arrhythmic medications such as amiodarone
- cardioversion.

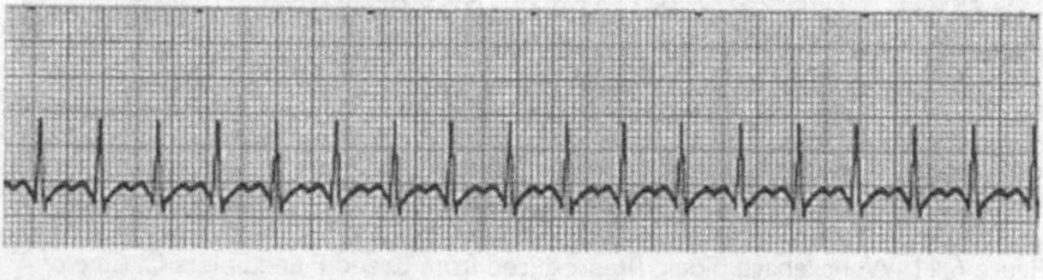

Figure 6.9 Supraventricular tachycardia. (Reproduced from Creed F and Spiers C, *Care of the Acutely Ill Adult: an essential guide for nurses*, 2010, with permission from Oxford University Press.)

Heart blocks

Definition

Heart blocks are caused by a conduction delay between the atria and ventricles, and may be referred to as atrioventricular (AV) block. Different types of block occur, including:

- first-degree heart block (see Figure 6.10)
- second-degree heart block:
  - Wenckebach (see Figure 6.11)
  - Mobitz type 2 (see Figure 6.12)
- third-degree or complete heart block (see Figure 6.13).

Third-degree heart block usually requires clinical intervention. The other forms may or may not be asymptomatic. First- and second-degree blocks can precipitate third-degree block.

Assessment findings

Patients may or may not be symptomatic. If symptomatic, they may present with:

- hypotension
- breathlessness
- syncope.

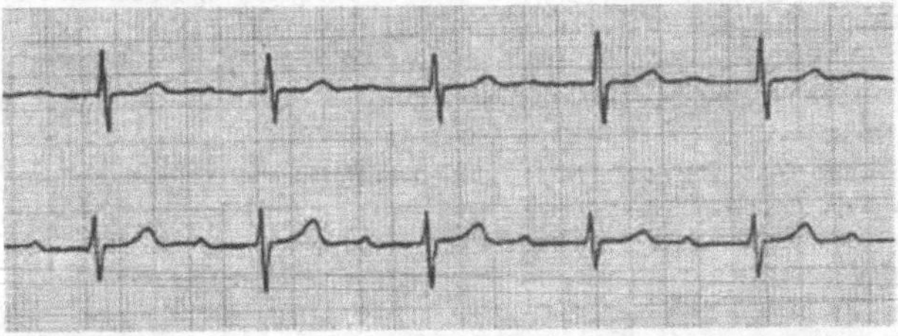

Figure 6.10 First-degree block. (Reproduced from Creed F and Spiers C, *Care of the Acutely Ill Adult: an essential guide for nurses*, 2010, with permission from Oxford University Press.)

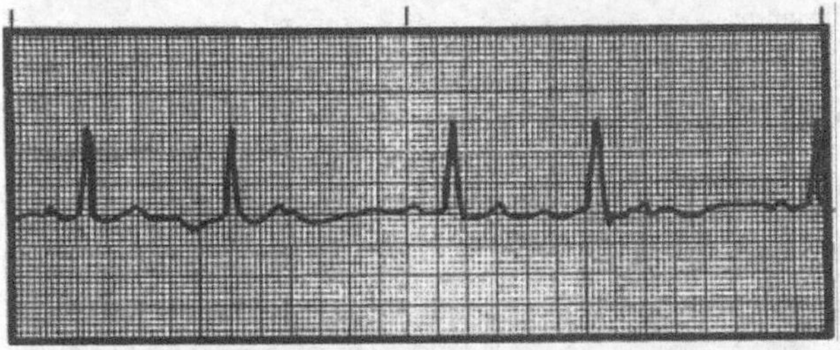

Figure 6.11 Wenckebach block. (Reproduced from Creed F and Spiers C, *Care of the Acutely Ill Adult: an essential guide for nurses*, 2010, with permission from Oxford University Press.)

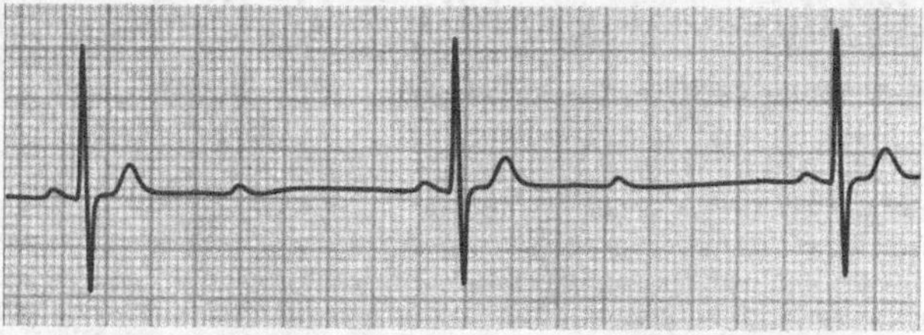

Figure 6.12 Mobitz type 2 block. (Reproduced from Creed F and Spiers C, *Care of the Acutely Ill Adult: an essential guide for nurses*, 2010, with permission from Oxford University Press.)

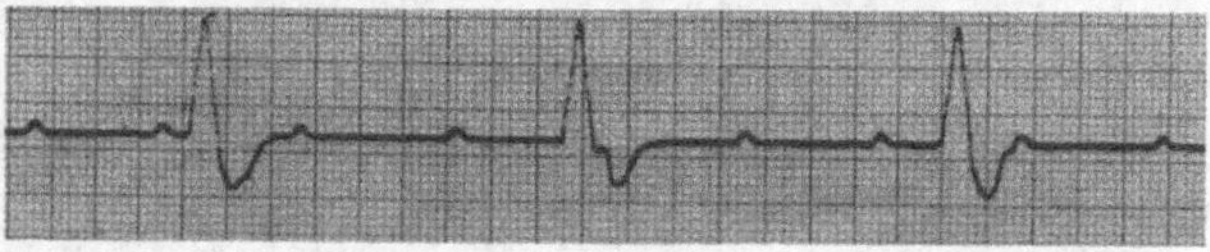

Figure 6.13 Complete heart block. (Reproduced from Creed F and Spiers C, *Care of the Acutely Ill Adult: an essential guide for nurses*, 2010, with permission from Oxford University Press.)

The ECG changes are summarized in Table 6.4.

Table 6.4 ECG changes associated with heart block

Heart block	Changes seen
First degree	Prolonged PR interval Regular rhythm
Wenckebach (second degree)	Progressive lengthening of PR interval until a beat is dropped Regularly irregular rhythm
Mobitz type 2 (second degree)	Varying conduction to ventricle leading to 2:1 or 3:1 block. The PR interval and QRS complex are constant
Complete (third degree)	There is no conduction between the atria and ventricles, so no distinguishable relationship between P waves and QRS complexes

Treatment

Treatment depends on the haemodynamic consequences of the block. Third-degree block may require temporary or permanent pacing.

References

12 Spiers C. Cardiovascular assessment and care. In: F Creed and C Spiers (eds) *Care of the Acutely Ill Adult: an essential guide for nurses*. Oxford University Press: Oxford, 2010. pp. 59–104.

13 National Institute for Health and Care Excellence (NICE). *Atrial Fibrillation: the management of atrial fibrillation*. CG180. NICE: London, 2014. www.nice.org.uk/guidance/cg180

Life-threatening cardiac arrhythmias

Ventricular tachycardia and ventricular fibrillation

Definition

All ventricular arrhythmias are potentially life-threatening and require urgent medical intervention. Ventricular tachycardia (VT) is a ventricular arrhythmia that most commonly occurs in patients with serious cardiac disease and in other critically ill patients. Ventricular fibrillation (VF) is a cardiac arrest scenario. In cases of VT and VF, immediate medical attention and resuscitation are required.

Assessment findings

In VT, the ECG (see Figure 6.14) shows no discernible P waves, and the QRS complexes are wide and bizarre. The patient may have lost consciousness and have no cardiac output (cardiac arrest), or they may demonstrate signs of severe haemodynamic compromise.

In VF, the ECG shows irregular chaotic waveforms with no discernible P waves or QRS complexes (see Figure 6.15). The patient will be unconscious and present with no cardiac output.

Treatment

For details of treatment for cardiac arrest, see ➔ p. 406.

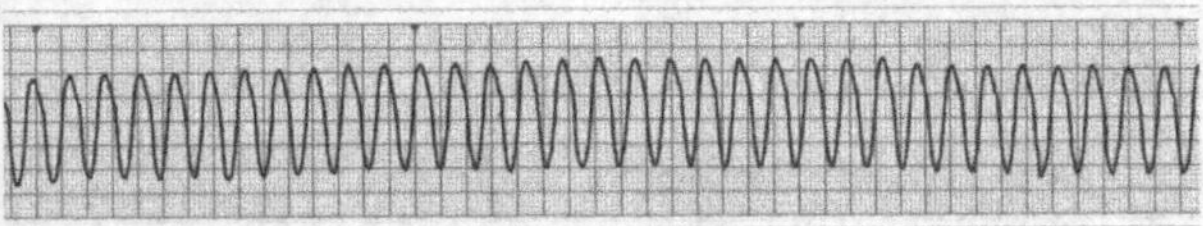

Figure 6.14 Ventricular tachycardia. (Reproduced from Creed F and Spiers C, *Care of the Acutely Ill Adult: an essential guide for nurses*, 2010, with permission from Oxford University Press.)

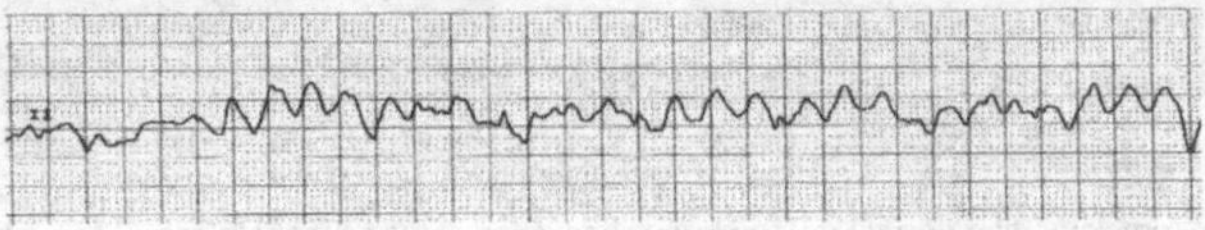

Figure 6.15 Ventricular fibrillation. (Reproduced from Creed F and Spiers C, *Care of the Acutely Ill Adult: an essential guide for nurses*, 2010, with permission from Oxford University Press.)

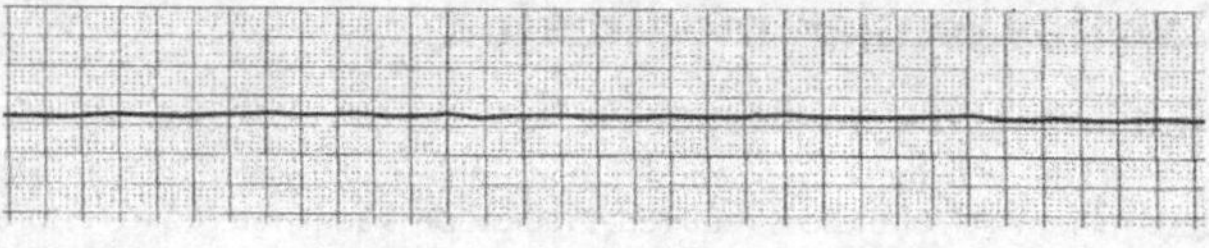

Figure 6.16 Asystole. (Reproduced from Creed F and Spiers C, *Care of the Acutely Ill Adult: an essential guide for nurses*, 2010, with permission from Oxford University Press.)

Asystole

Definition

Asystole is a cardiac arrest situation in which there is no electrical activity in the heart.

Assessment findings

The ECG will show an apparently flat line that may be undulating in nature (see Figure 6.16). A completely 'flat line' normally indicates detachment of the ECG leads. The patient will be unconscious, with no cardiac output.

Treatment

For details of treatment for cardiac arrest, see ➔ p. 406.

Pulseless electrical activity

Definition

Pulseless electrical activity (PEA) is a cardiac arrest situation in which there is electrical activity in the heart but no mechanical contraction associated with the electrical activity.

Assessment findings

The ECG will show a normal ECG complex with a defined P wave, QRS complex, and T wave. The ECG rate may be slower than normal. The patient will be unconscious, with no cardiac output.

Treatment

For details of treatment for cardiac arrest, see ➔ p. 406.

Cardiovascular medication

Anti-arrhythmic medications

Several anti-arrhythmic medications are available, and the medical team will determine which of these is required. Medication is administered to restore the heart to a regular rhythm. Anti-arrhythmic medications are classified according to their effect on the cardiac action potential and whether they block sodium, potassium, or calcium channels or β-adrenoreceptor sites.

- Class 1 anti-arrhythmic medication (sodium-channel blockers)—this is further subdivided into types i, ii, and iii. All types block the sodium channel and thus affect action potential duration. Class 1 drugs are not generally used, as they may cause life-threatening arrhythmias.[14] Examples include quinidine, disopyramide, and flecainide.
- Class 2 anti-arrhythmic medication (β-adrenoreceptor blockers)—this class has an effect on β-adrenoreceptor sites and is considered the best type of anti-arrhythmic drug for general use. Examples include propranolol and esmolol.
- Class 3 anti-arrhythmic medication (potassium-channel blockers)—drugs in this class lengthen the action potential and thus increase the refractory period. Examples include amiodarone and ibutilide.
- Class 4 anti-arrhythmic medication (calcium-channel blockers)—drugs in this class inhibit the inward movement of calcium ions and lengthen repolarization. Examples include verapamil and diltiazem.
- Unclassified anti-arrhythmic medication—this category includes medications with other mechanisms of action. Examples include adenosine, atropine, digoxin, and magnesium sulfate.

Antihypertensive medication

It may be necessary to treat potentially life-threatening hypertension, or hypertension that may be detrimental to the patient's health. Several antihypertensive agents are available, and the medical team will determine which antihypertensive is required. There is no evidence to suggest optimal drug therapy, so different medications may be used. Medications that may be utilized include the following.

Sodium nitroprusside

- This is a vasodilator that has an immediate effect on blood pressure.
- It is given intravenously, and care must be taken to avoid a profound drop in blood pressure.
- It may cause cerebral vasodilatation and hence may raise ICP.
- Ideally it should not be administered for more than 24 h, as it may cause metabolic acidosis.
- Side effects include headache, palpitations, dizziness, and nausea.

Glyceryl trinitrate (GTN)

- This is a vasodilator that, when given intravenously, takes effect within 1–2 min.
- Nitrates cause arterial and venous vasodilatation, and may also lead to cerebral vasodilatation and a risk of increased ICP.
- Side effects include headache, tachycardia, and nausea.

Hydralazine

- This is a peripheral vasodilator that, when given intravenously, will take effect within 15–30 min.
- Side effects include nausea, headaches, palpitations, and flushing.

Labetalol

- This acts by blocking α- and β-adrenergic receptors.
- It is given intravenously and will take effect within less than 5 min.
- Side effects include headache, rashes, and nausea.

Esmolol

- This is a short-acting selective β-adrenergic blocker.
- It is given by continuous infusion as it has a short half-life.
- When given intravenously it takes effect immediately.
- Side effects include bronchospasm, bradycardia, nausea, and vomiting.

Enalapril

- This is an angiotensin-converting enzyme (ACE) inhibitor.
- It takes effect within 10–15 min.
- Its mechanism of action includes:
    - inhibition of the conversion of angiotensin I to angiotensin II
    - reduction in secretion of aldosterone
    - increased peripheral vasodilatation.
- Side effects include hyperkalaemia, angioedema, cough, and sometimes profound hypotension.

Reference

14 Morton PG and Fontaine DK. *Critical Care Nursing: a holistic approach*, 10th edn. Lippincott Williams & Wilkins: Philadelphia, PA, 2012.

Chapter 7

Cardiovascular support

Cardiac monitoring

The critically ill patient may require complex monitoring during their episode of critical illness.

Monitoring tools that may be used include:

- continuous ECG monitoring
- 12-lead ECG recordings
- blood pressure monitoring
- central venous pressure monitoring
- cardiac output monitoring.

A combination of certain or all of these tools may be required, depending on the severity of critical illness. It is vital that the nurse understands:

- why the patient requires that form of monitoring
- how to utilize the monitoring tools
- the advantages of the tools
- the limitations of the tools.

Continuous ECG monitoring

[illegible] ECG monitoring. [illegible] ... heart rate [illegible] ... about the speed and amplitude of the pulse.

ECG [illegible] electrical activity of the heart. [illegible] electrodes are placed on the [illegible] and these detect the electrical activity of the heart. [illegible] the electrode will produce [illegible] positive deflection [illegible] away from the electrode will produce a negative deflection.

The basic [illegible] QRS [illegible] (see Figure 7.1).

Figure 7.1 [illegible]

Monitoring systems [illegible]

The 3-lead ECG system

- The 3 [illegible] leads I, II and III.
- [illegible]
- [illegible] commonly monitored using lead II.

The 5-lead ECG system

- [illegible]
- Electrodes [illegible]
- [illegible]

Continuous ECG monitoring

It is usual for most patients who are admitted to critical care units to have continuous ECG recording. This enables continuous observation of heart rate and rhythm, and also facilitates the setting of alarm parameters to warn of any disturbances to heart rate. ECG monitoring does not replace the need to take the pulse manually, as manual recordings will provide information about the strength and amplitude of the pulse.

The ECG provides a graphical representation of the electrical activity of the heart. Monitoring electrodes are placed on the patient's chest, and these detect the electrical activity of the heart. Activity moving towards the electrode will produce an upward or positive deflection, whereas activity moving away from the electrode will produce a downward or negative deflection.

The basic ECG waveform is labelled PQRST (and U) (see Figure 7.1).

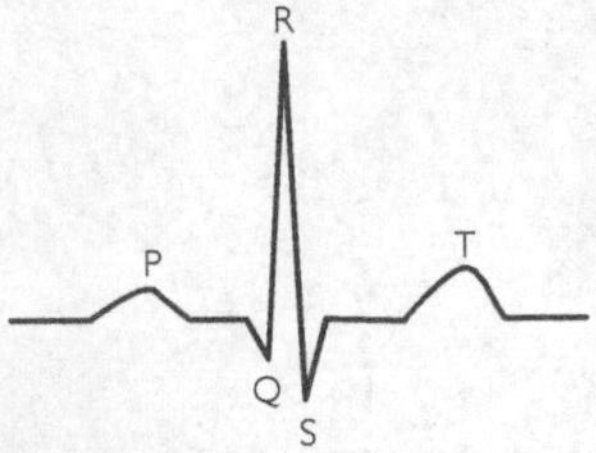

Figure 7.1 Basic ECG complex.

Monitoring systems may be either 3-lead systems or 5-lead systems.

The 3-lead ECG system

- The 3-lead systems allow monitoring of leads I, II, and III.
- Electrodes are placed on the patient's chest towards the right arm (RA), left arm (LA), and left leg (LL) (see Figure 7.2).
- It is most usual for patients to be monitored using lead II.

The 5-lead ECG system

- The 5-lead ECG system allows monitoring of any of the 12 leads, and usually two more leads may be displayed on the monitor at any one time (multi-channel ECG).
- Electrodes are placed towards the right arm (RA), right leg (RL), left arm (LA), left leg (LL), and a central chest lead (C).
- The clinical situation will normally determine which leads are viewed on the monitor, and discussion with the medical team may be required.

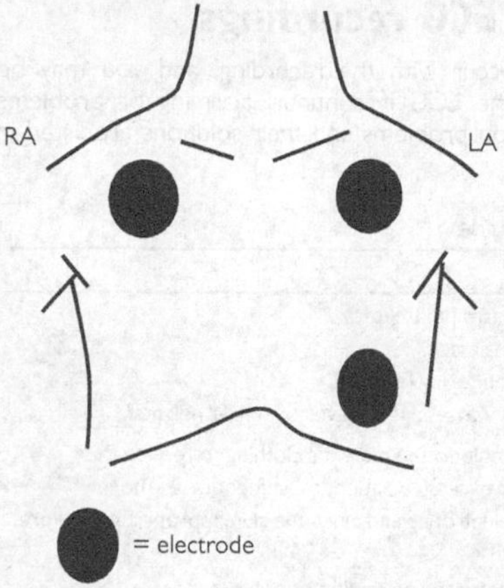

Figure 7.2 Three-lead ECG electrode positioning. RA, right arm; LA, left arm. (Reproduced from Adam SK and Osborne S, *Critical Care Nursing: science and practice*, Second Edition, 2005, with permission from Oxford University Press.)

Troubleshooting ECG recordings

Occasional problems may occur with the recording, and you may be required to 'troubleshoot' the ECG if continual alarming or problems with the trace occur. Common problems and their solutions are listed in Table 7.1.

Table 7.1 Troubleshooting guide

Problem	Solution
Excessive triggering of alarms	Review alarm parameters Check sensitivity Check monitoring lead Are the R waves and T waves of similar heights?
Wandering or irregular baseline	Clip the cable to the patient's clothing to reduce this Check for excessive patient movement or tremor Reapply electrodes and clean the skin appropriately before application
Intermittent trace	Check electrode connection to skin Check electrode connection to cable Check cable connection to monitor Check whether cable is damaged
No ECG trace	Adjust gain to see if it is set appropriately Check that cables are connected properly to the patient and the monitoring system Has the appropriate lead selector been utilized?

12-lead ECG monitoring

Recording a 12-lead ECG

Recording of a 12-lead ECG may be required in order to provide a more comprehensive view of the heart.

- Ten electrodes are placed on the patient to enable the monitoring system to view the heart from 12 views (hence '12-lead' ECG).
- One electrode is placed on each of the limbs, and six electrodes are placed on the patient's chest.
- The electrodes should ideally be placed over areas of least muscle mass to minimize electrical interference.

The 12-lead ECG is therefore composed of:

- three limb leads—I, II, and III. These form a hypothetical triangle with the heart at the centre
- three augmented (or modified) limb leads—augmented view left (aVL), augmented view right (aVR), and augmented view foot (aVF).
- six precordial or chest leads (V1–V6).

Twelve-lead ECGs may be recorded using a continuous system or may be serially recorded using a separate 12-lead ECG system. When serial ECGs are being recorded it is vital that the patient's electrodes are placed in the same position to allow comparison. There is often difficulty in placing the chest electrodes correctly (correct placement is shown in Figure 7.3). The anatomical positions for chest electrode placement are described in Table 7.2.

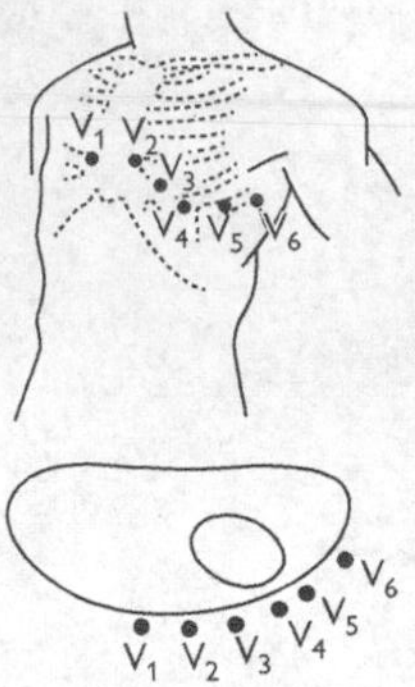

Figure 7.3 Diagram of chest electrode placement. (Reproduced from Chikwe J, Cooke D, Weiss A, *Oxford Specialist Handbook of Cardiothoracic Surgery*, Second Edition, 2013, with permission from Oxford University Press.)

Table 7.2 Anatomical positions for chest electrode placement

Chest lead	Anatomical position
V1	Fourth intercostal space to the right of the sternum
V2	Fourth intercostal space to the left of the sternum
V3	Midway between V2 and V4
V4	Fifth intercostal space, mid-clavicular line
V5	Anterior axillary line at the level of V4
V6	Mid-axillary line at the level of V4

Interpretation of the 12-lead ECG

This is complex and requires appropriate training. Therefore 12-lead ECGs should always be reviewed by a suitably qualified nurse or doctor. A systematic tool is required for the interpretation of the 12-lead ECG, as the latter needs to be reviewed in a logical manner.

Blood pressure monitoring

The accurate monitoring of blood pressure is an essential element of monitoring the critically ill patient. Occasionally this may be performed using non-invasive blood pressure systems, but more frequently a tranduced arterial monitoring system is used.

Non-invasive blood pressure recordings

A non-invasive system may be used for monitoring blood pressure in the early stages of critical illness if an arterial line is not deemed appropriate, or it may be used temporarily until an arterial line has been inserted.

Non-invasive systems are usually a reliable method of recording the patient's blood pressure, but if used frequently may cause excessive disturbance and discomfort to the patient.

- Attention should be paid to the size of the cuff, as an incorrectly sized cuff can cause false readings.
- The cuff bladder width should be 40–50% of the upper arm circumference. The bladder should encircle 80% of the upper arm.
- The cuff should be at the level of the heart to maintain a true zero level.
- Repeat interval times should be determined by the severity of the patient's condition.

Transduced arterial line recordings

Arterial lines allow the continuous monitoring of the systemic arterial pressure, and also provide vascular access for arterial blood sampling. They are generally used for the majority of critically ill patients. The use of transduced arterial monitoring is essential for:

- unstable patients
- patients on vasoactive infusions
- patients who require frequent arterial blood sampling
- patients for whom therapeutic decisions require an accurate blood pressure measurement.

The arterial line is normally situated in the radial artery, but may be located in other arteries (e.g. the brachial or femoral artery). The patient should ideally undergo an Allen's test to check for adequate collateral circulation prior to insertion.

There are a number of safety issues to be noted, as there are several risks associated with arterial lines and arterial monitoring. These include:

- bleeding
- infection
- thrombosis
- accidental disconnection
- occlusion of distal blood flow.

In order to maintain the safety of the line it is vital to be able to:

- regularly assess skin colour, temperature, and pulses distal to the cannula
- observe the site easily
- set alarm limits appropriately to facilitate early detection of disconnection
- clearly label and date the line to prevent accidental injection
- check connections to prevent accidental disconnection.

The transducer system

The transducer system works by transmitting pressures from the intravascular space through a fluid-filled non-compliant tube to a transducer. The transducer then converts this into an electrical signal which is in turn converted by the monitor into a trace and a digital reading.

It is essential that the transducer system is consistently situated as levelled to an external reference point to ensure accurate readings. The reference point will depend upon local policy, but it is usual to use either the phlebostatic axis or the sternal notch.

Once the reference point has been determined, the transducer should be zeroed prior to use and intermittently during use (frequency should be guided by local policy). Zeroing or recalibration is performed by:

- turning off the three-way tap to the patient
- opening the transducer to the atmosphere
- selecting the appropriate zeroing area on the monitor
- zeroing the transducer according to the manufacturer's guidelines
- closing the three-way tap to the atmosphere
- opening the three-way tap to the patient.

Arterial waveforms

The arterial waveform should be clearly displayed on the cardic monitor at all times. The normal waveform is represented in Figure 7.4 and consists of:

- a rapid upstroke—produced by the ejection of blood from the left ventricle into the aorta
- a dicrotic notch—produced by the closure of the aortic valve that marks the end of systole
- a definitive end point.

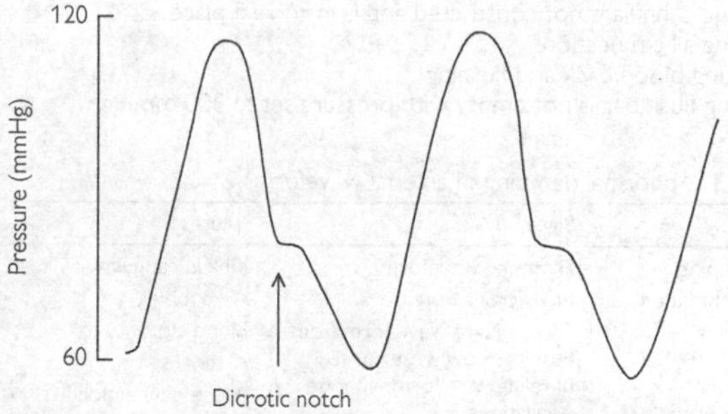

Figure 7.4 Normal arterial waveform. (Reproduced from Chikwe J, Beddow E, Glenville B, *Oxford Specialist Handbook of Cardiothoracic Surgery*, 2006, with permission from Oxford University Press.)

The pressures generated by the arterial monitoring include:
- systolic blood pressure
- diastolic blood pressure
- mean arterial pressure (MAP) = diastolic + (systolic-diastolic)/3.

Abnormal arterial waveforms

Variation in systolic blood pressure

Normally, there is only a minimal variation in systolic blood pressure during inspiration and expiration despite changes that occur in intra-thoracic pressure during the breathing cycle. Pulsus paradoxus is when a non-ventilated patient has more than 10 mmHg drop in systolic blood pressure during inspiration as compared to expiration. Reverse pulsus paradoxus, often referred to as a 'swing' in the arterial waveform, occurs when the systolic blood pressure of a mechanically ventilated patient increases during inspiration and decreases with expiration. The most common cause of a variation in systolic blood pressure is hypovolaemia. Other possible causes include tamponade, pericarditis, large pulmonary embolus, and tension pneumothorax.

Damping

Accurate arterial blood pressure monitoring requires a monitoring system which is optimally damped and is confirmed by:
- normal arterial waveform with a dicrotic notch
- comparable invasive blood pressure readings as the non-invasive blood pressure measurement
- after square wave form from flushing, only 1-2 oscillations occur before quickly returning to normal waveform.

Overdamping and underdamping may affect the reliability of the continuous blood pressure results (see Table 7.3). Troubleshooting actions for a problem with damping abnormalities include:
- checking cannula is not constricted and is in correct place
- checking all connections
- aspirating blood back and flushing
- ensuring flush bag is not empty with pressure set to 300 mmHg.

Table 7.3 Abnormal damping of arterial waveforms

Problem	Signs	Causes
Overdamping (Underestimation of systolic and overestimation of diastolic)	Flattened waveform No dicrotic notch After square wave form from flushing, slowly returns to baseline waveform without oscillations	Kink in cannula Air bubbles Blood clot Arterial spasm Loose connection
Underdamping (Falsely high systolic and falsely low diastolic)	Overshooting of systolic waveform (whip) After square wave form from flushing, multiple oscillations (ringing) occur before returning to baseline	Catheter artefact Stiff tubing High cardiac output Tachycardia Arryhthmias

Removal of an arterial line

The cannula may be removed if there are problems associated with its use (e.g. poor distal perfusion) or if it is no longer required. It is vital that care is taken to minimize complications associated with removal. Care should be taken to apply adequate pressure for sufficient time to ensure haemostasis.

Further reading

Nirmalan M and Dark PM. Broader applications of arterial pressure wave form analysis. *Continuing Education in Anaesthesia, Critical Care and Pain* 2014; 14: 285-90.

Romagnoli S et al. Accuracy of invasive arterial pressure monitoring in cardiovascular patients: an observational study. *Critical Care* 2014; 18: 644.

Central venous pressure monitoring

The central venous pressure (CVP) is recorded by using a central line that is normally inserted into either the internal jugular vein or the subclavian vein.

The tip of the line is situated in the superior vena cava and reflects the pressure in the right atrium. It is theoretically suggested that in a healthy patient this provides information about intravascular blood volume and right ventricular end diastolic pressure, although a recent meta-analysis questions the reliability of this.[1] See ➲ p. 52.

Nevertheless, the CVP may be used as a guide to treatment, but it is important to remember that *no single measurement* should be used to guide patient treatment. An overview of the trend in the patient's assessment results is much more likely to be clinically useful in relation to guiding fluid management.

There are a number of safety issues to be noted, as there are several risks associated with CVP monitoring, and complications may occur in up to 15% of patients. These include problems during insertion, such as:

- pneumothorax
- trauma to the surrounding tissue
- arrhythmias
- incorrect positioning
- air emboli.

Problems may also be noted after insertion. These include:

- infection
- thrombosis
- air embolism
- acting upon inaccurate CVP results.

Transducing the CVP

It is essential that the transducer system is adequately zeroed to an external reference point to ensure accurate readings. The reference point will depend upon local policy, but it is usual to use either the phlebostatic axis or the sternal notch.

Once the reference point has been determined the transducer should be zeroed prior to use and intermittently during use (frequency should be guided by local policy). Zeroing or recalibration is performed by:

- turning off the three-way tap to the patient
- opening the transducer to the atmosphere
- selecting the appropriate zeroing area on the monitor
- zeroing the transducer according to the manufacturer's guidelines
- closing the three-way tap to the atmosphere.

CVP values and waveforms

Normal CVP is considered to be in the range 2–10 mmHg (positive pressure ventilation and addition of PEEP will increase CVP values).

The normal waveform consists of an A, C, and V wave (see Figure 7.5). Each of these waves represents a different part of the cardiac cycle.

- A wave represents atrial contraction, and the downward slope represents arterial relaxation.
- C wave represents tricuspid valve closure.
- V wave represents the pressure generated to the right atrium during contraction of the right ventricle.

The CVP may be altered by changes in the patient's condition, but it is important that these are viewed alongside other clinical data from the CVS assessment.

Conditions that may cause CVP to rise include:

- right ventricular failure
- pericardial tamponade
- fluid overload
- pulmonary hypertension
- tricuspid regurgitation
- pulmonary stenosis
- peripheral vasoconstriction
- superior vena cava obstruction
- pulmonary embolism.

Conditions that may cause CVP to fall include:

- hypovolaemia
- excessive diuresis
- vasodilatation.

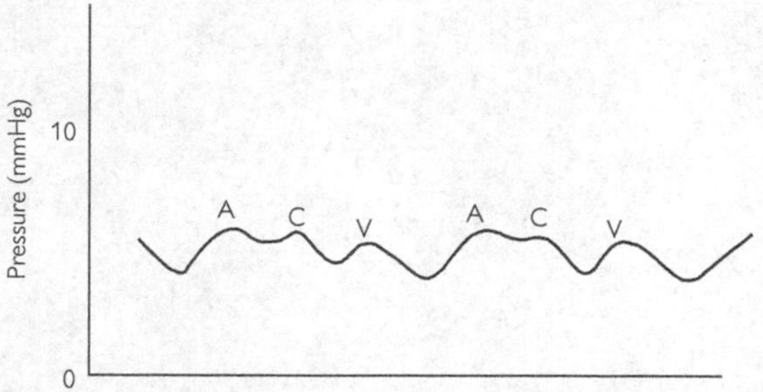

Figure 7.5 Normal CVP waveform. (Reproduced from Adam SK and Osborne S, *Critical Care Nursing: science and practice*, Second Edition, 2005, with permission from Oxford University Press.)

Removal of a CVP line

It may be necessary to remove the CVP line in order to replace it if there are signs of infection. A new line will need to be inserted prior to the removal of the old line if vasoactive or other infusions are utilizing the CVP line. The patient may also no longer require the line.

It is vital that no complications arise from the removal of the CVP line. Therefore, if the patient's condition permits, the procedure should be performed as follows:

- The patient should be positioned lying flat or with their head at a downward angle.
- Infusions through the CVP line should be discontinued.
- The catheter should ideally be removed during expiration to prevent air emboli.
- The catheter should be slowly withdrawn.
- Once the catheter has been removed a sterile occlusive dressing should be applied.
- It may be necessary to send the catheter tip to the microbiology lab (local policy should be followed).

Reference

1 Marik PE and Cavallazzi R. Does the central venous pressure predict fluid responsiveness? An updated meta-analysis and a plea for some common sense. *Critical Care Medicine* 2013; 41: 1774–81.

Cardiac output monitoring

The last decade has seen a significant increase in the number of cardiac output measurement tools available in critical care. Some units may utilize a variety of systems, whereas in other units [illegible] only one or a limited number available. Different cardiac output systems will provide additional data to estimation of cardiac output. The choice of a cardiac output measurement tool is dependent on:

- the equipment available in the local unit
- the measurements required for the patient
- the severity of the patient's illness.

For a long time, the main means of cardiac output measurement was the pulmonary artery catheter, but [illegible] have [illegible] a variety of other, more [illegible] to measure cardiac output. Many of the newer systems are less invasive than [illegible] and [illegible] use systems such as the [illegible] device:

- pulmonary artery catheter
- pulse contour cardiac output (PiCCO)
- lithium dilution cardiac output (LiDCO)
- transoesophageal Doppler system.

Pulmonary artery (PA) catheter

The [illegible] cardiac output and [illegible] measurements [illegible] right and left sides of the heart [illegible] used to measure:

- right atrial pressure (RAP)
- right ventricular pressure (RVP)
- pulmonary artery pressure (PAP)
- [illegible] pulmonary artery wedge pressure (PAWP).

[illegible] include:

- [illegible]
- [illegible]
- [illegible]
- [illegible] (SVO)
- [illegible]
- [illegible]
- [illegible]
- [illegible]
- [illegible]

Cardiac output monitoring

The last decade has seen a significant increase in the number of cardiac output measurement tools available in critical care units. Some units may utilize a variety of systems, whereas in others there may be only one tool or a limited range available. Different cardiac output systems will provide additional data to estimation of cardiac output. The choice of cardiac output measurement tool is dependent on:

- the equipment available in the local unit
- the measurements required for the patient
- the severity of the patient's illness.

For decades the pulmonary artery catheter has been regarded as the gold-standard tool for cardiac output monitoring. However, increasingly a variety of other tools are being utilized to measure cardiac output. Many of the newer systems are less invasive than traditional methods. The critical care nurse may use systems such as the following:

- pulmonary artery catheter
- pulse contour cardiac output (PiCCO)
- lithium dilution cardiac output (LiDCO)
- trans-oesophageal Doppler system.

Pulmonary artery (PA) catheter

This is used to measure cardiac output, and also provides other measurements that may be useful in clinical practice. The pulmonary artery catheter is situated in the right side of the heart and enters the pulmonary artery. It is therefore able to measure:

- right atrial pressure (RAP)
- right ventricular pressure (RVP)
- pulmonary artery pressure (PAP)
- indirectly, left atrial pressure (pulmonary artery occlusion pressure, PAOP, which is also known as pulmonary artery wedge pressure, PAWP).

Cardiac output is measured using thermodilution. Other variables are also calculated, including:

- systemic vascular resistance (SVR)
- pulmonary vascular resistance (PVR)
- oxygen consumption (VO_2)
- mixed venous oxygen saturations (SVO_2).

The pulmonary artery catheter typically consists of four lumens.

- The distal lumen (located in the pulmonary artery) is attached to the transducer for the measurement of cardiac output, and measures PAP. Mixed venous blood may be withdrawn from this lumen.
- The proximal lumen (located in the right atrium) may be used for measurement of RAP.
- The thermistor detects the patient's blood temperature and receives input from a thermistor at the tip of the catheter.
- The balloon inflation lumen is used to inflate the balloon for measurements of PAOP.

Insertion of a PA catheter

The nurse's role is to assist with insertion, and a strict aseptic technique is required. The catheter is inserted through a large vein (subclavian or internal jugular vein). The catheter is advanced through the right side of the heart into the pulmonary artery and eventually into the 'wedged' position. The nurse may need to observe the monitor during insertion to advise about waveform alterations and monitor for signs of cardiac arrhythmias. It is important that the balloon is deflated after insertion, and that the line is secured firmly to the patient.

Complications related to PA catheter insertion and use include:

- CVP line insertion complications (see ➔ p. 46)
- ventricular arrhythmias
- air embolism
- misplaced catheter or knotting of the catheter
- pulmonary artery rupture
- pulmonary artery ischaemia or infarction
- rupture of the right atrium
- valve damage
- infection.

Measuring cardiac output

Thermodilution

Older pulmonary artery catheter systems determine cardiac output by thermo dilution.

- A measured volume of cold fluid (normally saline) is injected into the PA catheter in the appropriate port.
- The temperature changed is sensed by a thermistor at the catheter tip and cardiac output is calculated from a temperature change curve that is generated by the computer as the cold fluid is injected.
- Techniques used should follow manufacturer guidelines to ensure accuracy of cardiac output measurement.

Thermofilament

Newer pulmonary artery catheter systems allow for continual cardiac output monitoring without the need for insertion of cold fluid.

- Distal section of catheter has a 10 cm thermal filament.
- Catheter emits pulses of heat from the filament resulting in a change in blood temperature which is measured to generate cardiac output value.
- Computes cardiac output over successive 3 minute intervals and then averaged out for continuous monitoring.

Measurement of pulmonary artery occlusion pressure

It may be necessary for PAOP (wedge pressure) to be measured from time to time, as this provides an indication of left atrial pressure and indirectly reflects left ventricular end diastolic pressure. This measurement is obtained by inflation of the balloon, and is best recorded at the end of expiration. It is essential that the correct technique is used.

- Only use specific syringe which has a maximum of 1.5 ml capacity.
- Inflate the balloon slowly until the trace flattens.
- Once the trace has flattened, stop inflating the balloon, to prevent over-inflation.

- Freeze the monitor and deflate the balloon (do not inflate the balloon for more than 15 s).
- Move the cursor on the monitor to allow calculation of PAOP at the end of expiration.
- When PAOP has been calculated, unfreeze the trace.

Normal values for PA catheter measurements

- Stroke volume: 60–100 mL.
- Cardiac output: 4–6 L.
- Cardiac index: 2.5–4 L.
- PAOP: 6–12 mmHg.
- Mixed venous O_2: 70–75%.
- SVR: 800–1200 dyne/s/cm.[5]

Pulse contour analysis

The pulse contour system allows cardiac output studies to be recorded without the need for additional line insertion. The system is able to record continuous cardiac output by using data from the pulse contour of the arterial trace. Therefore cardiac output studies can be recorded without using additional monitoring lines such as a PA catheter.

However, some pulse contour systems do require the use of thermodilution techniques to recalibrate the system to ensure that the data provided are accurate. Some systems use pulmonary thermodilution to recalibrate the calculation system, and will therefore provide some continuous data and some 'one-off' measurements that are utilized to calculate other variables.

Because there is no necessity for a PA catheter, some of the measurements traditionally associated with PA studies cannot be recorded (e.g. PAOP). However, other variables that can have an impact on treatment plans can be recorded. Therefore data from pulse contour analysis differ from those produced by other cardiac output measurement systems.

Pulse contour variables that can be measured or calculated include:

- continuous pulse contour cardiac analysis
- cardiac index
- stroke volume
- stroke volume variation
- systemic vascular resistance
- index of left ventricular contraction.

In addition, some pulse contour systems utilize transpulmonary thermodilution to provide the following variables:

- transpulmonary cardiac output
- intrathoracic blood volume
- extravascular lung water
- cardiac function index.

The equipment required for studies using pulse contour systems varies depending upon the manufacturer. The two main systems are:

- PiCCO© system (PULSION Medical Systems)
- FloTrac/Vigileo© system (Edwards Lifesciences).

Table 7.4 PiCCO© and FloTrac© data variables

Measurement	PiCCO©	FloTrac©
Stroke volume variation	< 10%	< 13%
Intravascular blood volume	800–1000 mL/m²	—
Extravascular lung water	3–7 mL/kg	—
Cardiac function index	4.5–6.5 L/min	—
Global end diastolic volume	680–800 mL/m²	—
Stroke volume index	—	33–47 mL/beat/m²
Cardiac index	3–5 L/min/m²	2.5–4 L/min/m²

PiCCO© system

- This utilizes a specialized thermistor striped arterial line, placed in a distal artery to measure the arterial waveform morphology.
- An algorithm is used to calculate the cardiac output from the area under the curve of the arterial trace.
- Transpulmonary thermodilution ensures the accuracy of calculations and is required to recalibrate the system.

FloTrac© system

- This utilizes a blood flow sensor that is attached to a normal arterial line.
- Cardiac output is calculated using an algorithm every 20 s.
- This system does not require external calibration once it has been commenced.
- No additional lines are required.

Normal values can be found in the user manual for each system.

These systems provide additional data, and the normal values for the additional measurements are listed in Table 7.4.

Lithium dilution cardiac output

This method utilizes the injection of lithium chloride to calculate the cardiac output.

- Lithium is injected via a central or peripheral line.
- A sensor in the arterial line detects the presence of lithium and calculates a plasma concentration–time curve.
- This is used to calculate the blood flow.

The system is also able to generate continuous cardiac output by utilizing pulse power derivation, and is not dependent upon waveform morphology to calculate continuous cardiac output measurements.

Cardiac output is measured using the following equation:

$$\text{Cardiac ouput} = \frac{\text{lithium dose (mmol)} \times 60}{\text{area} \times \text{(1 – PCV) (mmol/s)}}$$

Table 7.5 LiDCO© data variables

Systolic pressure variation	< 5 mmHg unlikely to be preload responsive > 5 mmHg may be preload responsive
Pulse pressure variation	< 10% unlikely to be preload responsive > 13–15% may be preload responsive
Stroke volume variation	< 10% unlikely to be preload responsive > 13% may be preload responsive
Stroke volume index	3.3–4.7 mL/m^2/beat
Left ventricular stroke work	58–104 gm/m/beat
Right ventricular stroke work	8–16 gm/m/beat
Coronary artery perfusion pressure	60–80 mmHg
Right ventricular end diastolic volume	100–160 mL
Right ventricular end systolic volume	50–100 mL
Right ventricular ejection faction	40–60%

It is therefore essential to measure the patient's packed cell volume (PCV) to enable accurate measurements to be obtained.

Because the system utilizes the injection of lithium chloride to calculate the cardiac output, some precautions are necessary. These include:

- limiting the number of measurements to 12 per day
- not using the system on patients who:
  - are receiving lithium therapy
  - are receiving non-depolarizing NMBAs
  - weigh less than 40 kg
  - are in the first trimester of pregnancy.

The system has shown a good correlation with PA catheter thermodilution as long as there is no indicator loss and there is good blood flow. Repeated blood sampling of 3–4 mL of blood is needed, and concerns have been raised about the need for this in a critically ill patient.[2]

Variables calculated from the lithium dilution system (LiDCO©) are listed in Table 7.5.

Doppler cardiac output measurement

Cardiac output can also be estimated by using Doppler ultrasound to measure blood flow through the aorta, and utilizing this to calculate cardiac output. Generally most systems use a probe placed into the patient's oesophagus to measure blood flow in the descending aorta. Some systems are externally placed (truly non-invasive), and are positioned suprasternally to allow calculation or measurement of flow. However, the oesophageal probe is used most frequently. This system requires no invasive lines and can be utilized in areas outside of critical care by experienced practitioners such as critical care outreach teams.

The systems work by measuring ultrasound waves that are reflected off moving red blood cells.

- The movement of red blood cells causes a change in frequency proportional to the velocity of the red blood cells within the aorta.
- When the diameter of the blood vessel is known, it is possible to calculate blood flow using the flow/velocity waveform.
- A continuous real-time waveform is produced from the Doppler.
- Continuous wave-contour analysis produces information about the circulation.
- Continuous cardiac output is calculated using an algorithm based on the Doppler configuration and the patient's height, weight, and age.
- Peak velocity is determined by the amplitude of the wave.
- Flow time is calculated by measuring the width of the base of the waveform.
- This information can be used to guide and monitor interventions such as fluid therapy and inotropic support.

For the system to work accurately it is essential that the Doppler probe is positioned correctly and that the waveform produced by the Doppler is sharp and well defined. Doppler measurement is useful for most patients. However, caution is needed in the following situations:

- presence of an intra-aortic balloon pump
- presence of aortic pathology
- recent surgery to the mouth, oesophagus, or stomach
- severe coagulopathy
- presence of oesophageal varices.

Reference

2 Drummond KE and Murphy E. Minimally invasive cardiac output monitors. *Continuing Education in Anaesthesia, Critical Care & Pain* 2012; **12**: 5–10.

Vasoactive medications

The various monitoring tools discussed in this chapter highlight the need to manipulate blood pressure by using vasoactive medication. Therefore a knowledge of vasoactive drugs and their indications, contraindications, and mechanisms of action is essential for the critical care nurse.

A vasoactive medication is one that is generally used when fluid manipulation in the critically ill patient is unsuccessful. Put simply, a vasoactive medication may be defined as a drug that has the ability to change the diameter of a blood vessel. However, many vasoactive medications also have a direct effect on other elements of the cardiac system, so it is perhaps more appropriate to consider all of the effects of vasoactive medication. These include:

- vasodilation
- vasoconstriction
- inotropic effects
- chronotropic effects
- dromotropic effects.

These categories can be summarized as follows:

- **Vasodilators** are medications that relax the smooth muscle in the blood vessel wall, thereby facilitating vasodilation. Generally this leads to a decrease in arterial blood pressure, a reduction in cardiac preload, and a decrease in cardiac output.
- **Vasoconstrictors** are medications that contract smooth muscle in the blood vessel wall, thereby causing vasoconstriction. This leads to an increase in blood pressure by causing an increase in systemic vascular resistance, cardiac preload, and cardiac output.
- **Inotropes** are medications that increase the contractility of the cardiac muscle.
- **Chronotropes** are medications that increase the heart rate.
- **Dromotropes** are medications that increase conduction through the AV node.

The effects of vasoactive medications are predominantly mediated by the medication binding to a receptor that causes the effect. These include α- and β-receptors, and it is important to note that medications may bind to more than one type of receptor. The main receptor sites and effects are listed in Table 7.6.

The most common vasoactive medications used in critical illness include:

- adrenaline
- noradrenaline
- dobutamine
- dopexamine
- dopamine.

Each of these drugs will bind to one or more receptors, and this will result in changes to vasomotor tone, contractility of the heart muscle, and speed of contraction and thus heart rate. Table 7.7 lists the receptors for each of these key medications. Further information about each of these drugs is provided later in this chapter.

Table 7.6 Receptor sites and effects

Receptor	Location	Action
α_1	Vascular smooth muscle Heart	Vasoconstrictor Weak inotrope and chronotrope
α_2	Vascular smooth muscle Heart	Peripheral vasodilator Inhibits noradrenaline release
β_1	Heart	Inotropes increase cardiac contractility Chronotropes increase cardiac rate
β_2	Bronchial smooth muscle Vascular smooth muscle AV node	Bronchodilator Skeletal muscle vasodilator Dromotrope
Dopaminergic	Vascular smooth muscle	Renal and splanchnic vasodilator

Table 7.7 The effect of vasoactive medications on receptors

	α_1-receptor	β_1-receptor	β_2-receptor	Dopaminergic receptor
Adrenaline	++	+++	++	0
Noradrenaline	+++	++	0	0
Dobutamine	0	+++	+	0
Dopexamine	0	++	+++	+
Dopamine				
Low dose	0	0	0	+++
Moderate dose	0	++	+	0
High dose	+++	+++	0	0

Vasoactive medications may cause side effects, and it is important that the benefits of the medication are not outweighed by its side effects. Side effects may be dose dependent and include:

- cardiac arrhythmias
- myocardial ischaemia
- decrease in renal perfusion
- decrease in splanchnic perfusion
- peripheral ischaemia
- labile blood pressure
- lactic acidosis.

Overview of specific vasoactive medications

Noradrenaline

- Dominant effect on α_1-receptors.
- Increases blood pressure by vasoconstriction.
- Preferred medication for patients presenting with sepsis[3] (see ➲ p. 340).
- May cause a reduction in cardiac output as afterload increases.
- May reduce renal and splanchnic perfusion.
- May increase coronary blood flow as a result of increase in diastolic pressure.
- Requires careful titration to ensure that the correct dose is given to maximize effectiveness and minimize side effects.
- Adverse effects include:
  - arrhythmias
  - poor peripheral perfusion (at high doses)
  - chest pain
  - headache.

Adrenaline

- Acts on α- and β-receptors.
- At low doses predominantly affects β-receptors and causes increased cardiac contractility and heart rate.
- At higher doses predominantly affects α-receptors and causes increased blood pressure through vasoconstriction.
- Net effect is to increase heart rate, blood pressure, and cardiac output.
- Increases myocardial oxygen requirements as heart rate increases.
- May decrease renal and splanchnic perfusion at higher doses.
- May be given as a bolus in emergency situations (see Chapter 15).
- Increases blood glucose levels.
- Acts as a bronchodilator (acts on β_2-receptors).
- May cause vasodilation at some doses, as it acts on skeletal muscle β_2-receptors.
- May worsen acidosis as rate of metabolism increases.
- Requires careful titration to ensure that the correct dose is given to maximize effectiveness and minimize side effects.
- Adverse effects include:
  - arrhythmias
  - myocardial ischaemia
  - chest pain
  - headache
  - dizziness
  - increased anxiety and nervousness.

Dobutamine

- Acts on β_1-receptors.
- Effect is mainly inotropic, and causes increased contractility of cardiac muscle.
- Has some chronotropic properties and increases cardiac rate.

- Important to ensure adequate preload prior to commencing this medication, as it may cause tachycardia when given to a hypovolaemic patient.
- Has some effect on β_2-receptors and may cause vasodilation, and reduce SVR and left ventricular end diastolic pressure.
- Requires careful titration to ensure that the correct dose is given to maximize effectiveness and minimize side effects.
- Adverse effects include:
  - arrhythmias
  - tachycardia
  - headache
  - nausea.

Dopexamine

- A synthetic analogue of dopamine.
- Acts mainly on β-receptors.
- Has some effect on dopaminergic receptors.
- Improves blood flow to mesenteric, renal, cerebral, and coronary arteries.
- Has some effect on decreasing noradrenaline release.
- Useful inotrope for patients with acute heart failure.
- May be appropriate for attenuating the inflammatory response in patients with sepsis.
- Adverse effects include:
  - tachycardia
  - arrhythmias
  - nausea
  - vomiting
  - headaches.

Dopamine

- Acts on dopaminergic receptors and on α- and β-receptors.
- Effect is dose dependent.
- Low-dose dopamine is not advised because of negative effects on gastric motility, splanchnic oxygen consumption, and the immune system.
- Higher-dose dopamine is an effective vasopressor and is recommended as a substitute for vasopressor in sepsis in highly selected patients (i.e. those not at risk of tachyarrhythmias).[3]
- Moderate doses increase cardiac contractility.
- Adverse effects include:
  - tachycardia
  - arrhythmias
  - nausea
  - vomiting
  - hypertension.

Reference

3 Dellinger R et al. Surviving sepsis campaign: international guidelines for management of severe sepsis and septic shock. *Critical Care Medicine* 2013; **41**: 580–637.

Intra-aortic balloon pump

An intra-aortic balloon pump is a mechanical device that sits in the aorta and is used as a temporary measure to support acute heart failure.

The intra-aortic balloon pump uses counter pulsation to support the failing heart—that is, the balloon inflates during diastole and deflates during early systole. This causes volume displacement of blood within the aorta both proximally and distally. The volume displacement increases coronary blood flow and has the potential to subsequently improve systemic perfusion by increasing cardiac output.

The purposes of the balloon pump are to:
- increase myocardial oxygenation
- increase cardiac output
- increase oxygen delivery
- increase myocardial oxygen uptake.

It is usually used to support patients:
- with cardiogenic shock
- post cardiac surgery
- post myocardial infarction to support mechanical defects
- pre-operatively if they are awaiting surgery with unstable angina.

Intra-aortic balloon pumps are contraindicated in:
- severe aortic valve insufficiency
- aortic dissection
- aorta iliac occlusive disease.

The timing of the counter-pulsation therapy is critical, as it is vital that the balloon inflates after the aortic valve has closed and deflates before the opening of the aortic valve. Timings are normally coordinated by using either the ECG complex or the arterial waveform. Suboptimal timing of the counter-pulsation therapy can lead to haemodynamic instability. Therefore it is essential that the console is set up correctly by an expert practitioner.

Nursing care for the patient with an intra-aortic balloon pump involves:
- monitoring cardiovascular observations
- monitoring for side effects of the intra-aortic balloon pump
- psychological care.

Side effects include:
- distal ischaemia
- compartment syndrome
- development of embolisms
- renal problems
- aortic damage or dissection
- haemorrhage.

The device is normally removed once the patient is more stable. This may be indicated by a decreasing need for inotropic support and improved cardiac output. It is important that the intra-aortic balloon pump is gradually weaned, and the device should never be abruptly stopped as this may lead to thrombus formation.

Pacing

Cardiac pacing is frequently indicated when there are cardiac conduction problems. These may be related to cardiac ischaemia or damage, or may be [illegible] to other causes, or [illegible].

Pacing is commonly used:

- to treat heart blocks—usually [illegible] degree [illegible] (see Chapter 9, [illegible])
- to [illegible] arrhythmias and [illegible]
- [illegible] post cardiac surgery ([illegible] valve surgery)
- in [illegible] such as [illegible] syndrome [illegible]
- [illegible] in the event of prolonged [illegible]
- [illegible] medication.

[illegible] critical care is [illegible] temporary [illegible] although [illegible] systems may be required. Temporary pacing is [illegible]:

- [illegible]
- [illegible] with electrodes
- [illegible] may be:
- transvenous
- epicardial
- [illegible]

Transvenous pacing

- This [illegible] a [illegible]
- The [illegible]
- The [illegible] with [illegible]
- The [illegible]
- The [illegible] to the [illegible]
- The [illegible] that pacing is [illegible]
- A [illegible] should [illegible]

Epicardial pacing

- [illegible] during surgery on the epicardium [illegible]
- [illegible]
- [illegible]
- [illegible]
- [illegible] should [illegible]
- [illegible] may be removed [illegible] when they are [illegible] by the [illegible].

Pacing

Cardiac pacing is normally indicated when there are cardiac conduction problems. These may be related to cardiac ischaemia or damage, or may be linked to other aspects of critical illness.

Pacing is commonly used:

- to treat heart blocks—usually complete (third-degree) or Mobitz type 2 blocks (see Chapter 6, ➔ p. 202).
- to override arrhythmias and to treat asystole.
- prophylactically post cardiac surgery (especially valve surgery).
- non-cardiac diseases such as Guillain–Barré syndrome sometimes require pacing in the event of profound bradycardia that does not respond to medication.

Most pacing in critical care is of a temporary nature, although occasionally permanent systems may be required. Temporary pacing units usually consist of:

- a pulse generator
- pacing leads with electrodes.

Pacing systems may be:

- transvenous
- epicardial
- transcutaneous.

Transvenous pacing

- This type of pacing requires a bipolar venous catheter to be inserted through a large vein.
- The internal jugular and subclavian sites are preferred.
- The tip of the catheter is placed in contact with the endocardium of the right ventricular apex.
- The catheter has a positive proximal electrode and a negative distal electrode.
- These are connected to the respective generator terminals on the pulse generator.
- The pulse generator voltage threshold is set to ensure that pacing is adequate.
- A pacing spike should then be seen before each stimulated complex.

Epicardial pacing

- Pacing leads are placed during surgery on the epicardium.
- This approach is commonly used post cardiothoracic surgery as a temporary measure in the event of post-operative inflammation and complications.
- The wires are connected to an external temporary pulse generator.
- The threshold is set.
- A pacing spike should then be seen before each stimulated complex.
- Wires may be removed externally when they are no longer needed, as directed by the surgeon.

Transcutaneous pacing

- This type of pacing is generally only used in emergency situations.
- Large gel pads are placed directly on the chest wall.
- Normally they are positioned anteriorly to the left of the sternum and posteriorly on the patient's back.
- Transcutaneous pacing may be used to treat bradycardia where the patient is haemodynamically compromised, until another system can be inserted.
- The electrodes need to make good contact with the skin in order for the pacing system to capture effectively (capture refers to successful deporalisation after the pacing impulse has been delivered).
- An on-demand mode should be used in the patient with bradycardia, to prevent possible arrhythmias.
- This type of pacing has the potential to cause discomfort to the patient, so is reserved exclusively for emergency situations.

Overriding arrhythmias

Occasionally pacing may be used to 'override' fast arrhythmias. This involves the doctor setting the pacemaker to a faster rate than the patient's tachycardia (normally 10–15 beats/min faster). It may be used to suppress supraventricular tachycardia, atrial flutter, and ventricular tachycardia. However, it is not effective in suppressing atrial fibrillation or sinus tachycardia.

Chapter 8

Neurological care

Neurological assessment

If an actual or potential neurological abnormality has been identified during a general ABCDE assessment (see ➲ p. 18) or while monitoring the patient, a more detailed and focused neurological assessment can provide further information to guide clinical management.

Focused health history

Subjective information about the neurovascular history can be taken from the patient if they are awake, or from other sources (e.g. family, caregivers, or patient notes).

Neurological symptom enquiry

- Headaches.
- Dizziness.
- Vertigo.
- Fainting.
- Seizures.
- Numbness and tingling.
- Weakness.
- Visual disturbance.
- Hearing loss.
- Tinnitus.
- Balance problems.
- Memory change.
- Loss of sense of smell and/or taste.

Focused physical assessment

- Table 8.1 provides a summary of a neurologically focused assessment, although a full assessment is not relevant for sedated patients, in whom the findings could be potentially misleading.
- Table 8.2 lists the tests that relate to the cranial nerves.
- Only assess sedation level and pupil responses for sedated patients.

Table 8.1 Neurologically focused assessment

Higher functions	Cranial nerves	Motor–sensory
Mentation Speech Gait Coordination	Testing of cranial nerves I–XII (see Table 8.2)	Movement Sensation Reflexes

Mentation

- Assess consciousness:
  - alertness
  - awareness of self and surroundings
  - responsiveness.
- Assess cognition:
  - sensory input
  - orientation to person, place, and time
  - information storage (short- and long-term memory)
  - information processing (judgement, reasoning).
- Use tools and scoring systems such as the GCS (see ➔ p. 246), AVPU, and CAM-ICU (see ➔ p. 21) as appropriate to the clinical context.
- If the patient has long-term mentation dysfunction, consider whether there is further mental and functional decline due to a new and acute neurological abnormality.

Speech

- Clarity.
- Volume.
- Content.
- Ability to express thoughts.

Gait

- Posture—symmetry, ability to stay upright.
- Weight-bearing.
- Gait pattern—normal, limping, shuffling, uncoordinated.
- Head-to-toe gait.

Coordination

- Ask the patient to touch your finger and then to touch their nose.
- Opposition test—thumb tip touches each fingertip individually.
- Rapid alternating movements—flipping hand back and forth on opposite palm.
- Rub heel up and down opposite shin.

Motor–sensory

- Tone:
  - Assess the tonicity of arms and legs through passive movements.
  - Hypotonicity—flaccid muscles.
  - Hypertonicity—rigidity, contractures, spasticity, stiff muscles.
- Power:
  - Arm drift—ability to keep the arms stretched out with palms up and eyes closed.
  - Assess strength against resistance of arms and legs.
- Sensation:
  - Assess the ability to feel light touch without paraesthesia throughout the arms and legs.
  - Assess the ability to identify painful stimuli.

- Reflexes:
  - Assess for the presence of deep tendon reflexes using a tendon hammer—biceps, triceps, supinator, knee, and ankle.
  - Plantar reflex—rub an object from the heel of the foot up the outer edge and across to the big toe (the normal response in adults is downward flexion of the toes).

Table 8.2 Cranial nerve examination

Cranial nerve	Nerve name	Normal function	Tests
I	Olfactory	Smell	Ask if there are problems with smell or taste
II	Optic	Visual acuity Visual fields	Near and distant vision Confrontation test
II III	Optic Oculomotor	Pupils: sense Pupils: react	Pupils—equal, round reactive to light (direct and consensual)
III IV VI	Oculomotor Trochlear Abducens	Eye movements	Follow finger—H shape Check for nystagmus and ptosis
V	Trigeminal	Motor: jaw Sensory: face	Jaw movements Sensation in three facial divisions
VII	Facial	Face movements	Raise eyebrows, close eyes tight, puff cheeks, whistle, smile
VIII	Vestibulocochlear	Hearing Balance	Whisper test (ability to hear whispering) Romberg's test (stand with eyes closed)
IX X	Glossopharyngeal Vagus	Pharynx	Swallowing ability Check uvula is in midline
XI	Spinal accessory	Trapezium Sternocleido-mastoid	Raise shoulders and turn head against resistance
XII	Hypoglossal	Tongue movement	Stick out tongue Move tongue from side to side

Causes of key abnormalities
- Change in level of consciousness and/or cognition.
- Pupil abnormalities.
- Sensation abnormalities.

Laboratory investigations

The following blood and laboratory tests may be useful:
- FBC
- U&E
- LFTs
- clotting
- arterial blood gas analysis, including lactate
- glucose.

Glasgow Coma Scale (GCS)

Appropriate clinical assessment of neurological status provides the nurse with the most sensitive measure of neurological deterioration. The Glasgow Coma Scale (GCS) is the tool generally used by nurses in the UK to assess neurological function.

Unfortunately this tool becomes less reliable when the patient is artificially sedated with medication. However, it is essential that every critical care nurse has an adequate understanding of the GCS and its potential limitations in critical illness. It consists of three assessment areas—eye opening, verbal response, and motor function. Tables 8.3, 8.4, and 8.5 summarize the responses and their associated scores. The maximum possible score is 15 and the minimum possible score is 3.

Table 8.3 GCS: eye opening

Descriptor	Score	How to assess
Spontaneous	4	Eyes open spontaneously when beginning assessment No need to talk or touch the patient to stimulate eye opening
To speech	3	Patient opens their eyes to normal voice No need to raise voice or shout
To pain	2	Patient opens their eyes to painful stimuli. This should be either trapezius squeeze or supraorbital pressure (if the patient has no facial fractures)
None	1	No response

Table 8.4 GCS: verbal response

Descriptor	Score	How to assess
Orientated	5	Patient is orientated to time, place, and person and can therefore specify: • the month and year • where they are • who they are
Confused	4	Patient is unable to specify the above coherently, *but* can talk in sentences. Content may be inaccurate
Inappropriate words	3	Patient utters only occasional words, no sentences noted in speech, may use expletives
Incomprehensible sounds	2	No word formation is noted. Patient may moan, groan, or cry out
None	1	No verbal response; include tracheostomy and endotracheal patients in this category

Table 8.5 GCS: motor response

Descriptor	Score	How to assess
Obeys commands	6	Patient is able to obey a simple commend such as 'Squeeze my hand and let go' or 'Move your fingers.' Best response only is scored. No need to differentiate between left and right
Localizes to pain	5	When painful stimuli are applied to the trapezius muscle, patient moves their hand to above the area to localize the pain source
Flexion to pain	4	Similar to localization, but patient does not move hand above painful stimuli, but there is a movement towards stimuli
Abnormal flexion to pain	3	Patient flexes arm at elbow and rotates wrist simultaneously. Indicative of nerve damage
Extension	2	Represents severe damage at brainstem level. Patient extends or straightens limbs. Arms may be rotated inwards
None	1	No response. May indicate paralysis, deep coma, or drug-induced coma

Teasdale and Jennet[1] designed the GCS to be used alongside other neurological assessments. These include:

- pupil response
- comparative motor assessment
- physiological indicators.

It is important to note that once the patient is sedated the critical care nurse is more reliant on pupil changes and physiological status.

Pupil responses

Pupil changes are attributable to pressure on the third cranial nerve (oculomotor nerve), and normally indicate pressure that may be a result of the early stages of tentorial herniation. Initial changes occur ipsilaterally (on the same side as injury), but later changes are contralateral (on the opposite side to injury). Pupil changes tend to present progressively. Initial and later changes are as follows:

- Pupil shape becomes ovoid.
- Pupil begins to dilate ipsilaterally, *but still reacts to light.*
- Pupil fixes ipsilaterally.
- Contralateral changes occur.

Physiological changes

There is a pattern of physiological changes as intracranial pressure increases. This pattern is referred to as Cushing's triad, and represents the body's attempt to compensate for rising intracranial pressure and the effects of increasing pressure on the brainstem. Changes include:

- hypertension with a widening pulse pressure
- bradycardia caused by midbrain compression
- alterations to respiratory rate (may not be apparent in ventilated patients).

Comparative motor assessment

Motor assessment is part of the GCS, but during GCS assessment 'best motor function' is tested. Comparative motor function testing is observing for differentiation in sides; therefore this test is looking for signs of contralateral weakness or hemiparesis. Contralateral changes occur because the nerve fibres cross over at the decussation of pyramids in the medulla oblongata. Subjective assessment of limb power may be unreliable, so it is normally preferable to use an objective assessment. Details of an objective assessment are shown in Table 8.6.

Other signs of rising intracranial pressure

It is important that the critical care nurse also monitors the patient for other signs that may indicate a rising ICP, including fluid and temperature regulation problems.

Table 8.6 Objective limb assessment tests

Neurological classification	Criteria
Normal power	Patient can match resistance; therefore they are able to hold limb up despite moderate attempts to push limb down
Mild weakness	Patient can hold limb up against mild resistance, but this may be overcome if resistance is increased
Severe weakness	Patient is able to move limb, but not against resistance
Flexion, extension, no power	Tested as in GCS using painful stimuli

Diabetes insipidus

Diabetes insipidus may occur as the intracranial pressure rises. As tentorial herniation begins, pressure increases around the area of the hypothalamus and pituitary gland. Pressure on the posterior part of the pituitary gland inhibits the production of antidiuretic hormone, and massive diuresis occurs. Therefore it is important to observe for any increases in urine output that are not attributable to increased fluid intake (e.g. from volume resuscitation). Synthetic antidiuretic hormone may be administered to prevent hypovolaemia, which would worsen cerebral blood flow and potentially further increase ICP.

Pyrexia

Temperature increases may also reflect increasing pressure on the hypothalamus. However, they may also indicate the presence of infection, so should be viewed alongside the patient's white cell count and other markers of infection.

Reference

1 Teasdale G and Jennett B. Assessment of coma and impaired consciousness: a practical scale. *Lancet* 1974; 2: 81–4.

Monitoring

Alongside assessment of neurological status using the GCS and associated tools, some critically ill patients may require more advanced neurological monitoring. This is especially important once the patient is sedated, as traditional forms of assessment then become less reliable. A number of monitoring tools are available for this. They include:

- intracranial pressure monitoring
- cerebral (brain) oxygen monitoring
- transcranial Doppler monitoring
- electroencephalogram (EEG)
- sedation monitoring.

Intracranial monitoring

Intracranial pressure is the pressure exerted within the cranium by the brain, the blood, and the cerebrospinal fluid. Therefore if one of these three components changes, the pressure within the cranium (i.e. the ICP) will alter. Although the Monro–Kellie hypothesis describes the ability for some compensation to occur, this is relatively limited, so it is important to have an accurate reflection of ICP in some critically ill patients.

Normal ICP

- Normal ICP is generally considered to be < 10 mmHg.
- ICP of > 20 mmHg is normally treated in critical care.
- Prolonged increases in ICP are associated with increased neurological damage and increased mortality rates.

Cerebral perfusion pressure

Although ICP may be useful in the management of the critically ill patient, cerebral perfusion pressure (CPP) may provide a better guide to brain perfusion. CPP is calculated by the monitor if ICP measurement is *in situ*. The calculation generally used is CPP = MAP – ICP. Normal CPP is 70–90 mmHg.

ICP and CPP measurements are normally utilized to:

- diagnose cerebral pressure and perfusion problems
- monitor the effects of medical and nursing interventions on ICP
- enable calculation of CPP
- guide treatment plans.

ICP monitoring

Several types of monitoring tools are available. The gold standard is considered to be ventricular monitoring, where the ICP probe is inserted into the lateral ventricles. The benefit of intraventricular systems is that CSF drainage may be facilitated to reduce an increased ICP.

Other types of ICP monitoring include subdural monitoring and parenchymal monitoring.

Risks associated with ICP measurement include:

- infection
- haemorrhage
- poor positioning
- malfunction
- obstruction.

Brain tissue oxygenation monitoring

The need to monitor brain oxygen levels directly has led to the development of tools that can measure (among other parameters) brain tissue oxygen levels.

These tools provide values for the partial pressure of brain oxygen ($PbtO_2$). This gives more accurate information about oxygen delivery and demand, and may be used to measure local areas of oxygenation within the brain. This may then be utilized to guide therapy.

- Normal $PbtO_2$: 25–50 mmHg.
- Ischaemic $PbtO_2$: < 15 mmHg
- Brain cell death $PbtO_2$: < 5 mmHg.

These monitors are usually 'multimodal', and have the facility to measure local brain temperature and ICP.

When using systems that measure brain oxygenation it is important to remember that this information must be considered alongside other variables to provide a holistic picture of the patient's condition.

Transcranial Doppler

The transcranial Doppler is a non-invasive tool that utilizes ultrasound technology to measure blood velocity in the cerebral arteries (usually the middle cerebral artery, but it can also assess the anterior and posterior cerebral arteries, the ophthalmic artery, and the internal carotid artery).

The Doppler works by emitting a signal from a probe which generates a wavelength signal as it is reflected by the red blood cells. This in turn is converted to a waveform which provides important information about the blood flow in that vessel. The Doppler machine is able to provide information about systolic, diastolic, and mean blood flow velocity. It may be used in several different groups of patients to provide information to guide treatment. Uses include:

- assessment of vasospasm and hyper-perfusion states in patients with subarachnoid haemorrhage and traumatic brain injury
- estimation of cerebral perfusion pressure when invasive monitoring is not or cannot be used
- determination of the adequacy of collateral blood flow during carotid artery surgery
- assessment of embolisms in patients with stroke or transient ischaemic attack (TIA).

Electroencephalograms

The electroencephalogram (EEG) may be a useful tool for highlighting some problems in neurological patients. However, it is important to note that it does require skilled interpretation to determine changes to the patient. Put simply, the EEG measures voltage fluctuations within the brain. This activity is recorded by using surface or needle electrodes and is then converted to a trace on the EEG monitor. Within critical care areas it may be used:

- to monitor cerebral activity
- to monitor patients with epilepsy, especially when muscle relaxants are being used, as these may prevent outward signs of seizure activity
- to confirm the diagnosis of epilepsy
- to help to predict the outcome for a patient in a coma
- as an adjunct in determining brainstem death (not part of the formal process for determining brainstem death in the UK; see Chapter 19)
- to monitor cerebral activity when using barbiturates (thiopental, phenobarbitone, phenobarbital) in head injury patients.

Sedation monitoring

Sedation monitoring may be utilized within critical care to assess the patient's level of sedation. One of the most commonly used tools for sedation monitoring is the Bispectral Index (BIS).

In some neurological patients it may be desirable to keep the patient heavily sedated (especially during the acute phase when ICP management is a significant issue). However, increasingly it is becoming more desirable to keep sedation levels to a minimum to prevent complications associated with over-sedation. Over-sedation within critical care is associated with:

- an increased incidence of ventilator-associated pneumonia
- longer patient stays
- the development of acute delirium.

Traditionally, EEGs have been used in specialist areas to determine brain function, identify burst suppression, and provide an indication of levels of sedation. However, these require specialist interpretation and are time consuming to analyse correctly.

Sedation monitoring was originally used in operating theatres, to ensure that effective levels of sedation were maintained throughout surgical procedures. However, many critical care units now utilize this technology to asses sedation levels in critically ill patients.

Sedation monitoring provides a non-invasive method of assessing objective criteria for the effectiveness of sedation based on the EEG trace.

- For the purpose of simplification, three elements of the EEG trace (amplitude, frequency, and phase) are converted into a numerical value from 0 to 100 (see Box 8.1).
- This removes the need for specialist interpretation, and makes interpretation of the EEG data much easier.
- The numerical value (from 0 to 100) provides an indication of the level of sedation achieved by means of medication.

Measurement of sedation levels by sedation monitoring may therefore be useful for a number of purposes, including:

- avoidance of over-sedation
- monitoring burst suppression in patients with epilepsy
- monitoring burst suppression in patients on barbiturate infusions
- ongoing research into its value as an early prognostic tool for traumatic brain injury.

Box 8.1 BIS numerical values for sedation

100:	Awake
80:	Light or moderate sedation. May respond to loud commands or mild prodding/shaking
60:	General anaesthesia. Unresponsive to verbal stimulus
40:	Deep hypnotic state
20:	Burst suppression
0:	Flat line EEG

However, it is suggested that although sedation monitoring remains a useful indicator, there are a number of factors that may make the readings unreliable.[2] These include:

- interference from other medical devices
- changes induced by some medications
- some neurological pathologies.

Although sedation monitoring does provide some useful data which may enable decisions to be made about sedation levels in critically ill patients, Bigham and colleagues[2] suggest that figures derived from monitoring should not be used in isolation, and that other indicators should also be taken into account.

Reference

2 Bigham C, Bigham S and Jones C. Does the bispectral index monitor have a role in intensive care? *Journal of the Intensive Care Society* 2012; 13: 314–19.

Traumatic brain injury

Definition

Traumatic brain injury occurs when there is damage to the brain as a result of trauma. Trauma may be caused by:

- acceleration injuries, in which a moving object strikes the head
- acceleration and deceleration injuries, in which the head strikes a stationary object
- coup and contrecoup mechanisms of injury, in which the brain moves backward and forward within the cranial cavity
- rotational injuries, in which neurons within the brain are rotated and stretched
- penetration injuries, in which a sharp object penetrates the brain.

Head injuries are classified in several ways. A key classification is into primary and secondary injuries.

- Primary injury occurs at the time of trauma. The effects of primary injury may be irreversible.
- Secondary injury occurs after the initial event and worsens the initial damage. Secondary injury may be caused by hypoxia, hyercapnia, hypotension, infection, ischaemia, cerebral oedema, seizures, or hyperglycaemia. Much of the management of the head-injured patient is geared toward prevention of secondary damage.

Alongside the classification into primary and secondary injuries, head injuries may also be categorized according to the area affected.

- Extradural haematoma—a collection of blood between the skull and the outside of the dura, often as a result of middle cerebral artery laceration. Patients often present with a brief period of lucidity followed by rapid neurological deterioration. The arterial bleed may quickly compromise the patient and cause herniation. Therefore prompt treatment is required.
- Subdural haematoma—a collection of blood between the dura and the arachnoid layer, often caused by tearing of the bridging veins. It may present as an acute, subacute, or chronic injury. It has a worse prognosis than extradural haematoma.
- Contusions—caused by laceration of vessels in the microvasculature, which results in bleeding or bruising into the brain tissue. Cerebral contusions may develop into an intracerebral haematoma.
- Intracerebral or intraparenchymal haematoma—a collection of blood within the parenchyma. It may be caused by trauma or hypertension (stroke), and it can result in delayed neurological deterioration.
- Subarachnoid haemorrhage—a collection of blood within the subarachnoid space. It may be caused by an aneurysm or by tearing of the microvessels in the arachnoid layer as a result of trauma. The patient may require cerebral angiography to exclude an aneurysmal bleed.
- Diffuse axonal injury—caused by tearing of the neuronal axons. It is normally associated with rotational and acceleration–deceleration injury. It usually worsens during the first 12–24 hours. The patient may present in a deep coma with little alteration to the initial CT scan. Later scans may show severe cerebral oedema.

Assessment findings

Patients will present with:

- changes to neurological function noted from in-depth neurological assessment
- deteriorating levels of consciousness (those with a GCS score of < 8 normally require intubation)
- changes on the CT scan
- possible haemodynamic changes (hypertension, bradycardia).

Treatment

Treatment aims to prevent secondary injury and should follow an ABCDE approach.

- The patient's ability to maintain their airway should be assessed.
- The patient should be intubated if the GCS score is < 8.[3]
- Intubation may also be necessary if the patient requires scanning and cannot cooperate due to decreasing levels of consciousness. Intubation might also be deemed necessary for inter-hospital transfer to a specialist centre.
- Adequate respiratory assessment is vital in all patients. This group of patients may be susceptible to aspiration pneumonia, especially if consciousness was lost prior to hospitalization.
- Care should be taken to maintain oxygen saturations above 95%. This may require supplemental oxygen.
- Consideration must be given to other significant injuries that might have an impact on respiratory function.
- If the patient is intubated, mechanical ventilation will be required.
- Arterial blood gases may be manipulated using ventilation. High levels of CO_2 will increase ICP. Low levels will reduce cerebral blood pressure. Normal parameters are usually as follows:
  - PaO_2: 13 kPa
  - $PaCO_2$: 4.5–5 kPa.
- Ventilated patients should have optimum levels of sedation and analgesia to prevent increases in ICP.
- Chest physiotherapy and regular turning are required to reduce the likelihood of chest infection and associated hypoxia. Sedation may be required prior to the commencement of chest physiotherapy. Pre-oxygenation may be required prior to suctioning.
- Patients should be nursed at 30° to avoid VAP.
- Care should be taken with positioning if the patient has a suspected spinal injury.
- Cardiovascular and fluid assessment is required for all patients.
- Continuous cardiac monitoring should be commenced for all patients.
- Fluid replacement may be given to initially increase blood pressure. This should be isotonic in nature, and 5% glucose should be avoided (as it will increase blood glucose levels and potentially cause fluid shifts and/or the development of cerebral oedema).
- Fluid output should be monitored carefully. A sudden increase in output may be suggestive of diabetes insipidus.

- In patients with severe head injury, blood pressure is normally artificially elevated with inotropes to maintain cerebral perfusion pressure. In patients in whom CPP is not recordable (i.e. those without ICP monitoring) it may be desirable to aim for a higher mean blood pressure using inotropic support.
- Temperature should be monitored carefully. Pyrexia will increase oxygen demand and potentially worsen cerebral oedema.
- Manipulation of temperature using therapeutic hypothermia may be required in an attempt to reduce cerebral oedema.
- Blood electrolytes should be closely monitored for signs of abnormalities.
- VTE assessment and prophylaxis will be required.
- Regular neurological assessment using the GCS, pupil size, limb assessment, and cardiovascular changes should be conducted at least hourly for patients with a GCS score of > 9.
- Changes in neurological assessment findings should be escalated immediately.
- In patients who are sedated, neurological assessment will be dependent upon pupil assessment, cardiovascular changes, and potential changes in fluid output. Pupil assessment should be performed at least hourly, or more often if the patient's condition deteriorates.
- Patients should receive appropriate levels of sedation and analgesia. Boluses may be required prior to care delivery, but care should be taken to avoid sudden drug-related hypotension.
- When ICP monitoring is being used, care should be taken to maintain ICP and CPP within set parameters. If the ICP rises, a stepwise approach should be taken to determine the cause of the increase, and appropriate treatment to reduce the ICP should be initiated. Table 8.7 describes a stepwise approach to ICP reduction.
- Medical intervention should be sought if ICP remains elevated despite attempts to reduce it.
- Quick and timely intervention should be provided if ICP remains high. Table 8.8 describes the emergency management of raised ICP.
- Care should be taken to ensure that consideration is given to other injuries that may have resulted from trauma. An advanced trauma life support (ATLS) survey (see ➔ p. 462) should have been conducted in the Emergency Department, and other specialists involved as required.
- Patients will require early establishment of nutritional support. This is likely to be enteral, and care should be taken to avoid nasogastric tube insertion in patients with skull fractures.
- Medication may cause a tendency to constipation, so early assessment of elimination needs and appropriate medication is essential.
- Psychological care and communication should be provided for the patient and their family.
- Pressure area assessment and appropriate interventions will be required.

Table 8.7 Stepwise approach to reducing ICP

Intervention	Rationale
Has pupil assessment changed?	May indicate worsening neurological status. Inform medical team. Consider emergency treatment such as mannitol/hypertonic saline
Has patient position changed?	Patients need to be nursed in neutral alignment to promote venous return from the cerebral circulation. Patient should be nursed at 30° head-up angle (unless contraindicated)
Are the endotracheal tapes too tight? Is the neck collar too tight?	This will restrict venous return and increase ICP
Is the patient showing signs of distress? Is the patient adequately sedated?	Consider increasing sedation to reduce ICP. Take care not to reduce blood pressure as a result of increasing sedatives
Is blood glucose level elevated?	Hyperglycaemia may increase cerebral oedema and should be avoided
Are arterial blood gases within set parameters?	Consider whether recent changes in ventilation have altered CO_2 levels. Liaise with anaesthetists to maintain within set parameters

Table 8.8 Emergency management of raised ICP following consultation with medical staff

Potential intervention	Rationale
Consider drainage of CSF if patient has appropriate ICP-monitoring system	Removal of CSF may reduce ICP. Lumbar puncture is not appropriate, as this may cause tentorial herniation
Manipulate arterial blood gases to reduce CO_2 levels	A reduced CO_2 level may reduce ICP. However, prolonged reduction will have a detrimental effect on cerebral blood and should be avoided
Administer osmotic diuretic	This may provide a short-term solution to cerebral oedema, but care should be taken to avoid hypotension due to fluid depletion. Serum osmolality should be monitored, as this intervention is unlikely to be effective if osmolality is high
Consider therapeutic hypothermia	Lowering the body temperature will reduce cerebral oxygen requirements
Consider barbiturate coma therapy	This may lower ICP, as it reduces cerebral oxygen requirements and may be neuroprotective. It is a longer-term solution, as barbiturate infusions have a long half-life
Consider decompressive craniectomy	Surgical intervention to reduce ICP has been shown to be effective. It is only available in specialist neurosurgical centres

Reference

3 National Institute for Health and Care Excellence (NICE). *Head Injury: triage, assessment, investigation and early management of head injury in children, young people and adults*. CG176. NICE: London, 2014. ℛ www.nice.org.uk/guidance/cg176

Subarachnoid haemorrhage

Definition

A subarachnoid haemorrhage is a collection of blood in the subarachnoid space. It may be caused by trauma (see ➔ p. 460) or be due to bleeding into the subarachnoid space. Bleeding is usually caused by rupture of a cerebral artery aneurysm, but may also be caused by arteriovenous malformation, hypertension, and tumours. At the time of the bleed, blood is forced into the subarachnoid space. Mortality and morbidity remain issues in the management of subarachnoid haemorrhage, and complications include:

- aneurysmal rebleeding
- cerebral vasospasm
- sodium imbalance (syndrome of inappropriate antidiuretic hormone or cerebral salt wasting)
- communicating hydrocephalus.

Assessment

Patients with subarachnoid haemorrhage may present with:

- a violent, sudden 'thunderclap' headache
- signs of cranial nerve dysfunction
- nausea and vomiting
- signs of meningeal irritation (neck stiffness, photophobia, pain in the back and neck, nausea and vomiting)
- neurological dysfunction. This may include:
  - hemiparesis or hemiplegia
  - cognitive deficits
  - speech disturbances
  - deteriorating GCS score
  - Cushing's triad related to cerebral oedema development.

Generally patients will be admitted to critical care if they:

- are at high risk of deterioration
- have a poor-grade aneurysm according to the World Federation of Neurosurgeons Scale (WFNS)[4]
- are presenting with deteriorating neurological function
- are unable to protect their own airway.

The WFNS (alongside other scoring systems)[4] is used to determine the severity of the bleed and to guide treatment and predict morbidity and mortality.

Additional assessments may include:

- CT scan
- CT angiography (CTA)
- MRI scan
- cerebral angiogram
- lumbar puncture (unless there is raised ICP).

Treatment

Definitive treatment is to secure the aneurysm to prevent rebleeding, as the mortality and morbidity rates are high. Statistical data suggest that as many as 30% of patients will rebleed.[5] Treatment may be endovascular or surgical, and includes:

- Guglielmi detachable coils (GDC)
- balloon remodelling
- surgical clipping of the aneurysm.

Following successful intervention to secure the aneurysm, care should be based on an ABCDE approach.

- The patient's ability to maintain an airway should be assessed.
- Generally, if the GCS score is < 8, intubation may be desirable.
- Adequate respiratory assessment is vital in all patients. Breathing may be compromised by the use of analgesia for pain control of the severe headache.
- Care should be taken to maintain oxygen saturations above 95%. This may require supplemental oxygen.
- If the patient is intubated, mechanical ventilation will be required.
- The patient may be at risk of developing neurogenic pulmonary oedema, so careful assessment and chest auscultation are essential.
- Arterial blood gases may be manipulated by the use of ventilation. A usual target gas would be PaO_2 13kPa and normal CO_2 value.
- Sedation and analgesia should be administered to reduce pain and promote patient comfort. Care should be taken not to decrease the blood pressure, as this may reduce cerebral perfusion pressures and increase the likelihood of complications.
- Once the aneurysm has been secured, the patient should be nursed at 30° to increase venous return and avoid VAP.
- Cardiovascular and fluid assessment is required in all patients. Patients are particularly at risk of sodium imbalances, especially hyponatraemia. Syndrome of inappropriate secretion of antidiuretic hormone (SIADH) is dilutional hyponatraemia due to water retention. Cerebral salt wasting (CSW) is hyponatraemia caused by fluid and sodium depletion. Correct diagnosis and treatment of SIADH and CSW are essential, and their symptoms and management are described in Table 8.9.
- Continuous cardiac monitoring should be commenced on all patients.
- Dehydration should be avoided. Fluid replacement should be given to maintain normal blood volume prior to intervention. Usual fluid intake following an aneurysmal bleed would be 3–4 L. This should be isotonic in nature, and 5% glucose should be avoided.
- ECGs may show ST-segment depression. The exact mechanism is not known, but care should be taken to initially eliminate a cardiac cause of ST depression.
- Regular neurological assessment using the GCS, pupil size, limb assessment, and cardiovascular changes should be conducted at least hourly. Early changes may be subtle but require medical attention (e.g. pronator drift).
- Changes in neurological assessment findings should be escalated immediately.

- In patients who are sedated, neurological assessment will be dependent upon pupil assessment, cardiovascular changes, and potential fluid output alterations. Pupil assessment should be performed at least hourly, or more often if the patient's condition deteriorates.
- ICP may be monitored in some critically ill patients. Quick and timely intervention should be provided if ICP remains high.
- Oral nimodipine should be administered to prevent the development of vasospasm.
- Patients should be carefully monitored for signs of vasospasm. There are several potential treatments for vasospasm, including:
  - induced hypertension (caution is needed with cardiac patients)
  - balloon angioplasty
  - intra-arterial vasodilator therapy
  - studies utilizing medication such as clazosentan, IV magnesium, and statins are ongoing.
- Patients should be monitored for signs of the development of communicating hydrocephalus.
- Regular pain assessment and management with appropriate analgesia are paramount.
- VTE assessment and prophylaxis will be required. However, low-molecular-weight heparin is not advisable until the aneurysm has been secured.

Table 8.9 Symptoms and management of SIADH and CSW

SIADH symptoms	CSW symptoms
High CVP	Low CVP
Low serum sodium levels	High urine output
Low urine output	Normal specific gravity
Normal specific gravity	High or normal serum osmolarity
Low serum osmolarity	Variable urine osmolarity
Normal urinary sodium levels	High urinary sodium levels
Absence of peripheral oedema	
SIADH management	**CSW management**
Fluid restriction flowing correct diagnosis of SIADH	Hypertonic saline
Care should be taken to increase the sodium levels slowly to avoid complications of fast correction, such as central pontine myelinolysis.	
During treatment the patient should be monitored closely for signs of cerebral vasospasm or neurological deterioration.	

References

4 Drake CG et al. Report of World Federation of Neurological Surgeons Committee on a universal subarachnoid hemorrhage grading scale. *Journal of Neurosurgery* 1988; **68**: 985–6.

5 Hickey J. *The Clinical Practice of Neurological and Neurosurgical Nursing*, 6th edn. Wolters Kluwer Health/Lippincott Williams & Wilkins: Philadelphia, PA, 2009.

Seizures (status epilepticus)

Definition

Status epilepticus is a clinical term that refers to:
- continuous seizures lasting at least 5 min
- two or more seizures without a period of consciousness between them.

The most common type of status epilepticus is generalized or tonic–clonic seizures. However, it is important to note that other seizure types may fit into this category.

Causes

There are many factors that may cause the patient to develop status epilepticus. These include:
- pre-existing epilepsy
- non-compliance with anticonvulsant therapy
- traumatic brain injury
- subarachnoid haemorrhage or stroke
- CNS infection
- cerebral tumours
- cerebral hypoxia
- metabolic abnormalities
- drug toxicity
- chronic alcoholism.

Assessment

The patient will present with signs of generalized seizures that either:
- are longer than 5 min in duration *or*
- involve no recovery of consciousness between seizures.

Treatment

Management should follow an ABC approach.
- The patient should be positioned lying on their side to maintain their airway.
- An artificial airway may be inserted, *but only if it is possible to do so without injuring the patient*. This will not be possible during the tonic phase of the seizure.
- Patients with refractory status epilepticus may require intubation.
- Suctioning may be required to maintain airway patency.
- High-flow oxygen should be administered.
- Respiration should be assessed, and if no respiration is apparent, appropriate respiratory resuscitation should be commenced.
- Patients who are intubated will require mechanical ventilation.
- Cardiovascular status should be evaluated with an appropriate CVS assessment.
- Intravenous access should be secured.
- IV fluids may be required.
- A neurological assessment should be conducted and the cause of the seizure identified where possible.
- Anti-epileptic drugs should be administered (see Table 8.10).

Table 8.10 Anti-epileptic drugs for status epilepticus, adapted from NICE guidelines[6]

Stage	Anti-epileptic drug
Early	Lorazepam IV (this may be repeated after 10–20 min) If patient normally takes regular anti-epileptic medication this should be administered
Established	The following drugs may be administered: Phenytoin Fosphenytoin Phenobarbital bolus
Refractory	General anaesthesia maintained with midazolam or propofol Thiopental infusion (up to 3 days) EEG monitoring Medication should be continued until 12 h after the last seizure noted on EEG

- It may be necessary to commence:
  - EEG therapy
  - vasopressors to increase ICP
  - ICP monitoring.
- Acidosis should be corrected if present.
- Appropriate critical care support should be provided until the patient is stable.

Reference

6 National Institute for Health and Care Excellence (NICE). *The Epilepsies: the diagnosis and management of the epilepsies in adults and children in primary and secondary care*. CG137. NICE: London, 2012. www.nice.org.uk/guidance/cg137/resources/guidance-the-epilepsies-the-diagnosis-and-management-of-the-epilepsies-in-adults-and-children-in-primary-and-secondary-care-pdf

Guillain–Barré syndrome

Definition

Guillain–Barré syndrome (GBS) is an acute inflammatory neuropathy. There are several subtypes of GBS, including:

- acute inflammatory demyelinating polyneuropathy
- acute motor axonal neuropathy
- acute motor and sensory axonal neuropathy
- Miller Fisher syndrome.

The neuropathy is caused by an acute demyelination process triggered by an autoimmune response. GBS has three phases:

- acute
- plateau
- recovery.

Causes

It is thought that a number of different factors may be responsible for triggering an autoimmune response. These include:

- acute viral illness
- *Campylobacter jejuni* infection
- post vaccination (rare).

Assessment findings

GBS is generally characterized by:

- bilateral motor weakness
- bilateral flaccid paralysis
- areflexia.

Patients may also present with:

- respiratory failure
- dysphagia
- pain
- autonomic dysfunction (arrhythmias, paroxysmal hypertension, urinary retention).

GBS has no effect on:

- levels of consciousness
- cognitive function
- pupillary signs.

Treatment

Treatment is largely supportive in nature, but patients may receive high-dose intravenous immunoglobulin or plasmapheresis in an attempt to shorten the duration of the illness. Intravenous immunoglobulin (IVIG) is usually the treatment of choice as it is easier to administer. Plasmapheresis may be undertaken in specialist centres. Supportive treatment will follow an ABCDE approach.

- Respiratory assessment is vital to detect early signs of respiratory failure.

- Tracheal intubation may be indicated if:
  - bulbar function is compromised
  - forced vital capacity is deteriorating
  - the patient is showing signs of respiratory failure or tiring.
- Early insertion of a tracheostomy is normally indicated to promote patient comfort and reduce the use of sedatives. Later the tracheostomy will be useful for facilitating weaning.
- Respiratory assessment is needed to monitor for complications of intubation, such as VAP.
- Careful CVS assessment should be undertaken to monitor for signs of autonomic dysfunction.
- Treatment for paroxysmal hypertension is not normally required.
- Fluid may be required to treat any hypotensive episodes.
- The patient may be prone to postural hypotension.
- Monitor for signs of arrhythmias (bradycardia or tachycardia).
- Careful fluid balance should be maintained.
- Excessive fluid loss from diaphoresis may require replacement.
- Neurological assessment is needed to determine signs of deteriorating or improving neurological function.
- Careful pain assessment is required, as the patient may experience severe pain. Often this may be neurogenic in nature and require appropriate neurogenic medication such as nortriptyline, amitriptyline, or pregabalin. Other analgesics such as paracetamol and non-steroidal anti-inflammatory drugs may be useful, although sometimes pain is refractory to these and stronger analgesia may be required.
- Perform careful assessment of the limbs to prevent secondary complications. Regular physiotherapy is essential. The patient may require limb splints or supports to promote normal posture and prevent complications.
- Sleep patterns should be monitored. Sleep deprivation may be caused by alterations to sleep pattern resulting from autonomic changes.
- Psychological support is essential, as the patient will be ventilated yet cognitively intact. As a result they often appear to be extremely anxious and agitated. The nurse's visible presence and positive reinforcement about the potential for recovery are essential.
- The patient should be referred to a speech and language therapist for support with communication.
- VTE assessment and appropriate prophylaxis are required.
- All necessary supportive care should be provided (see Chapter 3).

The patient should be monitored carefully for complications, which may include:

- urinary retention
- constipation
- paralytic ileus
- postural hypotension
- autonomic disturbances.

Myasthenia gravis

Definition

Myasthenia gravis is a chronic disease of the neuromuscular junction caused by an autoimmune response that destroys and therefore reduces the number of acetylcholine receptor sites at the postsynaptic membrane.

The severity of the myasthenia depends upon the number of sites destroyed. A decrease in the number of receptor sites will affect muscle contraction. This may result in some degree of muscle weakness, severe muscle weakness, or muscle fatigue.

The course of the illness is extremely variable, and in some patients muscle weakness may develop over a period of time, whereas others may present with rapid deterioration of muscle function.

When the intercostal muscles are affected, the patient develops dyspnoea and may require ventilation.

Diagnosis

Diagnosis is dependent upon:
- patient history and physical examination
- positive edrophonium test
- antibody titre for acetylcholine receptor
- repetitive muscle stimulation
- electromyography (EMG)
- MRI and/or CT scan of the thymus gland.

Causes

The exact cause of myasthenia gravis is uncertain. It is known to be caused by an autoimmune reaction, but it is not clear what triggers the autoimmune response. Studies have shown that a high proportion of patients with myasthenia gravis have an enlarged thymus gland or a thymus tumour.

Assessment findings

The patient will present with muscle weakness and fatigue. In myasthenia gravis, patients may develop gradual onset, the severity of which is classified from type 0 to 5. Patients are normally admitted to critical care units if they have any of the following:
- a myasthenic crisis (a sudden relapse of myasthenic symptoms)
- a cholinergic crisis (an event precipitated by the toxic effects of cholinergic inhibitor drugs used for the treatment of myasthenia)
- thymectomy for post-operative observation.

Patients with a myasthenic crisis will present with symptoms of:
- decreased bulbar functioning
- decreased function of the muscles of ventilation (intercostal and diaphragm)
- decreased muscle use in all muscles.

Therefore patients will have symptoms that include:
- increasing general weakness
- severe fatigue
- dysphagia
- neck muscle weakness
- respiratory muscle weakness

- decreased vital capacity
- respiratory failure.

Patients with a cholinergic crisis will typically present with:

- initial gastronintestinal problems such as cramping and diarrhoea (muscarinic effects)
- later signs (nicotinic effects) that are rapid in nature, and include:
  - severe muscle weakness
  - increased pulmonary secretions
  - acute respiratory failure.

A edrophonium test may be used to distinguish between myasthenic and cholinergic crises. However, if the patient is unable to cooperate it may not be appropriate. The edrophonium test should only be performed by a skilled healthcare professional, and atropine (antidote to edrophonium) must be available.

Treatment

Treatment is largely supportive in nature, but medical treatments may be given to reduce the time required in critical care.

Treatments for myasthenic crisis include the following:

- Immunosuppression—steroids and other immunosuppressant drugs may be given. Prednisolone is normally the drug of choice. It is normally given until the patient starts to show signs of improvement, and then gradually weaned to a maintenance dose. Azathioprine is usually given if prednisolone is contraindicated.
- Plasmapheresis or IVIG may be given. Plasmapheresis is usually only undertaken in specialist centres. IVIG is generally the treatment of choice as it is easier to administer.

Supportive care will utilize an ABCDE approach:

- In severely ill patients, priority is given to airway and respiratory assessment to determine the need for intubation and ventilation.
- An in-depth respiratory assessment including forced vital capacity should be undertaken.
- The quality of the patient's voice may also indicate the degree of deterioration.
- Intubation may be required if the patient has worsening bulbar function.
- Assessment for signs of aspiration pneumonia is important, especially in patients with decreased bulbar function.
- Cardiovascular assessment is necessary to determine the effect of the deterioration on CVS function.
- Fluid should be given to ensure that the patient remains hydrated.
- Accurate fluid balance should be noted.
- Neurological assessment is needed to determine the effects of the crisis on normal functioning. This may include:
  - assessment of motor function and strength in limbs
  - extra-ocular muscle assessment
  - head and neck strength
  - quality of voice (if extubated).
- Medication should be reviewed. Anticholinergic drugs should be given in the event of a myasthenic crisis, but withheld and gradually reintroduced in the event of a cholinergic crisis.
- VTE assessment and appropriate prophylaxis are required.
- All supportive care should be provided (see Chapter 3).

Meningitis

Definition

Meningitis is acute inflammation of the meninges caused by an infectious agent. It involves the pia and arachnoid layers of the meninges, the subarachnoid space, and the CSF within the subarachnoid space. Causative bacterial organisms include:

- *Streptococcus pneumoniae*
- *Neisseria meningitidis*
- *Haemophilus influenzae*
- *Listeria monocytogenes*.

Patients may also develop viral meningitis, but this is often a mild form and very rarely requires admission to critical care. Most patients who are admitted to critical care will present with bacterial meningitis. The mortality rate for bacterial meningitis remains high, and many patients who survive are left with significant morbidities, including hydrocephalus, deafness, blindness, cognitive deficits, and epilepsy.

Causes

Meningitis occurs when bacteria gain access to the meninges. This may result from contamination through:

- blood-borne routes
- spread of nearby infection (e.g. ear or sinus infection)
- CSF contamination during medical or surgical procedures (e.g. lumbar puncture, ICP monitoring).

Assessment findings

The initial signs of meningitis are associated with meningeal irritation, and include:

- severe headache
- stiff neck
- signs of meningeal irritation
- altered level of consciousness
- photophobia
- nausea and vomiting
- hypersensitivity
- seizures
- changes in electrolyte levels (especially sodium).

Later signs of meningitis are linked to increasing ICP and the development of sepsis. Signs of increasing ICP include:

- hypertension
- bradycardia
- changes to respiration.

Signs of sepsis include:

- raised body temperature (> 38°C)
- increased white cell count
- increased C-reactive protein levels
- increased serum lactate levels
- blood pressure changes, which may initially be masked by rising ICP.

Different types of meningitis may have noteworthy signs and symptoms.

Meningococcal meningitis

- Rapid deterioration of neurological status.
- Petechial rash.
- Areas of ecchymosis or skin discolouration.

Diagnosis

This may include:

- patient history
- lumbar puncture (contraindicated if ICP is rising)
- CT scan
- markers of infection and inflammation
- blood culture.

Treatment

Bacterial meningitis is a medical emergency and prompt intervention is needed. Patients require immediate treatment with intravenous antibiotics, and local protocols will dictate which antibiotics are used. Administration of antibiotic therapy should *not* be delayed until the results of CSF and blood cultures are known. The suspected causative organism should be treated with appropriate antibiotics until definitive results are available.

It may be necessary to isolate the patient to prevent the spread of the disease. Close family members and recent contacts may require prophylactic antibiotics. Hospital infection control policies should be followed in relation to isolation procedure, and appropriate advice provided to family members and recent contacts.

The management of patients with severe meningitis is complex, and requires collaborative assessment and management. Care planning should take into account the possible complications of:

- increased ICP
- rapidly deteriorating neurological status
- onset of severe sepsis
- respiratory failure
- seizures
- electrolyte imbalance
- hydrocephalus
- possible adrenal insufficiency (meningococcal infections).

Supportive care should adopt an ABCDE approach (see also ➔ p. 330 if the patient is presenting with signs of sepsis).

- The patient's ability to maintain their airway should be assessed.
- It is likely that the patient will require intubation and ventilation.
- Ventilation management should follow sepsis protocols (see ➔ p. 340).
- Manipulation of ventilation may be required to control ICP (see ➔ p. 251).
- The patient should be nursed with their head elevated to 30° to minimize the risk of VAP and reduce ICP.
- Regular respiratory assessment is needed to determine the impact of sepsis on the respiratory system.

- Regular chest physiotherapy is required to prevent complications associated with intubation.
- Cardiovascular and fluid assessment is required in all patients.
- Continuous cardiac monitoring should be commenced in all patients.
- Blood pressure should be carefully maintained within prescribed parameters with initial fluid resuscitation and/or vasopressors.
- Fluid balance should be closely monitored, and fluid resuscitation should follow sepsis guidelines if there is evidence of development of sepsis (see ➲ p. 339).
- If the patient is pyrexial, antipyretic medication should be given (once blood cultures have been taken) to reduce the body temperature and cerebral oxygen requirements.
- Assessment for disseminated intravascular coagulation (DIC) and other clotting abnormalities may be required.
- Regular neurological assessment using the GCS and limb assessment should be undertaken if appropriate. If the patient is sedated, ventilated pupil changes and other physiological signs of rising ICP should be noted.
- Changes in neurological assessment findings should be escalated immediately.
- In patients who are sedated, neurological assessment will be dependent upon pupil assessment, cardiovascular changes, and potential changes in fluid output. Pupil assessment should be performed at least hourly, or more often if the patient's condition deteriorates.
- Patients should receive appropriate levels of sedation and analgesia.
- Where ICP monitoring is being utilized, care should be taken to maintain ICP and CPP within set parameters. If ICP rises, a stepwise approach should be taken to determine the cause of the increase, and appropriate treatment to reduce ICP should be initiated.
- Medical intervention should be sought if ICP remains elevated despite attempts to reduce it.
- The patient should be assessed for signs of pain, and appropriate analgesia provided.
- Reduced lighting may be required if the patient has severe photophobia.
- All necessary supportive care should be provided (see Chapter 3).

Delirium

Definition

Delirium may be defined as an acute fluctuating disturbance of consciousness and cognition. Delirium generally develops over a short period of time and fluctuates over time. It is thought to occur in up to 80% of critically ill patients.

There are two main subtypes of delirium:

- hypoactive—characterized by withdrawal, lack of response, and apathy
- hyperactive—characterized by restlessness, agitation, and labile emotions.

Delirium may also exhibit mixed presentation—that is, both hypo- and hyperactive. This type is more difficult to identify in practice.[7]

Causes

A number of theories have been proposed to explain the pathophysiological development of delirium, including:

- neurotransmitter imbalance
- inflammatory processes
- cerebral oxygenation or metabolism
- amino acid concentration.

However, the exact pathophysiological cause is not yet known.

Risk factors have been identified, and these may be divided into host factors and illness factors (see Table 8.11).

Table 8.11 Risk factors for the development of delirium

Host factors	Illness factors
Age > 70 years	Acidosis
Substance misuse	Anaemia
Cognitive impairment	Fever, infection, sepsis
Depression	Hypotension
Hypertension	Metabolic dysfunction
Smoking	Respiratory disease
Visual impairment	High degree of severity of illness
Hearing impairment	Immobility
Alcohol abuse	Medications
Recreational drug abuse	Sleep deprivation
	Post-operative
	Increased bilirubin levels
	Increased urea levels
	Use of physical restraints

Assessment findings

Patients with delirium may present with:

- impaired concentration
- slow responses
- confusion
- visual and/or auditory hallucinations
- restlessness
- agitation
- sleep disturbances
- lack of cooperation
- withdrawal
- mood disturbances
- altered communication.

Most clinical areas will use an assessment tool such as the Confusion Assessment Method (CAM) (see ➔ p. 21). In critical care areas it is more helpful to use the CAM-ICU to help to confirm the diagnosis.

Treatment

Initial treatment should focus on trying to establish the cause of delirium. It is helpful to rule out obvious causes of delirium, such as:

- acute infection
- neurological causes (e.g. cerebral oedema)
- electrolyte disturbances
- metabolic abnormalities
- renal impairment
- medication side effects
- alcohol withdrawal.

Management will then focus on preventing harm to the patient and developing effective communication strategies.

Prevention of harm may require:

- verbal de-escalation processes
- non-verbal de-escalation processes
- management of psychosis.

Communication and reorientation strategies may include:

- regular reorientation to time, place, and person
- contact with familiar people (family and friends), photos, and other significant objects
- minimizing confusing stimuli
- reducing isolation
- correcting visual and hearing impairments
- use of clearly visible clocks
- early mobilization
- attempts to maintain circadian rhythm
- avoiding the use of physical restraints.

It may be necessary to medicate patients who are at risk of harm if other strategies fail. NICE[7] recommends the short-term use of medications such as haloperidol or olanzapine. They advise that medication, if required, is started at the lowest clinically appropriate dose and titrated cautiously according to symptoms.

Reference

7 National Institute for Health and Care Excellence (NICE). *Delirium: diagnosis, prevention and management*. CG103. NICE: London, 2010. www.nice.org.uk/guidance/cg103

Further reading

Brummel NE and Girard TD. Preventing delirium in the intensive care unit. *Critical Care Clinics* 2013: 29: 51–65.
www.icudelirium.org
www.icudelirium.co.uk

Chapter 9

Renal care

Acute kidney injury (AKI)

Acute kidney injury (AKI) can be defined as a rapid reduction in renal function (within 48 h) resulting in a failure to maintain fluid, electrolyte, and acid–base balance. The clinical outcomes of AKI include increased length of stay, critical care admission, higher mortality, and long-term dialysis. A worse outcome is linked to post-admission AKI.

AKI is usually associated with *oliguria*, which is due to a sudden and sustained drop in renal perfusion causing the glomerular filtration rate (GFR) to fall, resulting in a decrease in urine output. The kidneys are highly susceptible to ischaemia and/or toxins. The resultant vasoconstriction, endothelial injury, and inflammatory changes contribute to loss of glomerular or tubular function, interstitial oedema, and reabsorption of toxins.

Causes of acute kidney injury

Pre-renal conditions

These are conditions that decrease blood flow to the renal artery.

- **Hypovolaemia**—for example, haemorrhage, burns, gastrointestinal losses, excessive diuresis, and third spacing (ascites, pancreatitis).
- **Hypotension**—low cardiac output states, such as myocardial dysfunction, arrhythmias, valvular dysfunction, and obstructive states (pulmonary embolus, pericardial tamponade).
- **Sepsis**—septic changes to renal vasculature lead to reduced GFR despite increased cardiac output. Septic AKI has a greater likelihood of recovery compared with non-septic causes of AKI.

Intra-renal conditions

These are conditions that produce a direct ischaemic or toxic effect.

- **Hepatorenal syndrome**—seen in advanced cirrhosis without significant glomerular or tubular abnormalities.
- **Cortical necrosis**—nephrotic syndrome, renal artery occlusion or thrombosis, glomerulonephritis, vasculitis (see ➲ p. 378).
- **Acute tubular necrosis**—nephrotoxins (e.g. radiographic contrast, aminoglycosides, rhabdomyolysis).
- **Acute interstitial nephritis**—drugs including penicillins and NSAIDs.
- **Vascular**—emboli.

Post-renal conditions

These are conditions that hinder urine flow to the remainder of the urinary tract.

- **Raised intra-abdominal pressure**—impedes renal venous drainage.
- **Intra-ureteral conditions**—calculi, tumour, blood clot.
- **Extra-ureteral conditions**—retroperitoneal fibrosis, tumour, aneurysm.
- **Bladder obstruction**—prostatic hypertrophy, bladder tumour, blood clot, calculi, functional neuropathy.
- **Urethral obstruction**—stricture, phimosis, blocked urinary catheter.

Specific disorders associated with AKI

Acute glomerulonephritis

This refers to a specific set of renal diseases in which an immunological mechanism ...

Causes of acute glomerulonephritis

Systemic causes

- Wegener's granulomatosis—necrotizing vasculitis affecting small- and medium-sized vessels of the kidney, lung, and nasopharynx.
- Collagen vascular diseases (e.g. SLE) ... renal deposition of immune complexes.
- Hypersensitivity vasculitis—often associated with ...
- Polyarteritis nodosa ...
- Henoch–Schönlein purpura ...
- Goodpasture's syndrome ...
- Drug-induced ...
- Cryoglobulinaemia ...

Infectious causes

- ... endocarditis ...
- ...

Renal diseases

- Berger's disease—IgA glomerulonephritis ...
- Membranoproliferative glomerulonephritis ...
- Idiopathic rapidly progressive glomerulonephritis.

Hepatorenal syndrome

...

Specific disorders associated with AKI

Acute glomerulonephritis

This refers to a specific set of renal diseases in which an immunological mechanism triggers inflammation and proliferation of glomerular tissue. This can result in damage to the basement membrane or capillary endothelium. Sudden-onset haematuria, oliguria, and proteinuria accompany renal dysfunction. Granular red cell casts are present in the urine. Clinically it is associated with hypertension and peripheral oedema.

Causes of acute glomerulonephritis

Systemic causes

- **Wegener's granulomatosis**—necrotizing vasculitis affecting small and medium-sized vessels in the kidneys, lungs, and nasal cartilage.
- **Collagen vascular diseases** (e.g. systemic lupus erythematosus)—causes renal deposition of immune complexes.
- **Hypersensitivity vasculitis**—often associated with eosinophilia.
- **Polyarteritis nodosa**—causes vasculitis of the renal arteries.
- **Henoch–Schönlein purpura**—causes generalized vasculitis.
- **Goodpasture's syndrome**—antibodies to type IV collagen may rapidly result in oliguric renal failure and haemoptysis.
- **Drug-induced** (e.g. gold, penicillamine).
- **Cryoglobulinaemia**—abnormally high plasma levels of cryoglobulin.

Post-infectious causes

- **Group A streptococcal infection** (e.g. sore throat, upper respiratory tract infection)—usually occurs 1 week or more after the acute infection.
- **Other specific agents**—other bacteria, fungi, viruses, and parasites (e.g. malaria, filariasis), and atypicals (e.g. Legionnaire's disease).

Renal diseases

- **Berger's disease**—immunoglobulin-related nephropathy due to deposition of IgA and IgG.
- **Membranoproliferative glomerulonephritis**—deposition of complement causes expansion and proliferation of mesangial cells.
- **Idiopathic rapidly progressive glomerulonephritis.**

Hepatorenal syndrome

This is the development of AKI in patients with chronic liver disease presenting with ascites and portal hypertension. It may be caused by alterations in splanchnic circulatory tone and renal blood supply. The renin–angiotensin–aldosterone and sympathetic nervous systems are activated with profound renal vasoconstriction. It is associated with a high mortality. Liver transplantation is the definitive treatment, with normalization of renal function occurring soon after the transplant. Risk factors include:

- infection (e.g. bacterial peritonitis)
- acute alcoholic hepatitis
- large-volume paracentesis without albumin replacement
- gastrointestinal and variceal bleeding.

Rhabdomyolysis

This is the breakdown of striated muscle, resulting in release of myoglobin, which causes a combination of pre-renal, nephrotoxic, and obstructive renal failure.

Causes

- Direct trauma, crush injury, or burns.
- Muscle compression from prolonged immobility (e.g. surgery, coma).
- Metabolic illness (e.g. diabetic metabolic decompensation).
- Myositis or excessive muscle activity.
- Temperature extremes.
- Toxins—alcohol, solvents, drug abuse.
- Muscular dystrophies.

Substances released by damaged muscle

- Potassium, leading to hyperkalaemia, which may be resistant to glucose and insulin therapy and require urgent haemodialysis or haemodiafiltration (dialysis is more effect than filtration alone).
- Hydrogen ions, leading to metabolic acidosis (see ➔ p. 34).
- Phosphate, leading to hyperphosphataemia.
- Creatine, leading to elevated creatinine kinase activity (usually > 5000 IU/L).
- Myoglobin, leading to myoglobinuria; myoglobin is oxidized by hydroperoxides in the kidney, generating potent oxidizing ferryl-myoglobin. This is nephrotoxic, especially with coexisting acidosis and volume depletion, as it can obstruct renal tubules.

Management

- Maintain an effective circulating volume to meet perfusion needs (e.g. to ensure high urine output).
- Forced alkaline diuresis, with 6–10 L fluid/day to maintain urine pH > 6 using 1.24% sodium bicarbonate. Alkalinization stabilizes the oxidized form of myoglobin.
- Treat hyperkalaemia.
- Renal replacement therapy may be needed if AKI is established.
- Compartment syndrome may require treatment (referral to surgeons is needed) with decompression fasciotomy.
- Avoid NSAIDs and use opiate analgesia.
- Treat the underlying cause.

Further reading

Bagshaw S et al. Acute kidney injury in critical illness. *Canadian Journal of Anaesthesia* 2010; 57: 985–98.

Clec'h C et al. Multiple-center evaluation of mortality associated with acute kidney injury in critically ill patients: a competing risks analysis. *Critical Care* 2011; **15**: R128.

National Confidential Enquiry into Patient Outcome and Death (NCEPOD). *Acute Kidney Injury: adding insult to injury* NCEPOD: London, 2009. www.ncepod.org.uk/2009aki.htm

Identification and detection of AKI

Investigate by measuring serum creatinine concentration and comparing it with baseline values in *any* adult with acute illness if any of the following are likely or present:

- chronic kidney disease (adults with an estimated GFR of < 60 mL/min/1.73 m^2 are at particular risk)
- heart failure
- liver disease
- diabetes
- history of AKI
- oliguria (urine output < 0.5 mL/kg/h)
- neurological or cognitive impairment, which may mean limited access to fluids due to reliance on a carer
- hypovolaemia
- use of drugs with nephrotoxic potential (NSAIDs, aminoglycosides, ACE inhibitors, angiotensin II receptor antagonists, and diuretics) within the past week, especially if hypovolaemic
- use of iodinated contrast agents within the past week
- symptoms or history of urological obstruction, or conditions that may lead to obstruction
- sepsis
- deteriorating NEWS score
- age 65 years or over.

Urinalysis

Perform urine dipstick testing for blood, protein, leucocytes, nitrites, and glucose in all patients as soon as AKI is suspected or detected.

Assess the risk of AKI in adults before surgery. Be aware that increased risk is associated with emergency surgery, especially when the patient has sepsis or hypovolaemia, intraperitoneal dialysis, or chronic kidney injury. When adults are at risk of AKI, ensure that systems are in place to recognize and respond to oliguria.

Prevention

- Maintain effective blood pressure—MAP > 65 mmHg or patient specific, give inotropes as required.
- Maintain effective circulating volume—monitor fluid status, give IV fluids as required; avoid hydroxyethyl starches.
- Maintain effective cardiac output—monitor cardiac output and end-organ perfusion, give inotropes as required.
- Caution is needed with nephrotoxic medications—withhold or adjust the dose.

Detection of AKI

Detection of AKI is based on serum creatinine levels and urine output. The latest 2012 classification is from Kidney Disease Improving Global Outcomes (KDIGO),[1] which builds on the RIFLE and the AKIN criteria (see Table 9.1).

Table 9.1 AKI classification

Stage	Serum creatinine (within 48 h)	Urine output
1 Risk	Increase by ≥ 26 µmol/L *or* 1.5–1.9 times baseline	< 0.5 mL/kg/h for 6 h
2 Injury	2–2.9 times baseline	< 0.5 mL/kg/h for 12 h
3 Failure	Increase by ≥ 44 µmol/L *or* 3 times baseline	< 0.3 mL/kg/h for 24 h *or* anuria for 12 h

Reference

1 KDIGO. KDIGO clinical practice guideline for acute kidney injury. *Kidney International Supplements* 2012; 2 (Suppl.): 1–138.

Further reading

National Institute for Health and Care Excellence (NICE). *Acute Kidney Injury: prevention, detection and management of acute kidney injury up to the point of renal replacement therapy*. CG169. NICE: London, 2013. www.nice.org.uk/guidance/cg169/resources/guidance-acute-kidney-injury-pdf

Management of AKI

Airway and breathing

- Monitor respiratory rate and pattern (Kussmaul breathing is a pattern of rapid deep respirations that may develop secondary to acidosis).
- Monitor arterial blood gases.
- Respiratory failure, necessitating endotracheal intubation and ventilation, may develop secondary to:
  - deterioration in conscious level (secondary to uraemia)
  - pulmonary oedema (secondary to fluid overload).

Circulation

- Continuous monitoring, including ECG, CVP, and also cardiac output if necessary.
- Maintain adequate circulating volume, blood pressure, and cardiac output.
- Treat arrhythmias (secondary to hyperkalaemia).
- Monitor K^+ levels—treat hyperkalaemia promptly with 10 mL of 10% calcium gluconate to stabilize the myocardium, followed by 50 mL of 50% glucose containing 10 units of soluble insulin infused over 30 min and if necessary oral calcium resonium.

Fluid balance

- Monitor fluid input and output hourly. Avoid fluid overload.
- Suspect catheter blockage if sudden oligoanuria develops, and exclude by bladder irrigation and/or replacement of catheter. In patients with nephrostomies, stents, or urostomies, rule out the possibility of obstruction. In patients post-surgery or trauma, consider the possibility of blood clots causing obstruction, an anastomotic leak, or ureteric rupture.
- If obstruction has been excluded and the patient remains oliguric, optimize the circulating volume by giving a fluid challenge.
- Consider loop diuretics (e.g. furosemide) only to manage fluid overload or oedema, not just diuresis.
- If the circulating fluid volume has been optimized and the patient remains oliguric, fluid intake should be restricted to replace urine output and insensible losses only, and renal replacement therapy should be considered.

Nutrition

The patient with AKI is often catabolic, and nutrition should be commenced as soon as possible. Enteral nutrition is preferable to parenteral, as it has fewer complications (e.g. line-related sepsis) and maintains gut integrity. Special consideration should be given to the following:

- use of higher-concentration feeds if fluid restriction is required
- amino acid losses occur with haemofiltration
- B-group vitamins are water soluble and can be removed during renal replacement therapy
- electrolytes and trace elements should be administered either routinely or according to blood levels.

Other considerations

- Drug dosages or timings may need to be adjusted if they are renally excreted (e.g. penicillins, aminoglycosides, digoxin). A pharmacist should be consulted and blood levels measured.
- If the patient is anuric, remove the urethral catheter to reduce the risk of infection.

Renal replacement therapy: basic principles

Indications for renal replacement therapy

- Metabolic acidosis: pH < 7.3.
- Hyperkalaemia: > 6 mmol/L.
- Fluid overload.
- Pulmonary oedema.
- Severe uraemic symptoms: encephalopathy, pericarditis.
- Elevated urea (> 30 mmol/L) and creatinine (> 300 μmol/L).
- Clearance of nephrotoxins or other toxins.

Aims of renal replacement therapy

Discuss any potential indications for renal replacement therapy with the nephrologist and/or critical care specialist and the patient or carer. Include discussion and agreement on the escalation and ceiling of treatment, and the benefits and risks of commencing treatment.

The filter pore sizes are around 30 000 daltons. Molecules of low molecular weight (> 500 daltons) will pass freely through the filter, intermediate-molecular-weight molecules will move by diffusion or convection, and high-molecular-weight molecules will be retained. This will determine which if any molecules will require replacement or addition to the replacement fluid or dialysate (see Table 9.2).

Table 9.2 Molecular weight and solute removal guide

Molecule	Molecular weight in daltons
Sodium	33
Calcium	40
Urea	60
Creatinine	113
Uric acid	168
Dextrose	180
Vitamin B_{12}	1352
Myoglobin	17 000
Albumin	68 000
Globulin	150 000

Medications removed by renal replacement therapy

Drugs that are removed are those unbound to protein and those with a low molecular weight. They include:

- lithium
- methanol
- ethylene glycol
- salicylates
- barbiturates
- metformin
- aminoglycosides, metronidazole, carbapenems, cephalosporins, and most penicillins.

Medications not removed by renal replacement therapy

These include:

- digoxin
- tricyclics
- phenytoin
- gliclazide
- beta blockers (except atenolol)
- benzodiazepines
- macrolide and quinilone antibiotics
- warfarin.

Types of renal replacement therapy

- Continuous venovenous haemofiltration (CVVH).
- Continuous venovenous haemodialysis (CVVHD).
- Continuous venovenous haemodiafiltration (CVVHDF).
- Intermittent haemodialysis (IHD).
- Slow continuous ultrafiltration (SCUF).

A double-lumen cannula is inserted into a large vein (e.g. internal jugular, femoral, or subclavian vein). Blood is drawn from the patient through one lumen, while blood is simultaneously returned through the other lumen. This lumen enters the vein more proximally to prevent recirculation (see Figure 9.1). The therapy is continuous over a 24-h period to allow for gentle removal of fluid and solutes without causing dramatic fluid shifts or cardiovascular instability.

Physiological principles

Diffusion

- This is movement of solutes across a semi-permeable membrane from a high solute concentration to a low solute concentration (i.e. movement down a concentration gradient).
- Diffusion occurs when blood flows on one side of the filter membrane, and there is counter-current flow of dialysate solution on the other side.
- It is a passive transport mechanism, so is less predictable than convection in terms of solute clearance.
- Diffusion is affected by the resistance of the membrane, which is related to its thickness and the size and shape of the pores.
- Diffusion is utilized in haemodialysis and haemodiafiltration.

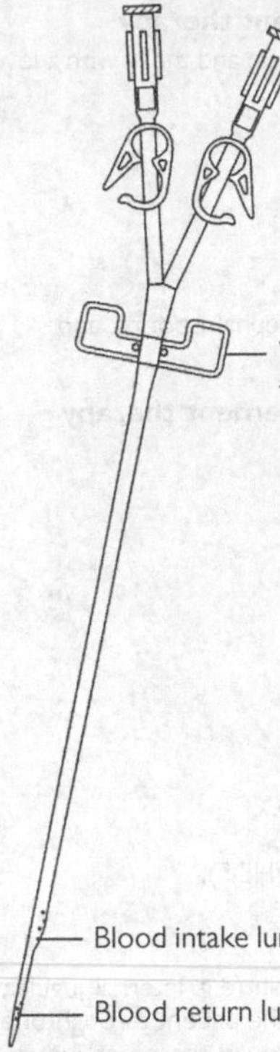

Figure 9.1 Vascular catheter for renal replacement therapy. (Reproduced from Adam SK and Osborne S, *Critical Care Nursing: science and practice*, Second Edition, 2005, with permission from Oxford University Press.)

Ultrafiltration

- This is the movement of fluid across a semi-permeable membrane under hydrostatic pressure.
- The hydrostatic pressure is generated to push water and small molecules across the semi-permeable membrane.
- Fluid removal occurs mainly by ultrafiltration, and minimal solute clearance occurs by convection during ultrafiltration.
- Ultrafiltration is utilized in haemofiltration and slow continuous ultrafiltration.

Convection

- This is the movement of fluid across a semi-permeable membrane by creating a solute drag.
- The pressure difference between the blood and the ultrafiltrate filters water, causing solvent drag as molecules move across the membrane with the water.
- It is an active transport mechanism, so solute clearance is predictable for a given amount of therapy and dependent on the substitution fluid flow rate.
- Solute clearance is affected by the amount of ultrafiltration, the solute concentration of plasma, and the size and shape of pores in the membrane.
- Convection is utilized in haemofiltration and haemodiafiltration.

Buffers (replacement fluid)

- To treat metabolic acidosis a buffer must be provided in either the dialysate fluid or the replacement fluid for haemofiltration.
- Lactate is commonly used as the buffer for haemofiltration, and is metabolized to bicarbonate in the liver. Excess lactate can cause a metabolic alkalosis, so a replacement fluid with a lower lactate content should be used. Conversely, in liver failure the lactate will not be metabolized, so serum lactate levels will increase.
- Bicarbonate itself can be used as a buffer for renal replacement therapy, but cannot be given with calcium because of the risk of chalk formation.

Pre-dilution

Replacement fluid is added to blood before passing through the filter.

Advantages

- It dilutes the blood, preventing an increase in haematocrit.
- It reduces the clotting risk.
- It increases filter-membrane efficiency.

Disadvantages

- It decreases the concentration of solutes removed.
- It decreases the clearance rate.

Post-dilution

Replacement fluid is added to blood after passing through the filter.

Advantages

- It increases the concentration of solutes removed.
- It increases the clearance rate.

Disadvantages

- It increases the haematocrit.
- It increases the clotting risk.
- It decreases filter-membrane efficiency.

Mixed dilution (i.e. pre- and post-dilution) may also be an option to consider. A *one-third pre-dilution and two-thirds post-dilution* split may be used both to achieve effective clearance and to extend the filter life.

Types of renal replacement therapy

Continuous venovenous haemofiltration (CVVH)

Filtrate is removed from the blood by convection using a replacement fluid, which is replaced either pre-dilution or post-dilution (i.e. before or after the blood passes through the filter). The blood on one side of the membrane exerts a hydrostatic pressure, causing solute molecules small enough to pass through the membrane to be dragged across with the water by the process of convection. The filtered fluid (ultrafiltrate) is discarded and the replacement fluid is added.

- **Goal:** solute removal and fluid management.
- **Indications:** uraemia, electrolyte imbalance, acid–base disturbance, removal of small and medium-sized molecules, low-molecular-weight proteins, and water.
- **Physiological principles:** ultrafiltration and convection.

Continuous venovenous haemodiafiltration (CVVHDF)

Filtrate is removed from the blood by diffusion using a dialysate solution running through the filter in a counter-current direction to the blood on the opposite side of the membrane, in order to maintain concentration gradients. Filtration still occurs because a pressure gradient exists, but diffusion can be utilized to facilitate the removal of solutes without the need to remove such large volumes of fluid. Therefore some fluid and solutes are removed by convection and then replaced post dilution. Fluid is also passed through the filter to create a concentration gradient for diffusion of solutes. When removal of water is required, the pressure on the blood side of the membrane has to be increased, forcing water molecules to pass into the dialysate.

- **Goal:** solute removal and fluid management.
- **Indications:** uraemia, electrolyte imbalance, acid–base disturbance, and removal of small molecules.
- **Physiological principles:** diffusion, ultrafiltration, and convection.

CVVHDF has the benefits of both techniques, but to a lesser extent than when either technique is used on its own.

General principles for renal replacement therapy

- Fluid balance recordings must be documented carefully to avoid confusion and prevent accidental hypo- or hypervolaemia.
- Blood flow through the circuit should be in the range 100–200 mL/min in order to reduce the clotting risk without damaging the filter with extreme pressures.
- Continuous anticoagulation of the circuit is usually necessary unless the patient is significantly auto-anticoagulated.
- Filters are usually hollow-fibre membranes made from biocompatible products (e.g. polyacrylonitrile).
- Vascular access should be in view or inspected regularly (particularly after a position change or patient movement).

- Adherence to infection prevention and control is essential, and aseptic non-touch technique must be used when accessing the vascular access device.
- Circuit tubing should be supported or clamped in position and checked for kinking, undue tension, or inadvertent disconnection.

Example of a prescription for renal replacement therapy

A typical prescription for a 75 kg patient requiring renal replacement therapy for AKI would be as follows:

Anticoagulation

- Unfractionated heparin—5000 IU bolus followed by a pre-filter infusion at 500 IU/h.
- Aim to anticoagulate the filter, but ensure that the activated partial thromboplastin time ratio (APTTR) is < 2.

Fluid balance over 24 h

- Aim for an even balance if the patient is euvolaemic.
- Aim for the appropriate negative balance if the patient is fluid overloaded (e.g. < 1500 mL/24 h).

Type of replacement fluid/dialysate

- Use solutions without potassium if serum potassium levels are high, but switch to potassium-containing solutions as serum potassium concentration normalizes.
- Use a bicarbonate-based buffer rather than a lactate-based buffer if there are concerns about lactate metabolism, or if serum lactate concentration is > 8 mmol/L.
- *Note: An intravenous bicarbonate infusion may be required if a lactate-based buffer is used.*

Exchange rate/treatment dose

- This should be 1500 mL/h (75 kg × 20 mL/kg/h). The treatment dose is usually prescribed as an hourly exchange rate, which is the desired hourly flow rate adjusted for the patient's weight. In CVVH, the exchange rate represents the ultrafiltration rate, whereas in CVVHDF it represents a combination of the ultrafiltration rate and the dialysate flow rate. In CVVHDF, the ratio of ultrafiltration to dialysate flow is often set at 1:1, but it can be altered to favour either the dialysis component or the filtration component.

Nursing interventions

Monitoring

- Haemodynamic monitoring should be continuous in order to detect hypovolaemia, hypotension, and arrhythmias.
- Monitor plasma potassium levels at least 4-hourly.
- Monitor core temperature and maintain at > 36°C. Heat loss from blood in the extracorporeal circuit and infusion of large volumes of room-temperature replacement fluid can reduce body temperature.
- Monitor circuit pressures and blood coagulation laboratory profiles.

Rest and sleep

Ensure that the patient is allowed adequate rest and sleep. Position the circuit tubing so as to prevent kinking and obstruction of blood flow, and thus avoid setting off machine alarms and increasing the risk of filter or circuit clotting.

Psychological care

The sight of large volumes of blood in the extracorporeal circuit can be frightening for the patient and their relatives. To reduce anxiety, discussion about renal replacement therapy as a treatment should be introduced before its commencement. A constant and reassuring nursing presence will also support the patient and their family.

Anticoagulation

- The aim is to prevent platelet and coagulation activation in response to contact of blood with a foreign surface (i.e. the filter or circuit).
- Too little anticoagulation can cause clotting in the filter. This is time-consuming to replace, expensive, and decreases efficiency as well as risking blood loss (a circuit contains 150–200 mL of blood).
- Too much anticoagulation can cause bleeding from cannula sites or spontaneous bleeds in the brain, bowel, or lung.
- Heparin is the most commonly used anticoagulant.
- Usually 5–20 IU/kg/h heparin is infused proximal to the filter.
- A pre-filtration heparin bolus of 2000–5000 IU may also be given if there are problems with filter clotting.
- If the patient has an adverse reaction to heparin (e.g. heparin-induced thrombocytopenia) or is at risk of bleeding (e.g. post-surgery), prostacyclin/epoprostenol (PG12) or alprostadil (PGE1) can be given at 2.5–10 ng/kg/min. Observe the patient for hypotension.
- Alternatively, citrate can be given in order to anticoagulate the circuit and filter without anticoagulating the patient. Citrate is both an anticoagulant and a buffer. It chelates ionized calcium, and the associated regional hypocalcaemia in the filter inhibits the generation of thrombin. The citrate is partially removed by filtration, and the remaining citrate is rapidly metabolized to bicarbonate in the liver, muscle, and renal cortex. Calcium infusion is required.

Anticoagulation tests required during heparin infusion

Activated clotting time (ACT)

ACT is normally maintained at 200–250 s for haemodialysis and 150–220 s for haemofiltration.

Whole blood partial thromboplastin time (WBPTT)

During haemodialysis the WBPTT must be maintained at the baseline value plus 40–80% (approximately 120–140 s), and during haemofiltration at the baseline value plus 50%.

Activated partial thromboplastin time (APTT)

- APTT should be checked 4–6 h after starting a heparin infusion.
- Aim for 1.5–2.5 times the control value.

Troubleshooting frequent filter clotting

- Ensure that the filter has been adequately primed prior to use.
- Check for kinking or obstruction of the double-lumen cannula.
- If arterial (outflow) circuit pressures are high, check the vascular access for signs of obstruction.
- If filter pressures are high, check the filter for signs of clotting, and if necessary reduce the blood flow rate if above 150 mL/min.
- Consider swapping access on the double-lumen cannula (this will result in recirculation of the blood between 20–40%).
- Consider changing the cannula if pressures remain high and filter clotting is likely.
- If repeated filter clotting occurs with full anticoagulation, consider pre-dilution using replacement fluid added prior to the filter to reduce viscosity (this will reduce filter efficiency).

Filtration fraction

This is the measure of filtrate removed as a percentage of blood flow. It indicates the haemoconcentration of the filter (i.e. how long the filter circuit will last). The lower the filtration fraction (FF), the longer the filter will last. To decrease the filtration fraction, increase the blood flow rate (BFR) or decrease the ultrafiltration rate (UFR). The ideal range for the filtration fraction is 20–30%. If the filtration fraction is higher than 30% there is an increased risk of clotting.

Filtration fraction formula:

$$FF(\%) = (UFR \times 100)/QP$$
$$QP = BFR \times (1 - Hct)$$

For example:

UFR = 1500 mL/h = 25 mL/min.

QP (filter plasma flow rate) = blood flow rate 150 mL/min × 0.6 (1 – 0.40 Hct) = 90 mL/min.

Therefore FF = (25 mL/min × 100)/90 mL/min = 27%.

Chapter 10

Gastrointestinal care

Gastrointestinal assessment

If an actual or potential gastrointestinal abnormality has been identified during a general ABCDE assessment (see ➲ p. 18) or while monitoring the patient, a more detailed and focused gastrointestinal assessment can provide further information to guide clinical management.

Focused health history

Subjective information about the gastrointestinal history can be taken from the patient if they are awake, or from other sources (e.g. family, caregivers, or the patient's notes). See ➲ p. 16 for an overview of history taking.

Gastrointestinal symptom enquiry

- Diet, indigestion, swallowing ability.
- Appetite, weight loss, weight gain.
- Nausea and vomiting.
- Diarrhoea, constipation, melaena.
- Abdominal pain.

Focused physical assessment

- Obvious signs of discomfort or distress.
- Inability to lie flat or cough due to abdominal pain.
- Nutritional assessment (see ➲ p. 24).
- Fluid assessment (see ➲ p. 24).
- Bowel assessment (see ➲ p. 305).
- Gastrointestinal-focused assessment of the face and abdomen (see Table 10.1).

Table 10.1 Gastrointestinal-focused assessment

	Normal	Abnormal
Inspection	Pink, moist mucous membranes White sclera Symmetrical, non-distended abdomen	Pallor Jaundice Dry mucous membranes Abdominal distension Abdominal asymmetry Abdominal wounds, drains, scarring, bruising
Palpation	Soft abdomen Non-tender abdomen	Firm abdomen Painful abdomen Mass
Percussion	Tympanic abdominal percussion note	Dullness on abdominal percussion
Auscultation	Bowel sounds present	Absent bowel sounds Hypoactive bowel sounds High-pitched, tinkling bowel sounds

Some authors suggest that auscultation should be performed prior to palpation, while others recognize that bowel sounds may not be a reliable assessment finding, due to normal sounds occurring with an abnormal abdomen, and vice versa.[1]

Abdominal landmarking
Any abnormal findings found during the health history and physical assessment should be documented and reported according to the specific quadrant of the abdomen in which the abnormality was identified (see Figure 10.1).

Causes of key abnormalities
- Jaundice—liver failure, gallstones.
- Abdominal distension—ascites, bowel obstruction, bleeding, sepsis, air (e.g. due to non-invasive ventilation without a nasogastric tube).
- Abdominal pain—abnormality of underlying structure (see Figure 10.1).
- Dullness on percussion—fluid, mass, faeces.

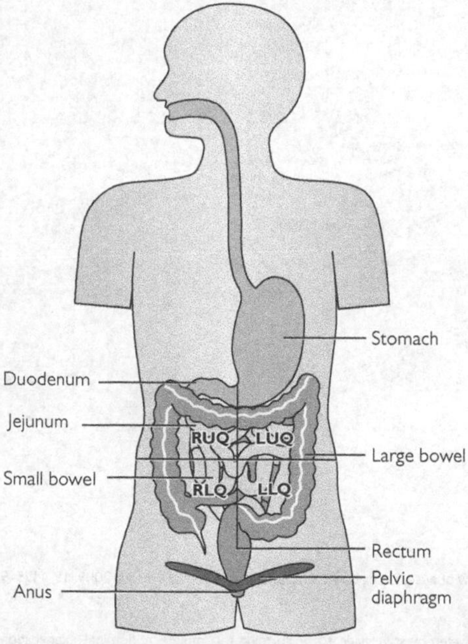

Figure 10.1 Abdominal quadrants. RUQ, right upper quadrant; LUQ, left upper quadrant; RLQ, right lower quadrant; LLQ, left lower quadrant. (Reproduced from Randle, Coffey, Bradbury, *Oxford Handbook of Clinical Skills in Adult Nursing*, 2009, with permission from Oxford University Press.)

- Absent bowel sounds—bowel obstruction.
- Hypoactive bowel sounds—bowel obstruction, opioids.
- High-pitched, tinkling bowel sounds—partial bowel obstruction.

Laboratory investigations

Blood tests which are relevant to check in a gastrointestinal review include:

- FBC and CRP
- U&E
- LFTs
- amylase and lipase.

Reference

1 Baid H. A critical review of auscultating bowel sounds. *British Journal of Nursing* 2009; **18**: 1125–9.

Further reading

Cox C and Stegall M. A step-by-step guide to performing a complete abdominal examination. *Gastrointestinal Nursing* 2009; **1**: 10–17.

Stayt L, Randle J and Coffey F. Gastrointestinal system. In: J Randle, F Coffey and M Bradbury (eds) *Oxford Handbook of Clinical Skills in Adult Nursing*. Oxford University Press: Oxford, 2009. pp. 397–454.

Gastrointestinal monitoring

Gastric residual assessment

[illegible]

Intra-abdominal pressure

[illegible]

[illegible]

[illegible]	[illegible]
[illegible]	[illegible]
[illegible]	[illegible]
[illegible]	[illegible]

Gastrointestinal monitoring

Gastric residual assessment

Gastric residual contents should be monitored regularly according to local protocol until enteral feeding has been established, or if significant abnormality of the gastrointestinal system is noted (see ➲ p. 308).

Gastric contents are observed for colour, consistency, and amount by aspirating fluid back from a large-bore oral or nasogastric tube. If the patient vomits, the same type of assessment can take place while observing the emesis. Table 10.2 provides an overview of normal and abnormal gastric content findings.

Intra-abdominal pressure

The pressure within the abdominal cavity can be estimated by obtaining a pressure measurement in the bladder. This is achieved by using either a Foley manometer or a Foley catheter which can be connected to a transducer (see Figure 10.2).

Intra-abdominal pressure (IAP) monitoring is indicated if the abdomen becomes distended, firm, or there is a risk of abdominal compartment syndrome (see ➲ p. 322). Normal and abnormal IAP values are listed in Box 10.1. High-pressure readings are most likely to be clinically significant if they show an upward trend within the context of other abnormal signs and symptoms indicating gastrointestinal dysfunction.

Table 10.2 Normal and abnormal gastric fluid content

Normal gastric content	Abnormal gastric content
Acceptable gastric residual volumes (see ➲ p. 308)	High gastric residual volumes
	Fresh blood
Normal gastric fluid colour	Coffee-grounds appearance
pH < 5.5	Faecal smell

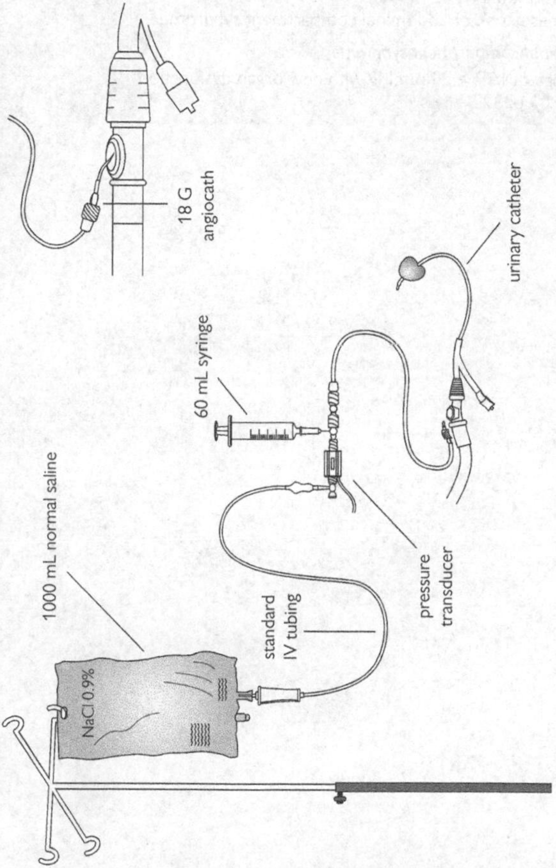

Figure 10.2 Intra-abdominal pressure monitoring: foley catheter transducer. (Drawing by Mark Gregory.)

Box 10.1 Normal and abnormal IAP values

- 5–7 mmHg
- < 12 mmHg not significant (may be due to COPD, obesity, or ascites)

Intra-abdominal hypertension (IAH)

- Constant IAP > 12 mmHg
- Increases risk of abdominal compartment syndrome

Abdominal compartment syndrome

- Constant IAP > 20 mmHg with new organ dysfunction
- See ➲ p. 322

Further reading

Delgado LA. Abdominal compartment syndrome: a guide for the gastrointestinal nurse. *Gastrointestinal Nursing* 2013; **11**: 42–8.

Desle et al. Intra-abdominal pressure measurement using the FoleyManometer does not increase the risk for urinary tract infection in critically ill patients. *Annals of Intensive Care* 2012; **2 (Suppl. 1)**: S10.

Lee RK. Intra-abdominal hypertension and abdominal compartment syndrome: a comprehensive overview. *Critical Care Nurse* 2012; **32**: 19–31.

Diarrhoea

Definition

[illegible]

Causes

Table 11.7 [illegible]

Assessment findings

- [illegible] a day
- [illegible]
- [illegible]
- Stool weight [illegible] 200 g/day

Management

- [illegible]
  - [illegible]
  - [illegible]
- [illegible]
- [illegible]
- [illegible]
- [illegible]
- [illegible]
- [illegible]
  - [illegible]

Table 11.7 [illegible]

Infective causes	[illegible]
[illegible]	[illegible]

Diarrhoea

Definition

Gastrointestinal dysfunction resulting in large amounts of frequent loose stools is commonly found in critically ill patients. Strategies for preventing diarrhoea include strict infection control precautions (see ➲ p. 44), appropriate use of antibiotics, and early enteral nutrition to maintain integrity of the gut mucosa.

Causes

Table 10.3 summarizes the infective and non-infective causes of diarrhoea. Medications with the potential to cause diarrhoea include antibiotics, laxatives (if overused), and sorbitol-containing drugs.

Assessment findings

- More than 3 stools a day.
- Watery, loose stools.
- Bristol Stool Chart—type 5, 6, or 7 (see Figure 10.3).
- Stool weight > 200 g/day.

Management

- Protect the skin from excoriation by means of:
  - careful washing
  - barrier cream or spray
  - a bowel management system (flexible rectal catheter with balloon seal and collection bag).
- Monitor electrolytes and treat imbalances.
- Monitor fluid status and treat fluid deficit (see ➲ p. 24).
- Review current medications and discontinue laxatives or other diarrhoea-inducing drugs that are not essential.
- Perform a rectal examination to rule out faecal impaction with overflow.
- Obtain stool specimens for:
  - MC&S (send three samples)
  - *Clostridium difficile* toxin.

Table 10.3 Causes of diarrhoea

Infective causes	Non-infective causes
Clostridium difficile	Medications
E. coli	Enteral feeding
Salmonella	Malabsorption
Tropical diseases	Inflammatory bowel disease
	Diverticulitis
	Overflow with faecal impaction

- Consider fibre-containing enteral feeds and probiotic additives.
- Provide appropriate antibiotic treatment if culture and isolation identify a bacterial cause (e.g. metronidazole or vancomycin for *C. difficile*).
- Take an abdominal X-ray if ischaemic or inflammatory bowel disease is suspected (or if there is bloody diarrhoea).
- Consider semi-elemental feeds if malabsorption is suspected.
- Use anti-motility agents (e.g. loperamide or co-phenotrope).

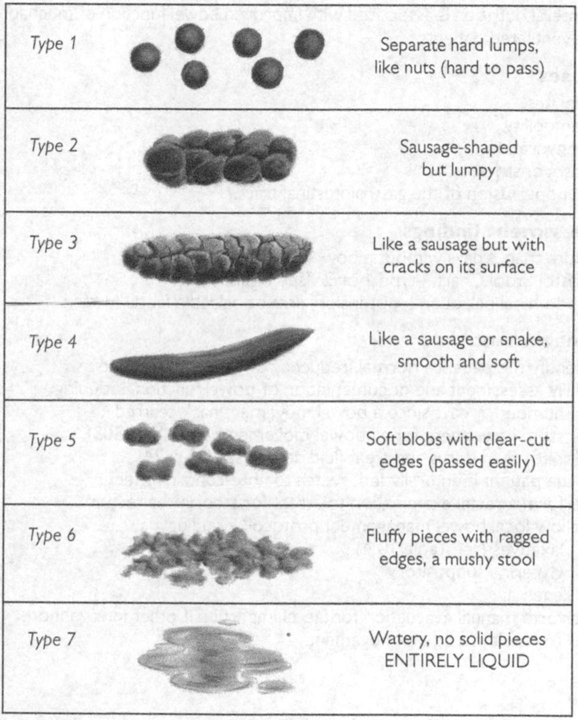

Type 1
Separate hard lumps, like nuts (hard to pass)
Type 2
Sausage-shaped but lumpy
Type 3
Like a sausage but with cracks on its surface
Type 4
Like a sausage or snake, smooth and soft
Type 5
Soft blobs with clear-cut edges (passed easily)
Type 6
Fluffy pieces with ragged edges, a mushy stool
Type 7
Watery, no solid pieces ENTIRELY LIQUID

Figure 10.3 Bristol Stool Chart. (Reproduced by kind permission of Dr. K. W. Heaton, Reader in Medicine at the University of Bristol © 2000 Norgine Pharmaceuticals Ltd.)

Constipation

Definition

The definition of constipation is subjective, but is usually considered to be more than 3 days without a bowel movement. However, in patients who are fed parenterally there may be minimal gastrointestinal content and waste for excretion, and expected bowel movements may be less frequent. Constipation occurs in up to 70% of critically ill patients, and early initiation of enteral nutrition is associated with improved bowel function of mechanically ventilated patients.[2]

Causes

- Opiates.
- Immobility.
- Dehydration.
- Vasoconstrictors.
- Hypoperfusion of the gastrointestinal tract.

Assessment findings

- More than 3 days without a bowel movement.
- Bristol Stool Chart—type 1 or 2[3] (see Figure 10.3).
- Abdominal palpation—distension, firm or palpable faecal matter.

Management

- Identify the patient's normal frequency of bowel movements.
- Daily assessment and documentation of bowel function, including:
  - number of days since a bowel movement has occurred
  - stool assessment for all bowel movements (see ➲ p. 305).
- Monitor fluid status and treat fluid deficit (see ➲ p. 24).
- If the patient is enterally fed, switch to fibre-containing feed.
- Perform a rectal examination to assess for stool in the rectum.
- Follow local bowel management protocol, including:
  - laxatives (see Table 10.4)
  - glycerine suppository
  - enema.
- Perform manual evacuation for faecal impaction if other interventions fail to result in a bowel movement.

Table 10.4 Laxatives

Type	Effect	Examples
Bulk-forming laxatives	Soluble fibres draw water into the gut and add bulk to the stool	Psyllium, bran, methylcellulose
Stimulant laxatives	Act by irritating and increasing the motility of the gut	Senna, docusate sodium, bisacodyl
Faecal softeners	Ease the passage of the stool by altering consistency	Liquid paraffin, seed oils
Osmotic laxatives	Draw water into the colon and increase volume and water content of stool	Lactulose, phosphate enema

References

2 Nassar AP Jr, da Silva FM and de Cleva R. Constipation in intensive care unit: incidence and risk factors. *Journal of Critical Care* 2009; **24**: 630.e9–12.

3 Lewis SJ and Heaton KW. Stool form scale as a useful guide to intestinal transit time. *Scandinavian Journal of Gastroenterology* 1997; **32**: 920–24.

Further reading

Bayón García C et al. Expert recommendations for managing acute faecal incontinence with diarrhoea in the intensive care unit. *Journal of the Intensive Care Society* 2013; **14** (Suppl.): 1–9.

McPeake J, Gilmour H and MacIntosh G. The implementation of a bowel management protocol in an adult intensive care unit. *Nursing in Critical Care* 2011; **16**: 235–42.

Masri Y, Abubaker J and Ahmed R. Prophylactic use of laxative for constipation in critically ill patients. *Annals of Thoracic Medicine* 2010; **5**: 228–31.

Hypomotility

Definition

When gastrointestinal motility becomes delayed, stomach contents accumulate, leading to abdominal distension, a high gastric residual volume (GRV), and the potential for vomiting and aspiration pneumonia to develop. Even patients with cuffed tracheal tubes are not completely protected from the risk of aspiration, as it is still possible for gastric contents to be aspirated past the cuff.

Normal gastrointestinal motility is indicated if a patient is tolerating enteral feeding which is confirmed by checking the GRV aspirated from a large-bore oro- or nasogastric tube. It is common practice to consider a GRV of up to 200–250 mL to be an indicator that enteral nutrition is being absorbed, although the REGANE study[4] concluded that a GRV of up to 500 mL may be a more appropriate threshold value. Another trial by Reignier and colleagues[5] indicated that mechanically ventilated patients in whom GRV was not checked were no more likely to develop ventilator-associated pneumonia than patients who received routine care. However, the findings of these studies may not be generalizable, particularly for surgical and severely ill patients. Until the debate about best practice for assessing and acting upon hypomotility of critical care patients has been clarified by further research, local interpretation of what constitutes a high GRV and local enteral feeding protocols should be followed.[6] Figure 10.4 shows a general template for the management of high GRVs.

Causes

- Medications—opiates, catecholamines, β-2 agonists.
- Post-operative ileus.
- Sepsis.
- Trauma.
- Increased ICP.
- Gastrointestinal ischaemia.
- Cellular cytokines and kinases released during reperfusion injury.
- Release of endotoxin or corticotropin (a stress response agent).

Assessment findings

- High GRV—as defined by local protocol, which typically considers a GRV of > a number between 200 and 500 mL to be high.
- Vomiting.
- Abdominal distension.
- Hypoactive or absent bowel sounds.

Management

- Monitor GRV according to local protocol.
- Continue low-volume enteral feeding.
- Semi-recumbent positioning (head-up angle of 35–45°).
- Prokinetics—metoclopramide, erythromycin.
- Post-pyloric feeding.

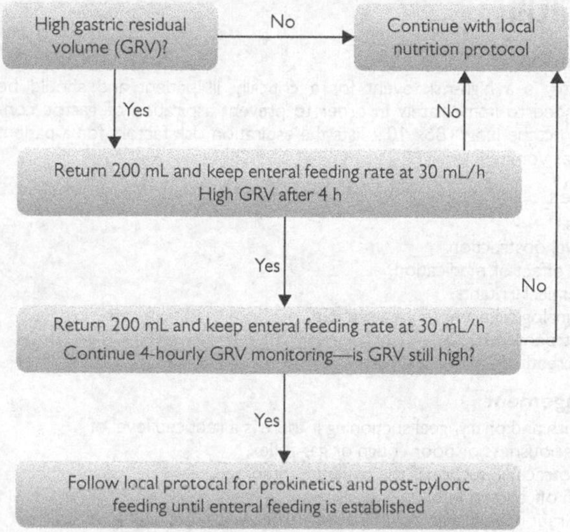

Figure 10.4 Management of high gastric residual volumes.

References

4 Montejo J et al. Gastric residual volume during enteral nutrition in ICU patients: the REGANE study. *Intensive Care Medicine* 2010; **36**: 1386–93.

5 Reignier J et al. Effect of not monitoring residual gastric volume on risk of ventilator-associated pneumonia in adults receiving mechanical ventilation and early enteral feeding: a randomized control trial. *Journal of the American Medical Association* 2013; **309**: 249–56.

6 Heyland D and Dhaliwal R. *Measuring Gastric Residual Volumes in Enterally Tube Fed Critically Ill Patients: the end of an era?* www.criticalcarenutrition.com/docs/qi_tools/Nibble%209%20-%20GRVs.pdf

Further reading

Ukleja A. Altered GI motility in critically ill patients: current understanding of pathophysiology, clinical impact, and diagnostic approach. *Nutrition in Clinical Practice* 2010; **25**: 16–25.

Vomiting

Definition

Vomiting is a high-risk event for a critically ill patient and should be responded to immediately in order to prevent aspiration of gastric contents into the lungs. Box 10.2 lists the aspiration risk factors for a patient who has vomited.

Causes

- Ileus.
- Bowel obstruction.
- Side effect of medication.
- Chemical irritants.
- Neurological event (e.g. raised ICP).
- Gastroenteritis.
- Pancreatitis.

Management

- Mouth and pharyngeal suctioning if there is a reduced level of consciousness or poor cough or gag reflex.
- Endotracheal suction if the patient is intubated.
- Turn off enteral feed.
- Aspiration with large-bore oro- or nasogastric tube, and leave on free drainage.
- Anti-emetics (e.g. metoclopramide, cyclizine, prochlorperazine, or ondansetron).
- Semi-recumbent positioning (head-up angle of 35–45°).
- Monitor electrolytes and treat imbalances.
- Monitor fluid status and treat fluid deficit (see ➲ p. 24).
- Review enteral feeding regime with doctor and dietitian.
- Provide mouth care.

Box 10.2 Aspiration risk factors

- Reduced level of consciousness.
- Diminished or absent cough or gag reflexes.
- Incompetent oesophageal sphincters.
- Delayed gastric emptying.
- Paralytic ileus.
- Displacement of enteral feeding tube (can be associated with vigorous coughing or retching).
- Presence of an enteral feeding tube.

Further reading

Collins AS. Postoperative nausea and vomiting in adults: implications for critical care. *Critical Care Nurse* 2011; 31: 36–45.

Acute abdomen

Definition

The phrase 'acute abdomen' is used to describe the rapid onset of clinically significant abdominal abnormalities when the underpinning problem is still unknown. There are numerous potential causes of an acute abdomen because the abdominal cavity contains a number of different organs and structures. Due to the potentially life-threatening nature of many of these causes, immediate medical referral is needed.

Causes

- Intestinal ischaemia.
- Peptic ulcer—perforation, gastrointestinal bleeding (see ➔ p. 318).
- Bowel obstruction.
- Cholecystitis.
- Pancreatitis (see ➔ p. 316).
- Appendicitis.
- Peritonitis.
- Abdominal aortic aneurysm.
- Ectopic pregnancy.

Assessment findings

- Severe sudden pain < 24 h in duration.
- Pain before vomiting.
- Raised temperature and heart rate.
- Distended, firm, tender abdomen.
- Raised WBC count.
- Bowel sounds—hypoactive, absent, or high-pitched/tinkling.
- Peritoneal signs—rebound tenderness, guarding, or rigidity.

Management

- Inform the doctor urgently and refer the patient to the surgical team as required.
- Give analgesia and anti-emetic for pain and nausea.
- Monitor gastric aspirates for amount and colour (see ➔ p. 308).
- Perform a rectal examination to assess for melaena.
- Give fluid resuscitation and haemodynamic support as required.
- Blood investigations:
  - FBC
  - U&Es
  - LFTs
  - clotting
  - glucose
  - amylase
  - arterial blood gas.
- Other investigations as appropriate to the assessment findings:
  - radiology—facilitate CT scan, ultrasound, or X-ray if ordered
  - urine—urinalysis, MC&S, pregnancy test
  - 12-lead ECG to rule out cardiac abnormality
  - intra-abdominal pressure monitoring.

Acute liver failure

Definition

Significant liver dysfunction with any degree of altered mentation (hepatic encephalopathy) in the absence of chronic liver disease indicates acute liver failure. Classification of acute liver failure is based on how fast encephalopathy develops after the initial signs of liver abnormality (see Table 10.5). Severe cases of acute liver failure may require transfer to a specialist liver intensive care unit for extracorporeal liver assist device (ELAD) therapy or transplantation.

Causes

- Paracetamol overdose.
- Acute viral hepatitis or other viruses.
- Hepatotoxic substances—drugs, excessive alcohol, mushrooms, chemicals, herbal remedies.
- Vascular causes—ischaemic hepatitis, Budd–Chiari syndrome.
- Pregnancy—acute fatty liver, HELLP syndrome.
- Autoimmune hepatitis.
- Metabolic causes—Wilson's disease, Reye's syndrome.

Assessment findings

- Hepatic encephalopathy (see Table 10.6).
- Cerebral oedema leading to raised ICP.
- Hypotension and tachycardia.
- Coagulopathy and bleeding.
- Jaundice and raised LFTs.
- Acute kidney injury.
- Metabolic disturbances.
- Infection.

Management

- Haemodynamic monitoring to assess for distributive shock.
- Fluid resuscitation, avoiding excessive volume overload.
- Vasoconstrictor if hypotension does not respond to IV fluids.
- Inotropic support as required.
- Antibiotics for prophylaxis or an identified infection.

Table 10.5 Classification of acute liver disease based on development of hepatic encephalopathy

Type of acute liver failure	Time between onset of liver dysfunction signs (e.g. jaundice) and encephalopathy
Hyperacute	0–7 days
Acute	7–28 days
Subacute	> 28 days

Table 10.6 Classification of hepatic encephalopathy

Grade	Clinical presentation
I	Mood change, slow mentation, disturbed sleep, usually alert and lucid
II	Drowsiness, inappropriate behaviour, easily arousable, conversant
III	Marked confusion and disorientation, agitation, stuporous but rousable
IV	Coma—unrousable to verbal or noxious stimuli, abnormal motor response to stimuli

- Blood components as required—FFP is only given if the patient is actively bleeding or prior to invasive procedures (INR is a highly sensitive marker of liver function and helps to monitor the progression and severity of liver injury).
- Give 50% glucose for hypoglycaemia.
- Renal replacement therapy for oliguria and/or significant acidosis.
  - Use bicarbonate-buffered replacement solution (see ➔ p. 291).
  - Avoid using heparin as anticoagulant if the patient has a low platelet count or is actively bleeding—use epoprostenol as an alternative.
- Blood investigations:
  - FBC
  - U&Es, phosphate, calcium, magnesium
  - LFTs
  - clotting
  - glucose
  - amylase
  - arterial blood gas and arterial ammonia
  - paracetamol level and toxicology screen
  - hepatitis screen
  - autoantibodies and immunoglobulins (autoimmune hepatitis).

Encephalopathy

- Avoid the use of sedatives, or give short-acting agents (e.g. propofol and fentanyl) if required for intubation or patient safety.
- Maintain cerebral perfusion pressure if cerebral oedema develops:
  - ICP monitoring is required in severe cases
  - see ➔ p. 251 for care of the patient with a raised ICP.

N-acetylcysteine infusion

- Paracetamol overdose (see ➔ p. 446).
- Consider for non-paracetamol-induced liver failure.[7]

Reference

7 Lee WM et al. Intravenous *N*-acetylcysteine improves transplant-free survival in early stage non-acetaminophen acute liver failure. *Gastroenterology* 2009; **137**: 856–64.

Further reading

Sargent S (ed.) *Liver Diseases: an essential guide for nurses and health care professionals.* Wiley-Blackwell: Chichester, 2009.

Chronic liver failure

Definition

Patients with chronic liver failure who are admitted to an intensive care unit have an overall hospital mortality rate of 55%, but those with cirrhosis, sepsis, and organ failure have an even higher mortality rate, ranging from 65% to 90%.[8] The intensive care management is not curative of the chronic liver disease itself, but is more supportive in nature, addressing secondary problems resulting from an acute on chronic episode. Common causes of acute on chronic liver failure are listed in Box 10.3.

Causes

- Alcoholic liver disease—progresses in severity through three stages:
  - fatty liver—fibrosis with recovery is still possible
  - alcoholic hepatitis—inflammation, necrosis, and fibrosis
  - cirrhosis—irreversible nodule formation due to hepatocyte destruction being more rapid than regeneration.
- Non-alcoholic fatty liver disease:
  - associated with metabolic syndrome (obesity, hyperlipidaemia, type 2 diabetes, and hypertension)
  - non-alcoholic steatohepatitis (NASH)—severe form with inflammation leading to fibrosis and cirrhosis.
- Viral causes—hepatitis, cytomegalovirus, Epstein–Barr virus.
- Metabolic cause—Wilson's disease.
- Autoimmune causes—primary biliary cirrhosis, autoimmune chronic hepatitis.
- Right-sided heart failure.

Box 10.3 Causes of acute on chronic liver failure decompensation

- Sepsis—respiratory, urinary, or ascites.
- Acute respiratory failure.
- Electrolyte imbalance.
- Variceal haemorrhage (see ➲ p. 318).
- Dehydration.
- Hepatocellular carcinoma.
- Hepatorenal syndrome:
  - acute kidney injury with acute or chronic liver disease in the absence of any other identifiable cause of renal pathology
  - thought to be related to reduced renal blood flow, and is often precipitated by bacterial peritonitis.[9]

Assessment findings

- Jaundice.
- Ascites.
- Hepatic encephalopathy (see Table 10.5).
- Coagulopathy.
- Gastrointestinal haemorrhage (see ➔ p. 318).
- Chronic signs—spider naevi, caput medusae, palmar erythema, asterixis, leukonychia, Dupuytren's contracture, and finger clubbing.

Management

- Haemodynamic monitoring, fluid resuscitation, and vasoconstrictor and inotropic support as required.
- Monitor for and treat acute respiratory failure secondary to abdominal distension or pleural effusions.
- Give 50% glucose for hypoglycaemia.
- Renal replacement therapy for oliguria and/or significant acidosis:
  - use bicarbonate-buffered replacement solution (see ➔ p. 291).
- Monitor for coagulopathy and gastrointestinal bleeding (see ➔ p. 318).
- Blood investigations:
  - FBC
  - U&Es, phosphate, calcium, magnesium
  - LFTs
  - clotting
  - glucose
  - amylase
  - arterial blood gas.

Ascites

- Paracentesis and IV fluid replacement as prescribed.
- Antibiotics for spontaneous bacterial peritonitis.
- Sodium restriction.
- Diuretics.

Encephalopathy

- Rule out other causes, such as sepsis, acidosis, uraemia, alcohol or drug withdrawal, and hypoxia.
- Avoid the use of sedatives, or give short-acting agents (e.g. propofol and fentanyl) if required for intubation or patient safety.
- Give lactulose—this osmotic laxative increases gastrointestinal motility, so there is less time for intestinal bacteria to metabolize protein to ammonia.
- A protein-restricted diet is no longer recommended.[10]

References

8 O'Brien AJ et al. Prevalence and outcome of cirrhosis patients admitted to UK intensive care: a comparison against dialysis-dependent chronic renal failure patients. *Intensive Care Medicine* 2012; **38**: 991–1000.

9 Wadei HM and Gonwa TA. Hepatorenal syndrome in the intensive care unit. *Journal of Intensive Care Medicine* 2013; **28**: 79–92.

10 Caruana P and Shah N. Hepatic encephalopathy: are NH_4 levels and protein restriction obsolete? *Practical Gastroenterology* 2011; **35**: 6–18.

Pancreatitis

Definition

Inflammation of the pancreas can result from an acute, chronic, or acute on chronic process. Pancreatic enzymes are prematurely activated in the pancreas instead of within the duodenum, leading to autodigestion. The localized injury resulting from this autodigestion triggers the release of cytokines, hormones, and other vasoactive substances as part of the inflammatory response. This leads to the development of oedema, bleeding, necrosis, pseudocysts, and abscesses (see Figure 10.5). Initially, systemic inflammatory response syndrome (SIRS) occurs, with the potential for sepsis and multi-organ dysfunction syndrome (MODS) to develop if the initial precipitating factor is not resolved and the pancreatitis becomes progressively more severe (see ➔ p. 328).

Causes

- Biliary disease—gallstones or common bile duct obstruction.
- Alcohol.
- Endoscopic retrograde cholangiopancreatography (ERCP).
- Medications—diuretics, sulfonamides, ACE inhibitors, valproic acid.
- Abdominal trauma.
- Infection.
- Idiopathic causes.

Assessment findings

- Nausea and vomiting without relief.
- Abdominal pain.
- Abdominal distension and tenderness.
- Fever.
- Jaundice.
- Elevated serum pancreatic enzymes—amylase and lipase.
- Raised WBC count, CRP, and lactate dehydrogenase (LDH).
- Raised bilirubin, AST, and PT (liver disease).
- Elevated alkaline phosphatase (biliary disease).
- Hyperglycaemia.

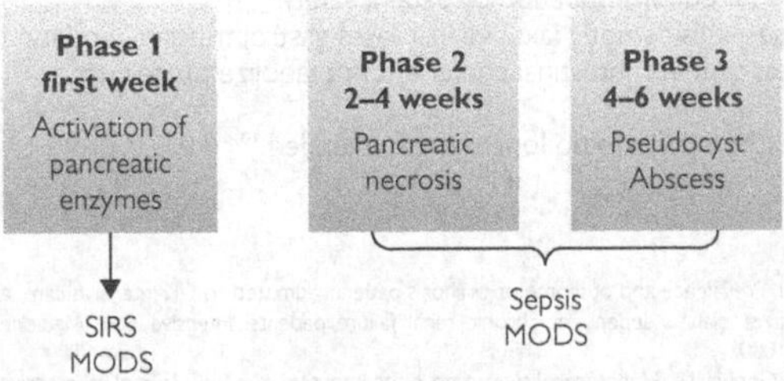

Figure 10.5 Progression of acute pancreatitis. SIRS, systemic inflammatory response syndrome; MODS, multi-organ dysfunction syndrome.

- Electrolyte imbalances.
- Metabolic acidosis.
- Retroperitoneal bleeding—Cullen's sign (bruising near the umbilicus) and Grey Turner's sign (flank bruising).
- Steatorrhoea —oily, foul-smelling, grey faeces secondary to excess fat in faeces.

Management

- Haemodynamic monitoring to assess for distributive shock from systemic inflammatory response syndrome (SIRS) (see ➲ p. 328).
- Fluid resuscitation, avoiding excessive volume overload.
- Vasoconstrictor if hypotension does not respond to IV fluids.
- Inotropic support as required.
- Monitor for and treat acute respiratory failure secondary to abdominal distension.
- Insulin therapy for hyperglycaemia.
- Renal replacement therapy for oliguria and/or significant acidosis.
- Analgesia and anti-emetics as required.
- Monitor electrolytes and treat imbalances.
- Antibiotics for an identified infection—the evidence for the effectiveness of their prophylactic use is inconclusive.[11]
- Confirm nutritional regime with doctor:
  - nasogastric or nasojejunal enteral feeding
  - total parenteral nutrition only if necessary—routine bowel rest is no longer recommended.[12]
- Blood investigations:
  - FBC
  - U&E, phosphate, calcium, magnesium
  - LFTs
  - clotting
  - glucose
  - amylase and lipase
  - arterial blood gas.
- ERCP or surgery as required.

References

11 Villatoro E et al. Antibiotic therapy for prophylaxis against infection of pancreatic necrosis in acute pancreatitis. *Cochrane Database of Systematic Reviews* 2010; Issue 5: CD002941.
12 Al-Omran M et al. Enteral versus parenteral nutrition for acute pancreatitis. *Cochrane Database of Systematic Reviews* 2010; Issue 1: CD002837.

Gastrointestinal haemorrhage

Definition

Bleeding can occur in either the upper or lower regions of the gastrointestinal tract. If there are significant amounts of continual haemorrhage, referral to endoscopy and/or general surgery will be required for definitive treatment.

Causes

- Peptic ulcers.
- Varices secondary to portal hypertension.
- Mallory–Weiss tear.
- Tumours.
- Ischaemic colitis.
- Crohn's disease.
- Ulcerative colitis.
- Diverticulitis.

Assessment findings

- Upper gastrointestinal bleeding:
  - bloody or coffee-ground gastric aspirates or emesis
  - melaena.
- Lower gastrointestinal bleeding—rectal passing of fresh blood or clots.
- Signs of hypovolaemic shock (see ➲ p. 175)—hypotension, tachycardia, prolonged capillary refill time, cool skin, and weak pulse.
- Abdominal distension and tenderness.
- Hyperactive bowel sounds.

Management

- Monitor gastric contents aspirated from oro- or nasogastric tube.
- Monitor bowel movements for melaena.
- Use semi-recumbent positioning (head-up angle of 35–45°).
- Haemodynamic monitoring to assess for hypovolaemic shock.
- Monitor fluid status and treat fluid deficit (see ➲ p. 24).
- Blood components as required (see ➲ p. 398).
- Gastric acid suppressive therapy—proton-pump inhibitor.
- Confirm with doctor the enteral feeding regime, depending on the amount of bleeding, cause of bleeding, and need for endoscopic investigation.[13]
  - Clarify whether enteral feeding should be initiated, continued at the same rate, or stopped.
  - Active bleeding may result in high gastric residual volumes, thus increasing the risk of pulmonary aspiration.
  - Low-rate enteral feeding may protect the gut mucosa and prevent further bleeding.

- Blood investigations:
  - FBC
  - U&E
  - LFTs
  - clotting
  - arterial blood gas
  - cross-matching.
- Use medication with a gastrointestinal vasoconstrictor effect—vasopressin, terlipressin, or octreotide.
- Endoscopy treatment—sclerotherapy or banding.
- Use balloon tamponade if bleeding is not controlled by medication or endoscopy treatment (see Table 10.7).
  - The Sengstaken–Blakemore tube contains three lumens (oesophageal balloon, gastric balloon, and a gastric aspiration port) (see Figure 10.6).
  - The Minnesota tube contains the same three lumens as a Sengstaken–Blakemore tube, but in addition has a fourth lumen for oesophageal aspiration.

Table 10.7 Nursing management of the patient with balloon tamponade*

Intervention	Rationale
Continuous monitoring	Balloon could burst or migrate to oropharynx
Sedation and analgesia	Nasogastric tube is uncomfortable and patient must remain still
Elevated head of bed	To prevent pulmonary aspiration of gastric contents
Aspiration or frequent suction of nasogastric tube	To monitor gastric content and prevent pulmonary aspiration
Irrigation of nasogastric tube	To maintain patency, as the tube may become blocked with clots
Deflate balloon every 6–8 h	To prevent oesophageal necrosis

*Traction is no longer recommended.[14]

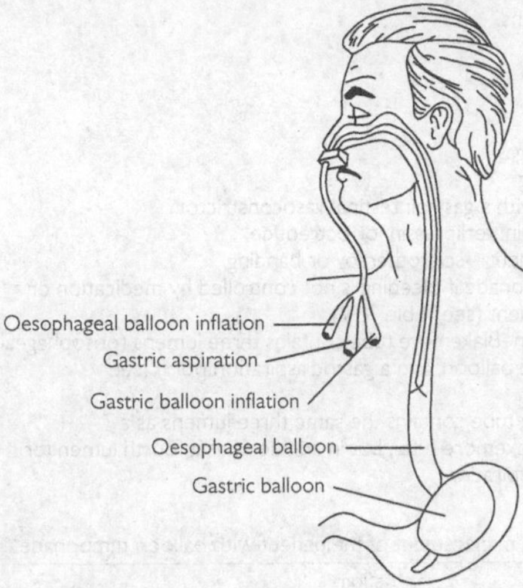

Figure 10.6 Balloon tamponade using a Sengstaken–Blakemore tube. (Reproduced from Waldmann, Soni and Rhodes, *Oxford Desk Reference: critical care*, 2008, with permission from Oxford University Press.)

References

13 Hébuterne X and Vanbiervliet G. Feeding the patients with upper gastrointestinal bleeding. *Current Opinion in Clinical Nutrition and Metabolic Care* 2011; **14**: 197–201.

14 Sargent S. *Liver Diseases: an essential guide for nurses and health care professionals*. Wiley-Blackwell: Chichester, 2009.

Further reading

Waldmann C, Soni N and Rhodes A. Gastrointestinal therapy techniques. In: *Oxford Desk Reference Critical Care*. Oxford University Press: Oxford, 2008. pp. 73–80.

Abdominal compartment syndrome

Definition

Abdominal compartment syndrome [illegible] abdominal fluid.

Increased pressure within the peritoneal [illegible] the walls of the intra-abdominal organs [illegible] output.

Causes

Capillary leakage/fluid resuscitation:

- [illegible] (SIRS)
- [illegible]
- [illegible]
- [illegible]

Increased abdominal contents:

- [illegible]

- [illegible]
- [illegible]
- [illegible]

Increased intraluminal contents:

- [illegible]
- Paralytic ileus
- [illegible]

Decreased abdominal wall compliance:

- [illegible]
- [illegible] PEEP
- [illegible]
- [illegible]

Assessment findings

- [illegible] mmHg
- Abdominal [illegible] and tenderness
- [illegible] vomiting
- [illegible]
- Acute kidney injury
- Acute respiratory failure
- Hypotension [illegible]

Abdominal compartment syndrome

Definition

Abdominal compartment syndrome is defined as a continuous intra-abdominal pressure reading of > 20 mmHg with new organ failure[15] (for an overview of intra-abdominal pressure monitoring, see ➲ p. 300). The underlying problem can be either a primary cause inside the abdomen itself, or a secondary issue outside the abdomen which results in the accumulation of intra-abdominal fluid.

Increased pressure within the peritoneal or retroperitoneal spaces causes ischaemia of the intra-abdominal organs along with secondary complications of dysfunction of the respiratory and cardiovascular systems. For example, as the pressure continues to rise, lung expansion becomes restricted and the vena cava becomes compressed, consequently reducing the return of blood to the heart and ultimately leading to a reduction in cardiac output.

Causes

Capillary leakage during fluid resuscitation

- Systemic inflammatory response syndrome (SIRS).
- Sepsis.
- Burns.
- Trauma.

Increased abdominal contents

- Haemorrhage within the abdominal cavity.
- Ascites.
- Liver disease.
- Pancreatitis.
- Peritonitis.
- Intra-abdominal mass.

Increased intra-luminal contents

- Gastroparesis.
- Paralytic ileus.
- Bowel obstruction.

Decreased abdominal wall compliance

- Patient–ventilator dyssynchrony.
- High levels of intrinsic or extrinsic PEEP.
- Prone positioning.
- Abdominal surgery with tight closure.

Assessment findings

- Intra-abdominal pressure > 20 mmHg.
- Abdomen distended, firm, and tender.
- Nausea and vomiting.
- High gastric residual volumes.
- Acute kidney injury.
- Acute respiratory failure.
- Hypotension, tachycardia, and reduced cardiac output.

Management

- Avoid excessive fluid resuscitation.
- Improve abdominal compliance:
  - Optimize mechanical ventilation settings.
  - Give sedation, analgesia, and neuromuscular block as required.
  - Optimize patient positioning—avoid prone positioning and hip flexion.
- Evacuate intraluminal and abdominal contents:
  - Aspirate oro- or nasogastric tube and leave on free drainage.
  - Give enema.
  - Give prokinetics
  - Drain ascites.
- Haemodynamic monitoring to assess preload and cardiac output (see ➔ p. 226).
- Vasoconstrictor to maintain a mean arterial pressure (MAP) sufficiently higher than the intra-abdominal pressure (IAP) to give an abdominal perfusion pressure (APP) of ≥ 60 mmHg:
  - APP = MAP – IAP.
- Renal replacement therapy for oliguria and/or significant acidosis.
- Surgical decompression.

Reference

15 Kirkpatrick AW et al. Intra-abdominal hypertension and the abdominal compartment syndrome: updated consensus definitions and clinical practice guidelines from the World Society of the Abdominal Compartment Syndrome. *Intensive Care Medicine* 2013; **39**: 1190–206.

Further reading

Lee RK. Intra-abdominal hypertension and abdominal compartment syndrome: a comprehensive overview. *Critical Care Nurse* 2012; **32**: 19–31.

Malbrain M and De Waele J. *Intra-Abdominal Hypertension: core critical care*. Cambridge University Press: Cambridge, 2013.

The Abdominal Compartment Society. www.wsacs.org

Refeeding syndrome

Definition

Malnourished patients are at risk of developing significant metabolic, electrolyte, and fluid shifts if standard feeding regimes are started too quickly or prior to correcting glucose and electrolyte abnormalities. Refeeding syndrome can be a consequence of either enteral or parenteral feeding, and the risk factors for this syndrome are summarized in Table 10.8.

Causes

- Rapid refeeding in patients who are malnourished due to:
    - prolonged starvation
    - anorexia nervosa
    - chronic alcoholism.
- Excessive dextrose infusion.
- Antacids.

Assessment findings

- Pulmonary oedema.
- Arrhythmias.
- Hypophosphataemia.
- Hypokalaemia.
- Hypomagnesaemia.
- Hypocalcaemia.
- Altered glucose metabolism.
- Vitamin deficiencies.

Table 10.8 Criteria for identifying high risk of refeeding syndrome

Patient has one or more of the following:	Patient has two or more of the following:
• BMI < 16 kg/m^2	• BMI < 18.5 kg/m^2
• Unintentional weight loss > 15% within the last 3–6 months	• Unintentional weight loss > 10% within the last 3–6 months
• Little or no nutritional intake for > 10 days	• Little or no nutritional intake for > 5 days
• Low levels of potassium, phosphate, or magnesium prior to feeding	• History of alcohol abuse or medication including insulin, chemotherapy, antacids, or diuretics

Source: NICE guidelines.[16]

Management

- The NICE guidelines[16] make the following recommendations :
  - Commence feeding at 10 kcal/kg/day, increasing the rate slowly to meet or exceed full needs by 4–7 days.
  - Give 5 kcal/kg/day in extreme cases (BMI < 14 kg/m^2 or negligible intake for > 15 days).
  - During the first 10 days of feeding give thiamine, vitamin B, and a balanced multivitamin and trace element supplement.
- Continuous ECG monitoring is required.
- Monitor fluid status and treat imbalances (see ➔ p. 24).
- Monitor electrolytes and treat imbalances prior to starting feeding.
- Coordinate the feeding regime as discussed with dietitian and doctor.

Reference

16 National Institute for Health and Care Excellence (NICE). *Nutrition Support in Adults: oral nutrition support, enteral tube feeding and parenteral nutrition*. CG32. NICE: London, 2006. www.nice.org.uk/guidance/cg32

Further reading

Adkins SM. Recognizing and preventing refeeding syndrome. *Dimensions of Critical Care Nursing* 2009; 28: 53–60.

Byrnes MC and Stangenes J. Refeeding in the ICU: an adult and pediatric problem. *Current Opinion in Clinical Nutrition and Metabolic Care* 2011; **14**: 186–92.

Chapter 11

Sepsis

Introduction

Despite an extensive amount of research aimed at understanding the pathogenesis of SIRS and sepsis and translating this into improved clinical management, mortality remains high, with up to 50% of patients still dying from severe sepsis and septic shock.[1] In the UK, sepsis accounts for 37 000 deaths each year, and also carries an annual financial cost of £2 billion.[2]

Although the prevailing view of the pathophysiology of SIRS is of an overwhelming and inappropriately exaggerated immune response to a trigger, more recent research has shown that there may be a variety of immunological responses.[3] These range from anti-inflammatory to hyper-inflammatory responses. When immunosuppression occurs as an anti-inflammatory response, there may be increased susceptibility to further infection. Stimulation of the inflammatory response will cause release and activation of a complex range of inflammatory mediators from white cells, concomitant activation of inflammatory pathways, and endothelial damage. These result in major alterations to fluid and blood flow redistribution, vasodilatation, microvascular obstruction, altered mitochondrial function, and increased or otherwise altered metabolic demand. The consequence of this may be organ dysfunction, which ranges from 'mild' to severe, and affects one or more organs. Box 11.1 lists the common triggers of SIRS.

Systemic inflammatory response syndrome (SIRS)

This is a non-specific generalized inflammatory response of the body to an extrinsic insult. It typically presents with two or more of the following:

- temperature >38°C or < 36°C
- heart rate > 90 beats/min
- respiratory rate > 20 breaths/min or hyperventilation with P_aCO_2 < 4.3 kPa (32 mmHg)
- WBC count > 12 000 cells/mm^3 or < 4000 cells/mm^3, or > 10% immature forms.

Sepsis

This is defined as SIRS when the trigger for the massive systemic inflammation is a suspected or identified infection.

Box 11.1 Common triggers of SIRS

- Infection
- Trauma
- Pancreatitis
- Major burns
- Major surgery without adequate organ perfusion
- Haemorrhage or major blood transfusion
- Ischaemic tissue
- Periods of inadequate perfusion followed by reperfusion
- Miscellaneous—drug related, near-drowning, pulmonary embolus

Severe sepsis

This is sepsis complicated by organ dysfunction or tissue hypoperfusion.

Septic shock

This is a type of distributive shock in which severe sepsis resulting in hypotension is unresponsive to fluid resuscitation (see ➲ p. 176).

Sepsis-induced hypotension

This is low blood pressure resulting from sepsis in the absence of other causes as evidenced by any of the following:

- systolic blood pressure (SBP) < 90 mmHg
- mean arterial pressure (MAP) < 70 mmHg
- drop in SBP by 40 mmHg compared with patient's baseline value.

Sepsis-induced tissue hypoperfusion

This is poor tissue perfusion as evidenced by any of the following:

- sepsis-induced hypotension
- hyperlactataemia
- oliguria.

References

1 Levy MM. Introduction. In: R Daniels and T Nutbeam (eds) *ABC of Sepsis*. Wiley-Blackwell: Chichester, 2010. pp. 1–4.
2 The UK Sepsis Trust. *Sepsis*. http://sepsistrust.org/sepsis/
3 Mitchell E and Whitehouse T. The pathophysiology of sepsis. In: R Daniels and T Nutbeam (eds) *ABC of Sepsis*. Wiley-Blackwell: Chichester, 2010. pp. 20–24.

Further reading

Daniels R et al. *Sepsis: a guide for patients and relatives*. UK Sepsis Trust: Sutton Coldfield, 2012. http://sepsistrust.org/wp-content/uploads/2013/10/Sepsis_A5_final1.pdf
Global Sepsis Alliance (GSA). http://globalsepsisalliance.com
Kleinpell R et al. Implications of the new international sepsis guidelines for nursing care. *American Journal of Critical Care* 2013; 22: 212–22.
UK Sepsis Group. www.uksepsis.org
UK Sepsis Trust. http://sepsistrust.org
US Sepsis Alliance. www.sepsisalliance.org
World Sepsis Day. www.world-sepsis-day.org

Sepsis presentation

The Surviving Sepsis Campaign[4] defines sepsis as a documented or suspected infection with some of the clinical variables outlined in the diagnostic criteria listed in Table 11.1. Because of this extensive list of associated clinical signs and symptoms, and the numerous types of microorganisms that can potentially cause an infection, sepsis is considered to be a syndrome rather than a specific disease.

Assessment findings

In addition to the clinical signs and symptoms listed in Table 11.1, other findings in a patient with sepsis may include:

- ↓ systemic vascular resistance (SVR)
- ↓ stroke volume
- ↓ central venous pressure (CVP)
- relative hypovolaemia despite oedema (third spacing)
- impaired tissue oxygen utilization (↑ lactate and ↑ SVO_2)
- ↓ SVO_2 if tissues are extracting high levels of oxygen
- acidosis.

Table 11.1 Clinical presentation of sepsis (adapted from the Surviving Sepsis Campaign guidelines[4])

Type of variable	Clinical findings
General	↑ or ↓ Temperature ↑ Heart rate > 90 beats/min ↑ Respiratory rate ↓ Blood pressure Altered mental status Oedema and positive fluid balance Hyperglycaemia in the absence of diabetes
Inflammatory	↑ or ↓ WBC count ↑ CRP ↑ Procalcitonin
Organ dysfunction	↓ PaO_2 and ↓ SpO_2 ↓ Urine output despite fluid resuscitation ↑ Creatinine Coagulation abnormalities Ileus (absent bowel sounds) Thrombocytopenia Hyperbilirubinaemia
Tissue perfusion	↑ Lactate ↓ Capillary refill or mottling

Table 11.2 Comparison of early and late sepsis

Early sepsis: hyperdynamic	Late sepsis: hypodynamic
Warm	Cool
Flushed	Clammy
Bounding pulse	Thready pulse
↑ Respiratory rate	Hypothermia
↑ Cardiac output (or normal)	↓ Cardiac output

Further physical assessment and haemodynamic monitoring findings depend on the progression of sepsis as the patient moves from the hyperdynamic state of early sepsis to a hypodynamic presentation (see Table 11.2). Early sepsis is typical of a distributive type of shock in which the initial clinical problem is a reduced afterload from the systemic vasodilation. Preload is relatively low as a result, and the cardiac output may be high or normal if the patient's cardiac function is capable of increasing inotropy as a compensation response.

If the infective cause of the sepsis is not resolved, the body's compensation mechanisms begin to fail. Myocardial depression may also result from the inflammatory processes of the SIRS response. As the sepsis progresses, the patient becomes cooler, with a reduced cardiac output.

Reference

4 Dellinger RP et al. Surviving sepsis campaign: international guidelines for management of severe sepsis and septic shock: 2012. *Critical Care Medicine* 2013; 41: 580–637.

Severe sepsis presentation

Sepsis is considered to be a critical and serious problem when the severity increases to the point of organ dysfunction or tissue hypo-perfusion.

The diagnostic criteria for severe sepsis in the guidelines of the Surviving Sepsis Campaign[5] include:

- sepsis-induced hypotension
- lactate levels above upper limit of laboratory normal reference range
- urine output < 0.5 mL/kg/h for > 2 h despite fluid resuscitation
- acute lung injury: $PaO_2/F_iO_2 < 250$ in the absence of pneumonia
- acute lung injury: $PaO_2/F_iO_2 < 200$ in the presence of pneumonia
- creatinine > 2.0 mg/dL (176.8 μmol/L)
- bilirubin > 2 mg/dL (34.2 μmol/L)
- platelets < 100 000/μL
- coagulopathy (INR > 1.5).

Reference

5 Dellinger RP et al. Surviving sepsis campaign: international guidelines for management of severe sepsis and septic shock: 2012. *Critical Care Medicine* 2013; **41**: 580–637.

Neutropenic sepsis

Neutropenia

A neutrophil is a type of white blood cell that plays an important role in the inflammatory response to fighting off microorganisms. Patients with a low neutrophil count ($< 1.0 \times 10^9/L$) are therefore significantly at risk of developing infections because of their immunocompromised state. If the infection of a patient with neutropenia results in sepsis, neutropenic sepsis occurs. The typical causes of neutropenia are listed in Box 11.2.

Box 11.2 Causes of neutropenia

- Chemotherapy
- Radiation therapy
- Infections (e.g. HIV, tuberculosis, Epstein–Barr virus)
- Leukaemia
- Aplastic anaemia
- Autoimmune disorders
- Congenital

Patients who are receiving chemotherapy have an even higher risk of neutropenic sepsis if any of the following circumstances are also present:[6]

- time period of 7–10 days after chemotherapy administration
- previous or multiple chemotherapy treatments
- haematological conditions
- invasive intravenous device
- elderly age group
- comorbidities
- advanced cancer
- general poor health
- patients on clinical drug trials.

Patients with neutropenic sepsis can initially present with quite vague symptoms and appear to be 'well' with only mild tachycardia or hypotension. However, once the compensation mechanisms begin to fail, severe sepsis and septic shock can develop extremely quickly because of the lack of neutrophils to manage the infection.

Reference

6 Barrett K and Dikken C. Neutropenic sepsis: preventing an avoidable tragedy. *Journal of Paramedic Practice* 2011; **3**: 116–22.

Further reading

National Institute for Health and Care Excellence (NICE). *Neutropenic Sepsis: prevention and management of neutropenic sepsis in cancer patients*. CG151. NICE: London, 2012. www.nice.org.uk/guidance/CG151

Sepsis 6

The Sepsis 6 is a list of key interventions for improving patient outcome. They should be completed in a timely manner, ideally within the first hour after sepsis is diagnosed. Based on the Surviving Sepsis Campaign guidelines, the Sepsis 6 offers a simplified pathway relevant to the ward setting, and serves as a reminder to critical care clinicians of the fundamental actions necessary to prevent the development of severe sepsis and septic shock.[7]

Sepsis 6 interventions

- High-flow oxygen.
- Blood cultures.
- Antibiotics.
- Lactate and FBC.
- IV fluid administration.
- Check urine output hourly.

Reference

7 Daniels R et al. The sepsis six and the severe sepsis resuscitation bundle: a prospective observational cohort study. *Emergency Medicine Journal* 2011; 28: 507–12.

Early goal-directed therapy

The concept of early goal-directed therapy was introduced in 2001 by Rivers and colleagues,[8] and involved actively attempting to correct preload, afterload, and contractility in patients with severe sepsis or septic shock. This was achieved by aiming for normal values of the specific resuscitation end points of $ScVO_2$, lactate, base deficit, and pH in an attempt to balance oxygen delivery with oxygen demand. The study by Rivers and colleagues[8] demonstrated that patients with sepsis who had early goal-directed therapy initiated on arrival at hospital had a reduced mortality ($P = 0.0009$) and less severe organ dysfunction ($P < 0.001$) compared with patients who received standard therapy. However, there has been criticism of their study because it was a single-centre trial and did not clearly show whether the results were due to the therapy as a whole or to individualized components.[9] Recently, three large multi-centred studies regarding the effectiveness of early goal directed therapy have shown different results to the Rivers study including: Protocolized management in sepsis (PROMISE)[10], Australasian resuscitation in sepsis evaluation (ARISE)[11] and Protocol-based care for early septic shock (ProCESS)[12]. In all three of these trials, aggressive early goal directed therapy care with specific protocols for sepsis did not improve patient outcomes compared with 'usual care'. What constitutes 'usual care' has changed greatly since the original Rivers study in 2001 because of the wide awareness of the Surviving Sepsis Campaign principles which may account for this lack of difference in outcomes.[13] Nevertheless, the findings from PROMISE, ARISE and ProCESS have prompted debate and re-evaluation of the role of early goal directed therapy for septic patients.

References

8 Rivers E et al. Early goal-directed therapy in the treatment of severe sepsis and septic shock. *New England Journal of Medicine* 2001; **345**: 1368-1377.

9 Marik PE. Surviving sepsis: going beyond the guidelines. *Annals of Intensive Care* 2011; **1**: 17.

10 Mouncey PR, Osborn TM, Power GS et al. Trial of early, goal-directed resuscitation for septic shock. *The New England Journal of Medicine* 2015; **372**: 1301–11.

11 The ARISE Investigators and the ANZICS Clinical Trials Group. Goal-directed resuscitation for patients with early septic shock *The New England Journal of Medicine* 2014; **371**: 1496–506.

12 The ProCESS Investigators. A randomized trial of protocol-based care for early septic shock. *The New England Journal of Medicine* 2014; **370**: 1683–93.

Sepsis care bundles

The Surviving Sepsis Campaign[13] has provided two different care bundles for patients with sepsis to standardize practice and ensure that priority actions are completed as early as possible. Time zero is considered to be the point at which the clinical findings of sepsis initially present.

Complete within the first 3 hours

- Lactate measurement.
- Blood cultures prior to antibiotics.
- Broad-spectrum antibiotics.
- Crystalloid 30 mL/kg for hypotension or lactate ≥ 4 mmol/L.

Complete within the first 6 hours

- Vasopressor for hypotension that is unresponsive to initial fluid resuscitation to maintain MAP at ≥ 65 mmHg.
- If hypotension persists despite volume resuscitation (septic shock) or initial lactate > 4 mmol/L, reassess volume status and tissue perfusion.
- Remeasure lactate if levels were previously high.

Reference

13 Dellinger RP et al. Surviving sepsis campaign: international guidelines for management of severe sepsis and septic shock: 2012. *Critical Care Medicine* 2013; 41: 580–637.

Management of severe sepsis

The Surviving Sepsis Campaign guidelines for the management of severe sepsis and septic shock provide a comprehensive overview of evidence-based care, which will now be summarized, highlighting the most relevant aspects for critical care nursing practice.

Initial resuscitation and infection issues

Initial resuscitation

During the first 6h of resuscitation, the goals of initial resuscitation of sepsis-induced hypoperfusion (hypotension or lactate [illegible]) should include all of the following:

- CVP 8–12mmHg
- MAP ≥65mmHg
- Urine output ≥0.5mL/kg/h
- $S_{cv}O_2$ ≥70% or S_vO_2 ≥65%
- [illegible] patients should [illegible] resuscitation [illegible] to normalize lactate level [illegible] appropriate to the patient's elevated lactate levels.

Screening and performance improvement

Early recognition of sepsis is [illegible] used to identify patients who have a potential [illegible] to allow [illegible] earlier [illegible] therapies. [illegible] performance improvement [illegible] initial [illegible] decision.

[illegible] performance improvement efforts [illegible] the implementation of [illegible] [illegible] education [illegible] protocols [illegible] and [illegible] related to sepsis management [illegible] is also important.

Diagnosis

Before the initiation of antibiotic therapy, cultures should be taken, ideally [illegible] of infection [illegible]:

- Blood (two sets [illegible] and [illegible] indwelling vascular access device [illegible] 48h)
- Sputum
- Urine
- Other potential sites [illegible] (e.g. wounds, CSF, pleural fluid)
- Imaging investigations to identify the site of infection may also be required (e.g. X-ray, CT scan, ultrasound).

Antimicrobial therapy

The administration of intravenous antimicrobial therapy [illegible] within the first hour [illegible] of septic shock and severe sepsis without septic shock [illegible] the first [illegible] therapy [illegible] against all likely pathogens and [illegible] into the [illegible] source of infection. [illegible] with [illegible] therapy [illegible] to [illegible] when [illegible] appropriate.

Management of severe sepsis

The Surviving Sepsis Campaign guidelines for the management of severe sepsis and septic shock[14] provide a comprehensive overview of various aspects of care, which will now be summarized, highlighting the most relevant aspects for critical care nursing practice.

Initial resuscitation and infection issues

Initial resuscitation

During the first 6 h of resuscitation of a patient with sepsis-induced hypotension, a protocolized approach may be used to guide care, which is aimed at achieving the following goals:

- CVP 8–12 mmHg
- MAP ≥ 65 mmHg
- urine output 0.5 mL/kg/h
- $ScVO_2 \geq 70\%$ or $SVO_2 \geq 65\%$.

Resuscitation should also be tailored to achieving a normal lactate level if hypoperfusion has caused an elevated lactate level.

Screening and performance improvement

Early recognition of sepsis is more likely if sepsis screening tools are used to identify patients who have a potential or actual infection. If sepsis is detected early on using this type of screening, the sepsis care bundles can then be initiated as soon as possible.

Performance improvement efforts in relation to multidisciplinary actions to improve outcomes for patients with sepsis can include activities such as sepsis-related education programmes, protocols, and auditing. Feedback for all members of the critical care team about local data related to septic patients and areas for further improvement of sepsis care is also important.

Diagnosis

Before the initiation of antibiotic therapy, cultures should be taken from potential sources of infection, such as:

- blood (two separate cultures for both aerobic and anaerobic bottles)
- urine
- sputum
- other potential areas of infection (e.g. wounds, cerebrospinal fluid).

Further investigations to identify an infection may also be required (e.g. X-ray, CT scan, ultrasound, or MRI).

Antimicrobial therapy

The specific antimicrobial agent that is needed for a particular patient with sepsis will depend on the type of pathogen that is causing the infection (e.g. bacteria, virus, or fungus). Antimicrobial therapy should begin within the first hour after identifying severe sepsis or septic shock, and should initially adopt an empirical anti-infective approach, until the laboratory results have confirmed the type and source of infection. Daily review of antimicrobial therapy is necessary to ensure discontinuation when clinically appropriate.

Source control

Once the location of the infection that is causing sepsis has been identified, interventions should be implemented that limit the impact and spread of the infection from this source (e.g. drainage of an abscess, debridement of necrotic tissue, or removal of invasive devices). Intravenous access devices in particular should be removed and re-sited if they are still required.

Infection control

Infection control precautions should be maintained at all times to reduce the spread of the infection to other patients, and to prevent the introduction of new microorganisms to the septic patient. See ➔ p. 44 for a review of infection control priorities in intensive care, including the role of selective oral decontamination and selective digestive decontamination.

Haemodynamic support

Fluid therapy

Initially, liberal amounts of intravenous fluids are typically required for sepsis-induced tissue hypoperfusion, due to the extensive vasodilation and leaky capillaries that occur as a result of the systemic inflammatory response. A 30 mL/kg crystalloid fluid challenge should be given, with further rapid administration of intravenous fluids provided as needed to achieve predefined goals (e.g. goals for pulse pressure, stroke volume variation, mean arterial pressure, heart rate, lactate concentration, and urine output). Hydroxyethyl starches should not be used, although albumin may have a role in patients who require large amounts of crystalloid fluid resuscitation (see ➔ p. 56). If multi-organ dysfunction syndrome (MODS) develops as the sepsis progresses, over-resuscitation can cause pulmonary oedema, acute kidney injury, and intra-abdominal hypertension. Cautious administration of intravenous fluids or fluid removal may be required for later stages of sepsis[15] (see Figure 11.1).

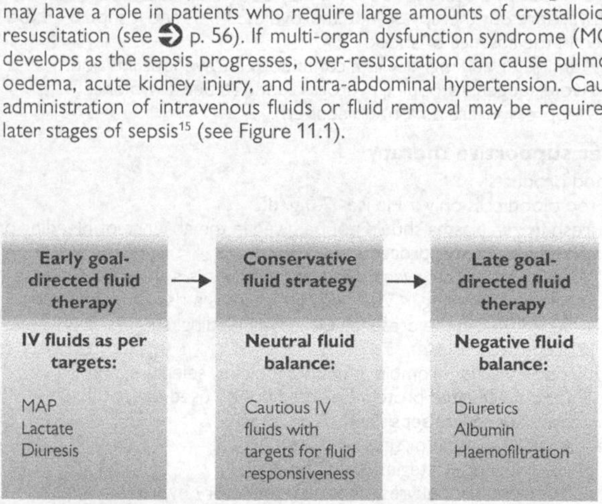

Figure 11.1 Fluid management in patients with severe sepsis. MAP, mean arterial pressure (adapted from the three-hit model and global increased permeability syndrome)[15].

Vasopressors

- The target mean arterial pressure (MAP) should initially be 65 mmHg, and then be evaluated to establish which MAP is needed to achieve resuscitation end points (e.g. lactate, signs of skin perfusion, mental status, urine output).
- Noradrenaline infusion is the vasopressor of choice for sepsis-induced hypotension.
- Adrenaline infusion can be considered if noradrenaline is insufficient to maintain an adequate MAP.
- Vasopressin infusion at 0.03 units/min can also supplement noradrenaline, either to help to reach the target MAP or to decrease the amount of noradrenaline needed.

Inotropic therapy

- Dobutamine infusion up to 20 mcg/kg/min should be administered if there is evidence of:
  - myocardial dysfunction (e.g. low cardiac output, increased cardiac filling pressures)
  - continual hypoperfusion even when the target MAP has been reached by using fluid resuscitation and vasopressor therapy.
- Inotropes should not be administered to elevate cardiac output to supranormal levels.

Corticosteroids

- Intravenous hydrocortisone should only be given if fluid resuscitation and vasopressor therapy do not improve the MAP, and it should not be given in the absence of shock.
  - Administer 200 mg/day as a continuous intravenous infusion.
  - Avoid suddenly stopping hydrocortisone (taper down once vasopressors are no longer required).

Other supportive therapy

- Blood products:
  - red blood cells only if Hb is < 7.0 g/dL
  - fresh frozen plasma should not be given in the absence of bleeding or scheduled invasive procedures
  - platelets should be given if the platelet count is $< 10 \times 10^9$/L in the absence of bleeding, $< 20 \times 10^9$/L if there is a risk of bleeding, or $< 50 \times 10^9$/L in the presence of active bleeding, surgery, or invasive procedures.
- Erythropoietin, antithrombin, immunoglobulins, selenium, and recombinant activated protein C should not be used as specific treatments for severe sepsis and septic shock.
- Mechanical ventilation of sepsis-induced ARDS:
  - protective lung strategies (see ➔ p. 157)
  - recruitment manoeuvres for severe refractory hypoxaemia
  - prone positioning for $PaO_2/FiO_2 \leq 100$ mmHg (see ➔ p. 158)
  - head of bed elevated to 30–45° if the patient is being mechanically ventilated
  - non-invasive ventilation as appropriate (see ➔ p. 142)

    - weaning protocol that includes regular spontaneous breathing trials and extubation as soon as clinically feasible (see ➲ p. 164)
    - pulmonary artery catheter should not be routinely used for sepsis-induced ARDS
    - conservative approach to fluid therapy in the absence of tissue hypoperfusion
    - β-2 agonists should not be used to treat sepsis-induced ARDS unless there is evidence of bronchospasm.
- Sedation, analgesia, and neuromuscular blockade:
    - sedation should be minimized and goal directed (see ➲ p. 77)
    - neuromuscular blocking agents (NMBAs) should be avoided if possible in the absence of ARDS, but are indicated for early sepsis-induced ARDS and $PaO_2/FiO_2 < 150$ mmHg (see ➲ p. 82)
    - train-of-four monitoring for patients who are receiving NMBAs (see ➲ p. 83).
- Insulin infusion to maintain blood glucose concentration at ≤ 10 mmol/L.
- Renal replacement therapy as required using continuous therapy for haemodynamically unstable septic patients (see ➲ p. 290).
- Bicarbonate therapy should not be used to improve haemodynamic status or for lactic acidosis with pH ≥ 7.15.
- DVT prophylaxis using low-molecular-weight heparin and compression devices or thromboembolic-deterrent (TED) stockings.
- Stress ulcer prophylaxis for patients with risk factors for gastrointestinal bleeding.
- Nutrition:
    - administer enteral or oral feeding as soon as possible, starting with low-dose feeding (up to 500 calories/day) and increasing caloric intake only as tolerated (see ➲ p. 62)
    - instead of total parenteral nutrition (TPN) alone, use glucose and enteral nutrition or supplemental parenteral nutrition (TPN and enteral) in the first week after severe sepsis or septic shock has been identified (see ➲ p. 66).
- Do not use nutrition with specific immunomodulating supplements.
- Set goals of care and discuss the prognosis with the patient and their family as early as possible, or at least within 72 h after ICU admission.

References

14 Dellinger RP et al. Surviving sepsis campaign: international guidelines for management of severe sepsis and septic shock: 2012. *Critical Care Medicine* 2013; **41**: 580–637.

15 Cordemans C et al. Fluid management in critically ill patients: the role of extravascular lung water, abdominal hypertension, capillary leak, and fluid balance. *Annals of Intensive Care* 2012; **2** (Suppl. 1): S1. http://www.ncbi.nlm.nih.gov/pmc/articles/PMC3390304/

Metabolic disorders

Diabetes mellitus

Definition

Diabetes mellitus is a chronic disease characterized by raised blood glucose levels. The disease has several different subtypes:

- **Type 1 diabetes**—thought to be related to autoimmune destruction of the beta cells in the pancreas. It commonly occurs in childhood or young adulthood, and patients require insulin replacement therapy.
- **Type 2 diabetes**—the most common form of diabetes. The World Health Organization predicts that there will be a doubling in the number of people with type 2 diabetes by 2030. It normally occurs as a result of the development of insulin resistance and a reduction in the ability of the pancreas to produce sufficient insulin. It may be controlled by dietary modification, oral hypoglycaemic medication, or insulin, depending on the severity of the disease. The increasing number of patients with type 2 diabetes in developed countries is thought to be due to lifestyle factors such as poor diet and obesity.
- **Gestational diabetes**—this can occur as a result of pregnancy, and the patient's health status may return to normal after delivery, or gestational diabetes may precede the development of type 2 diabetes.

Patients with diabetes may be admitted to critical care because of poor glucose control, which may be caused by:

- diabetic ketoacidosis
- hyperglycaemic hyperosmolar states
- hypoglycaemia.

Diabetic ketoacidosis

Definition

Diabetic ketoacidosis (DKA) is a complex metabolic disorder [illegible]

- hyperglycaemia
- acidosis
- ketonaemia.

[illegible] in patients with type 1 diabetes [illegible] patients with type 2 diabetes. The incidence is [illegible] members of the population [illegible] over the past two decades [illegible]

Assessment findings

The patient should be assessed [illegible]

[illegible]

Management

[illegible]

Management is based on:

[illegible]

Monitoring

[illegible]

Diabetic ketoacidosis

Definition

Diabetic ketoacidosis (DKA) is a complex metabolic disorder characterized by the presence of:

- hyperglycaemia
- acidosis
- ketonaemia.

It is more likely to occur in patients with type 1 diabetes, but is increasingly being seen in patients with type 2 diabetes. The incidence is approximately 4–8 episodes per 1000 members of the population of patients with diabetes. Mortality rates have fallen significantly over the past two decades, and represent about 2% of all cases.

Assessment findings

The patient should be assessed using a systematic framework such as ABCDE (see ➲ p. 18) to evaluate the effect of DKA on the body's systems. Patients who present in critical care with DKA are likely to have a combination of the following symptoms on admission:

- blood ketone level > 6 mmol/L
- bicarbonate level < 5 mmol/L
- arterial pH < 7.0
- decreased GCS score (< 12)
- reduced oxygen saturations
- hypotension secondary to hypovolaemia (excessive diuresis)
- tachycardia
- anion gap > 16 mmol/L.

Management

Management should follow a recognized care bundle. The Joint British Diabetes Societies Inpatient Care Group[1] recommends that care bundles are split into four time zones in the first 24-h period:

- hour 1—immediate management
- 1–6 hours
- 6–12 hours
- 12–24 hours.

Management is based on:

- stabilization
- restoration of adequate circulation
- glucose control
- electrolyte replacement.

Stabilization

The patient's ability to maintain an airway should be assessed. If the patient's GCS score is low, intubation and mechanical ventilation are likely to be needed.

- Self-ventilating patients will require oxygen to maintain normal saturations.
- Frequent ABG measurements should be recorded to monitor O_2, CO_2, and pH levels.

Restoration of adequate circulation

- Water deficits are likely to be high (estimated at 100 mL deficit/kg).
- Significant fluid replacement may be required.
- Crystalloid fluid replacement is recommended. Current guidelines suggest 0.9 % saline with added premixed KCl. Care should be taken to monitor for hyperchloraemia.
- Rapid fluid replacement with care is recommended for adults. Rapid fluid replacement is not recommended for children and small young adults. Table 12.1 shows the suggested rates for a previously well 70 kg adult.[1]
- Target blood pressure is normally a systolic pressure of > 90 mmHg.
- CVS monitoring and invasive fluid assessment (e.g. CVP) may be required.
- Fluid balance should be closely monitored. The patient will require urinary catheterization.
- Patients with a history of CVS, renal impairment, or comorbidities will require extra vigilance during the assessment of fluid status.

Glucose control

- A fixed-rate IV insulin infusion (FRIII) should be commenced, and this should be related to weight, with the exception of obese patients, for whom a modified scale is recommended.
- Give an insulin infusion of 50 units of soluble insulin in 50 mL of 0.9% saline.
- Current guidelines suggest that a fixed rate of 0.1 unit of insulin/ kg/h should be infused (e.g. 7 mL/h). Suggested weight-related infusion rates are shown in Table 12.2.[1]
- Regular blood glucose monitoring is essential.
- If the blood glucose concentration is > 20 mmol/L or 'high' on point-of-care testing (POCT), specimens should be sent to the main laboratory.
- The blood glucose concentration should decrease by 3 mmol/h. Failure to achieve this target requires urgent review.

Table 12.1 Saline and potassium replacement regime[1]

Fluid	Volume
0.9% sodium chloride	1000 mL over first hour
0.9% sodium chloride with potassium chloride	1000 mL over next 2 h
0.9% sodium chloride with potassium chloride	1000 mL over next 2 h
0.9% sodium chloride with potassium chloride	1000 mL over next 4 h
0.9% sodium chloride with potassium chloride	1000 mL over next 4 h
0.9% sodium chloride with potassium chloride	1000 mL over next 6 h
Reassessment of CVS status is mandatory at 12 h. Further fluid may be required	

Table 12.2 Weight-related doses for fixed-rate IV insulin infusion (FRIII)

Patient weight (kg)	Insulin dose (units/h)
60–69	6
70–79	7
80–89	8
90–99	9
100–109	10
110–119	11
120–129	12
130–139	13
140–149	14
> 150	15 (refer to diabetic team)

- If the glucose concentration falls below 14 mmol/L in the first 6 h, IV glucose may be required.
- Blood ketones should be assessed regularly. If this is not possible, venous bicarbonate levels may be assessed. Ketone monitoring should be continued until ketoacidosis has been corrected.
- If the patient takes long-acting insulin this may still be administered subcutaneously if the local protocol permits.
- FRIII should be discontinued once the patient is stable. Normal medication administration should then be commenced following discussion with the medical team.

Electrolyte replacement

- Administration of IV insulin *will* reduce serum potassium levels. Therefore close observation is needed.
- The recommended target range for potassium levels is 4–5 mmol/L.
- Potassium replacement should be given as standard (see Table 12.1). If potassium levels are outside the normal reference range (high or low), medical review should be urgently sought.
- Monitor for signs of cardiac arrhythmias linked to potassium abnormalities.
- There is no evidence to support the routine use of sodium bicarbonate or phosphate administration.
- Regular assessment of other electrolytes is recommended, and treatment in line with normal local protocols.

Complications associated with DKA

Several complications may arise following the management of DKA. These include the following:

- **Hypokalaemia and hyperkalaemia**—these are potentially life-threatening. Careful management during the acute episode should prevent them from occurring.
- **Hypoglycaemia**—severe hypoglycaemia is associated with cardiac arrhythmias, acute brain injury, and death. Care should be taken to closely monitor blood glucose levels, and replacement glucose should be provided once the blood glucose concentration falls to 14 mmol/L and FRIII is continuing. Close monitoring for signs of hypoglycaemia is essential. Note that signs will be masked in the sedated ventilated patient.
- **Cerebral oedema**—this is uncommon in adults with DKA. Children are more likely to develop cerebral oedema, and therefore separate guidance is available for the management of DKA in children.
- **Pulmonary oedema**—this is unlikely to occur, and if it does may be linked to iatrogenic fluid overload. Care should be taken with fluid replacement in vulnerable groups (i.e. patients with cardiac or renal impairment, or comorbidities). Additional monitoring and assessment may be required in these patient groups.

Reference

1 Joint British Diabetes Societies Inpatient Care Group. *The Management of Diabetic Ketoacidosis in Adults*. Diabetes UK: London, 2013.

Hyperglycaemic hyperosmolar state

Definition

There is not a universally accepted definition of hyperglycaemic hyperosmolar state (HHS), and it is argued that any such definition would be an arbitrary one. Nevertheless, this is a specific problem associated with diabetes that requires specific management. It is more common in elderly patients with type 2 diabetes, but may also be seen in younger patients. The mortality rate is significantly higher, at around 15–25% of patients who present with HHS. The condition tends to manifest over a period of days (unlike DKA), resulting in severe dehydration and hyperosmolar states. Other respects in which HHS differs from DKA include:

- high osmolarity
- hyperglycaemia without severe ketoacidosis
- severe dehydration
- an extremely unwell patient.

Assessment

The patient should be assessed using a systematic framework such as ABCDE (see ➔ p. 18) to evaluate the effect of HHS on the body's systems. Patients who are admitted to level 2 or 3 care tend to present with:

- serum osmolality > 350 mOsm/L
- serum sodium concentration > 160 mmol/L
- pH < 7.0
- hypo- or hyperkalaemia
- deteriorating GCS score or cognitive impairment
- reduced oxygen saturations
- low blood pressure
- tachycardia or bradycardia
- oliguria
- serum creatinine concentration > 200 µmol/L
- hypothermia
- other serious comorbidities.

Management

Management should follow a recognized care bundle. The Joint British Diabetes Societies Inpatient Care Group[2] recommends that care bundles are divided into four time zones in the first 24-h period:

- hour 1—immediate management
- 1–6 h
- 6–12 h
- 12–24 h.

The goals of treatment are to:

- stabilize the patient
- normalize serum osmolality
- restore circulating volume
- normalize blood glucose levels
- restore electrolyte balance.

Stabilization

The patient's ability to maintain an airway should be assessed. If the patients's GCS score is low, intubation and mechanical ventilation are likely to be needed.

- Self-ventilating patients will require oxygen to maintain normal saturations.
- Frequent ABG measurements should be recorded to monitor O_2, CO_2, and pH levels.

Normalization of serum osmolality

- Patients will present with extreme fluid loss It is estimated that HHS causes fluid depletion in the range of 100–220 mL/kg.
- Serum osmolality requires close monitoring and should be measured hourly. (If POCT is not available, this may require calculation using the following formula: serum osmolality = $2Na^+$ + glucose + urea.) It may be useful to plot the results graphically to see the trend in levels.
- Rapid changes in osmolality may be harmful because rapid correction of osmolality may cause significant fluid shifts, so fluid replacement should be performed cautiously to provide a gradual decline in serum osmolality.

Restoration of circulating volume

- Cautious fluid replacement is required to prevent significant fluid shifts and complications of HHS.
- Current recommendations are that 0.9% sodium chloride should be used as principal fluid replacement. If the patient's osmolality is not falling despite fluid replacement, hypotonic solutions such as 0.45% sodium chloride may be used.
- The aim of treatment is to replace approximately 50% of volume lost in the first 12 h, and the remainder in the following 12 h.
- The suggested fluid regime is 1 L of 0.9% sodium chloride in the first hour, followed by 0.5–1 L/h in the next 6 h. The target is to achieve a positive balance of 2–3 L within 6 h.
- Care should be taken with vulnerable groups (i.e. patients with cardiac or renal impairment, and those with comorbidities).

Normalization of blood glucose levels

- Fluid replacement alone will reduce blood glucose levels as serum osmolality decreases during the initial stages.
- Care should be taken to ensure that insulin therapy is commenced *after* initial fluid resuscitation, to avoid fluid shifts to the intracellular space.
- Insulin may be required earlier in the management of the patient if they have significant ketonaemia.
- If insulin is required, a fixed-rate IV insulin infusion (FRIII) should be started at 0.05 units/kg/h (e.g. 4 units in an 80 kg patient).
- The aim is to reduce blood glucose levels slowly, at a rate of 5 mmol/L/h.
- Higher doses of insulin may be required if the initial doses of insulin and fluid do not decrease blood glucose levels.

Restoration of electrolyte balance

- Sodium and potassium levels should be closely monitored.
- Sodium levels may increase slightly during initial fluid resuscitation.
- Further fluid resuscitation may be required if sodium levels continue to rise.
- Sodium levels should not be decreased too quickly. *The decrease should not exceed 10 mmol in 24 h.*
- Potassium shifts are less pronounced than in DKA.
- Potassium levels should be monitored and potassium replaced if necessary.
- Hypophosphataemia and hypomagnesaemia are common in HHS.
- There is little evidence to support replacement of phosphate and magnesium unless this is clinically indicated.

Complications of HHS

Complications are associated with a higher mortality rate in this group of patients. They include:

- vascular complications:
  - myocardial infarction
  - stroke
  - venous thromboembolism
- seizures
- cerebral oedema
- central pontine myelinolysis.

The cerebral complications are normally associated with a rapid shift in osmolality levels. Therefore it is important to correct osmolality carefully and gradually.

Reference

2 Joint British Diabetes Societies Inpatient Care Group. *Management of the Hyperosmolar Hyperglycaemic State (HHS) in Adults with Diabetes*. Diabetes UK: London, 2013.

Hypoglycaemia

Definition

Hypoglycaemia is the commonest side effect of insulin and sulfonylurea medications. Other treatments for diabetes are less likely to cause hypoglycaemia. Hypoglycaemia may be defined as a blood glucose concentration below 4 mmol/L.

Risk factors for critically ill patients developing hypoglycaemia include:
- tight glycaemic control
- severe liver failure
- renal replacement therapy
- reduction in feeding or carbohydrate intake
- Addison's disease
- hypo- and hyperthyroidism
- misreading the patient's prescription, or medication error
- inadequate blood glucose monitoring.

Assessment

Common signs of hypoglycaemia may be masked in the sedated and ventilated critically ill patient. The patient should be assessed using a systematic framework such as ABCDE (see ➔ p. 18) to evaluate the effect of hypoglycaemia on the body's systems. Symptoms include the following:

Autonomic signs
- Sweating.
- Palpitations.
- Shaking.
- Hunger.

Neuroglycopenic signs
- Confusion.
- Drowsiness.
- Odd behaviour.
- Speech difficulty.
- Incoordination.

General malaise
- Headache.
- Nausea.

In addition, hypoglycaemia can cause:
- coma
- hemiparesis
- seizures
- permanent neurological deficits
- death.

Management

Prompt management is essential to prevent neurological damage. An ABCDE assessment (see ➲ p. 18) will identify the priorities of care. The patient may require high-flow oxygen or increased oxygen during the hypoglycaemic episode. Management includes the following:

- immediate cessation of any IV insulin until the patient has stabilized
- increasing blood glucose levels (the three options are shown in Table 12.3)
- reassessment and close monitoring of blood glucose levels following a hypoglycaemic episode
- checking blood glucose levels more regularly following a hypoglycaemic episode
- establishing whether there was a reason why hypoglycaemia occurred.

Table 12.3 Methods of increasing blood glucose levels

Drug	Method of administration
Glucagon	Useful for patients without IV access May take up to 15 min to work Mobilizes glycogen from the liver Less effective if patient is taking sulfonylurea, or if patient has liver failure or chronic malnutrition
20% or 10% glucose	75–85 mL over 10–15 min (20%) 150–160 mL over 10–15 min (10%) Given intravenously Rapid response Blood glucose levels should be checked after 10 min Repeated doses may be required Extravasion may cause tissue damage Central access is preferred route May be given peripherally in an emergency (unlicensed route) May cause pain or phlebitis if given peripherally May cause rebound hyperglycaemia

Further reading

Joint British Diabetes Societies Inpatient Care Group. *The Hospital Management of Hypoglycaemia in Adults with Diabetes Mellitus*. Diabetes UK: London, 2013.

Diabetes insipidus

Definition

Diabetes insipidus (DI) is caused by insufficient secretion of antidiuretic hormone (ADH). In the absence of ADH the kidneys secrete too much water, leading to significant fluid loss and hypovolaemia. High sodium levels are caused by the removal of excessive water, and serum osmolality will rapidly increase. DI can be triggered by nephrogenic or neurogenic causes. It may also be triggered by pregnancy (gestational DI).

Nephrogenic DI causes the kidneys to fail to respond to the presence of ADH. It can be triggered by:

- genetic disorders
- renal diseases:
  - pyelonephritis
  - post transplantation
- systemic diseases:
  - sickle-cell anaemia
  - polycystic disease
- medication side effects:
  - lithium
  - gentamycin.

Neurogenic or central DI may be triggered by:

- cerebral oedema following traumatic brain injury
- damage to the pituitary gland (e.g. due to trauma, surgery, or stroke)
- tumours of the posterior pituitary gland, or removal of tumours of the pituitary gland.

Assessment

The patient should be assessed using a systematic framework such as ABCDE (see ➔ p. 18) to evaluate the effect of hypoglycaemia on the body's systems. Symptoms include:

- polyuria
- polydipsia (if the patient is conscious)
- signs of dehydration
- hypotension
- tachycardia
- increased capillary refill time
- decreased CVP.

Laboratory results may show:

- reduced levels of ADH
- high sodium levels
- high serum osmolality
- low urine osmolality
- low urinary specific gravity.

Management

Management is linked to:

- prevention of dehydration
- correction of sodium imbalance
- prevention of further complications.

Nursing and medical management

- Careful recording of fluid intake and output is essential.
- Accurate fluid balance is needed to enable calculation of likely fluid requirements. The free water (FW) deficit may be calculated using the following formula:

  $$\text{FW deficit} = 0.6 \times \text{weight (kg)} \times (\text{current Na} \div 140 - 1).$$

- Regular cardiovascular assessment is needed to determine the effect of fluid loss on cardiac output.
- Fluid replacement is needed to prevent dehydration and hypovolaemic shock. Significant fluid replacement may be required if diuresis is excessive. Fluid replacement will be guided by blood results and the patient's condition.
- Neurogenic DI (central DI) responds well to administration of vasopressin, and this should be given as required to reduce urine output.
- Nephrogenic DI will not respond to vasopressin, and may require the use of thiazide diuretics to attempt to regulate water and sodium excretion.
- A rapid return to normal osmolality may cause worsening of cerebral oedema in patients with traumatic brain injury, and care should be taken to closely monitor serum osmolality.

Complications of DI

- Cardiovascular compromise.
- Seizures.
- Encephalopathy.

Further reading

Morton PG and Fontaine DK. *Essentials of Critical Care Nursing: a holistic approach.* Lippincott Williams & Wilkins: Philadelphia, PA, 2013.

Hyperthyroidism

Definition

Hyperthyroidism is a medical condition caused by excessive levels of thyroid hormones. Graves' disease is the most common form of hyperthyroidism. Over-secretion of thyroid hormones leads to increased cellular metabolism throughout the body, and symptoms may include:

- weight loss
- tachycardia
- hyperactivity
- fatigue
- gastrointestinal hypermotility
- muscle tremor
- anxiety
- exophthalmos.

A rare but life-threatening form of hyperthyroidism is thyrotoxicosis (sometimes referred to as a thyroid storm). Thyrotoxicosis normally occurs in untreated or undertreated patients with hyperthyroidism. It may be triggered by:

- severe infection
- pregnancy
- trauma
- withdrawal or non-compliance with anti-thyroid medication
- iodine therapy.

Assessment

The patient should be assessed using a systematic framework such as ABCDE (see ➔ p. 18) to evaluate the effect of hormone excess on the body's systems. Symptoms include:

- pyrexia (often > 40°C)
- tachycardia
- arrhythmias
- hypertension
- hypotension
- cardiac failure
- fluctuations in consciousness (agitation, confusion, or coma)
- seizures
- diarrhoea, vomiting, and abdominal pain
- unexplained jaundice.

Management

Management of the patient should focus on four main areas:

- supportive therapy
- reduction of plasma thyroid concentration
- blockade of the peripheral effects of thyroxine
- isolation of causative factors.

It is usual to measure thyroid-stimulating hormone, and free and total T_3 and T_4.

- Airway and breathing assessment is needed to determine the adequacy of ventilation and oxygenation.
- Oxygen should be administered in self-ventilating patients to maintain normal saturations (above 94%).
- Cardiovascular assessment is needed to determine the effects of excessive thyroxine on the cardiovascular status.
- Continuous monitoring is needed to identify and allow prompt management of cardiac arrhythmias.
- Anti-arrhythmic medication may be required.
- Blood pressure and cardiac output should be monitored and heart failure treated if necessary.
- Temperature regulation should be monitored and appropriate action taken to treat hyperpyrexia.
- Sedation may be required if the patient is excessively agitated. However, care should be taken that the sedative medication does not suppress respiratory function.

Medical management

Various medical regimes may be used to control acute episodes. Treatment is aimed at blocking the synthesis, release, and conversion of thyroxine and reducing the effects of thyroxine on the cardiovascular system. This is achieved as follows:

- Anti-thyroid medication to prevent the synthesis of thyroxine will normally be administered.
- Iodine to inhibit the release of thyroxine may also be administered.
- Beta blockade is used to inhibit the peripheral effects of excessive thyroxine and reduce stress on the cardiovascular system.
- Steroids may also be administered to inhibit the conversion of T3 to T4. Hydrocortisone or dexamethasone may be used.

A final consideration is the isolation and management of the cause.

- If infection is likely, appropriate antimicrobial treatment should be commenced.
- Trauma or other suspected contributing factors should be managed accordingly.

Further reading

Carroll R and Matfin G. Endocrine and metabolic emergencies: thyroid storm. *Therapeutic Advances in Endocrinology and Metabolism* 2010; 1: 139–45.

Hypothyroidism

Definition

Hypothyroidism or myxoedema is a medical condition caused by decreased levels of thyroid hormones—T3 (liothyronine sodium) and T4 (thyroxine sodium). Patients with hypothyroidism present in hospital with symptoms related to under-secretion of hormones. These may include:

- bradycardia
- hypotension
- fatigue
- oedema
- increased weight.

Myxoedema coma is a rare but life-threatening condition linked to decreased thyroid function. This group of patients will normally require critical care management. Myxoedema coma occurs in patients with hypothyroidism, and may be triggered by:

- infection
- stroke
- trauma
- gastrointestinal bleeds
- use of some sedatives.

It may also be triggered in critically ill patients if their maintenance dose of thyroxine is omitted. Patients may also present in an acute coma with previously undiagnosed hypothyroidism.

Assessment

The patient should be assessed using a systematic framework such as ABCDE (see ➔ p. 18) to evaluate the effect of hormone deficiency on the body's systems. Symptoms include:

- decreased level of consciousness
- seizures
- hypoxia and hypercapnia secondary to hypoventilation
- hypotension
- bradycardia
- heart blocks and arrhythmias
- fluid retention
- hyponatraemia
- decreased gut motility
- nausea, vomiting, and constipation
- hypothermia
- hypoglycaemia.

Management

Immediate stabilization of the patient presenting with myxoedema coma is essential alongside drug therapy to correct decreased thyroxine levels.

- Airway assessment is required, as decreased level of consciousness may necessitate intubation.
- Ventilation or respiratory support may be required to maintain adequate gaseous exchange.

- Acid–base balance should be monitored with ABG sampling.
- Thorough assessment of cardiovascular status is required to monitor the effects of electrolyte imbalance on the cardiovascular system.
- Continuous cardiac monitoring will be required, especially if the patient has severe bradycardia or heart block.
- Fluid balance should be monitored and fluid and electrolytes replaced accordingly. Cautious fluid replacement may be used to maintain diuresis.
- Care should be taken not to increase sodium imbalance too quickly because of the risk of central pontine myelinolysis (damage to the myelin sheath of neurons in the brainstem). This may cause life-threatening neurological disturbances such as unconsciousness, seizures, and cessation of respiratory function.
- Blood glucose monitoring and supplementation of glucose may be required (see ➔ p. 354).
- Central temperature should be monitored, as the patient may require gradual rewarming.
- Neurological status should be closely monitored. Seizures should be monitored and treated accordingly.
- The cause of the crisis should be identified and treated.
- Drug therapy (I.e. thyroxine replacement) will be required. This should be administered either orally or intravenously, depending on the patient's condition. Thyroxine levels should be monitored carefully. A sudden increase in thyroxine levels may cause angina, arrhythmias, and myocardial infarction, so should be avoided.

Further reading

Mathew V et al. Myxedema coma: a new look into an old crisis. *Journal of Thyroid Research* 2011; 2011: 493462.

Phaeochromocytoma

Definition

A phaeochromocytoma is a rare endocrine tumour of the chromaffin cells that causes excessive secretion of catecholamines and is associated with signs and symptoms of catecholamine excess. Patients with phaeochromocytoma may be admitted to critical care units because of:

- a hypertensive crisis triggered by the tumour
- the need for pre-optimization before surgery (specialist centre)
- post-operatively, following excision of tumour (specialist centre).

Assessment

Signs and symptoms are related to excessive amounts of circulating catecholamines. Patients may present with:

- palpitations or tachycardia
- headache
- sweating
- severe hypertension (sustained or paroxysmal)
- nausea and other abdominal symptoms
- chest pain
- hyperglycaemia.

Diagnosis is based on a number of assessment tools, including:

- measurement of urinary and serum metanephrines (formed by the breakdown of catecholamines); this may not be useful in critical care patients
- CT scan
- MRI
- PET scan.

Management

Initial management may be medical in nature and focus on stabilization of the patient if a hypertensive crisis occurs. It is likely that short-acting antihypertensive medication will be administered in a hypertensive crisis.

Management of hypertension

Patients in a hypertensive crisis will require:

- constant cardiovascular monitoring
- administration of short-acting antihypertensive medication
- careful titration of medication to prevent significant swings in blood pressure.

Surgery is usually the main treatment for this tumour, and may be performed laparoscopically. Management may relate to pre-operative and post-operative considerations.

Pre-operative considerations

Surgery may cause a massive release of catecholamines, and it is usual practice to attempt to reduce the problems associated with surgery by adequate pre-operative preparation. This may involve the following:

- Thorough cardiovascular assessment (echocardiogram, blood pressure measurement, ECG, etc.). Pre-existing cardiac disease will be adversely affected by sudden release of catecholamines.
- Administration of alpha blockade to minimize the risk of an intra-operative hypertensive crisis. Calcium-channel blockers may also be used.
- Low-dose beta blockade may also be administered to minimize the potential tachycardia reflex response.
- An acute pre-operative hypertensive crisis may be managed with short-acting antihypertensive medication such as nitroprusside or magnesium sulphate.

Post-operative considerations

Surgery can potentially cause the patient to become unstable, and blood pressure instability and tachycardia are common, as is hypoglycaemia. Removal of the tumour may precipitate marked vasodilatation that may not respond to vasopressors because of pre-operative alpha blockade which persists for more than 36 h. Patients may require:

- constant cardiovascular monitoring
- fluid resuscitation to maintain blood pressure
- monitoring of blood glucose levels (due to rebound hypoglycaemia)
- monitoring for a potential Addisonian crisis (in patients with hypotension and hypoglycaemia)
- hypertension can occur, and the underlying cause should be determined and treated (e.g. pain, autonomic instability, volume overload).

Further reading

Därr R et al. Pheochromocytoma—update on disease management. *Therapeutic Advances in Endocrinology and Metabolism* 2012; 3: 11–26.

Addison's disease

Definition

Addison's disease is a relatively rare disorder caused by primary adrenal cortisol insufficiency. It usually occurs as a result of autoimmune destruction of the adrenal cortex, but may also be triggered by cancers, tuberculosis, infection, and as a side effect of some medications (e.g. ketoconazole). In addition, it may occur secondary to hypothyroidism, surgical removal of the pituitary gland, or a sudden withdrawal from high-dose glucocorticoid therapy.

Assessment

Signs and symptoms are related to the decreasing levels of glucocorticoids and mineralocorticoids. Two of the primary roles of these hormones are to help to regulate fluid and electrolyte balance and blood glucose levels.

Acute development of adrenal cortisol insufficiency can trigger an Addisonian crisis (a life-threatening condition which may manifest with little warning). This may follow severe infection, trauma, or major surgery where the demand for cortisol and aldosterone exceeds supply.

The patient will quickly deteriorate and cardiovascular collapse will occur if prompt management is not instigated. The patient should be assessed using a systematic framework such as ABCDE (see ➔ p. 18) to evaluate the effect of hormone deficiency on the body's systems. Symptoms include:

- fluid and electrolyte loss
- hypovolaemia
- hyponatraemia
- hypoglycaemia
- hyperkalaemia
- hypercalcaemia
- leukocytosis
- possible acidosis
- possible abdominal pain, nausea, and vomiting.

Management

Immediate management of an Addisonian crisis is necessary to ensure that essential metabolic function is maintained. Crawford and Harris[3] have highlighted the need to target the 5 S's:

- salt replacement
- sugar replacement
- steroid replacement
- support of physiological functions
- search for the causative factor.

This will necessitate the following:

- thorough assessment of the patient's cardiovascular status to monitor for the effects of fluid loss and electrolyte imbalance of the cardiovascular system
- rapid fluid replacement using crystalloids; inotropic support may be required if cardiovascular compromise is severe
- continuous ECG monitoring because of hyperkalaemia

Box 12.1 Administration of hydrocortisone and fludrocortisone

Initial treatment	Later treatment
Hydrocortisone:	Fludrocortisone:
Mimics the effects of normal corticosteroids, and achieves similar results May have some immuno-suppressive effects and may alter the metabolism of fats, carbohydrates, and proteins	Used for its mineralocorticoid properties. It binds to the aldosterone receptors and increases fluid retention and sodium retention, thus increasing extracellular volume. It also facilitates excretion of potassium, thus reducing hyperkalaemia

- correction of hyperkalaemia using insulin and dextrose to prevent cardiac arrhythmias
- strict fluid balance to note fluid losses and replacement
- strict blood glucose monitoring, and replacement of glucose if serum blood glucose levels are low (see ➲ p. 354)
- administration of hydrocortisone (immediate drug therapy) and fludrocortisone (once the patient is stable) (see Box 12.1)
- investigations to identify and rectify the possible cause
- vigilance for signs of infection (linked to immunosuppression by IV steroids).

Reference

3 Crawford A and Harris H. Adrenal cortex disorders: hormones out of kilter. *Nursing 2011 Critical Care* 2011; 7: 20–35.

Chapter 13

Immunology

Components of the immune system

Lymphatic system

Lymphatic plexuses

These networks of lymphatic vessels are located in the tissue intercellular spaces that drain tissue fluid into lymph.

Lymphatics

These are a collection of lymphatic vessels that originate from lymphatic plexuses along which lymph nodes are located.

Lymph nodes

These small masses of lymphatic tissue collect and filter lymph and transport it to the circulation.

Lymphatic ducts

These larger lymphatic vessels combine to form the ducts that drain lymph from all areas of the body into the venous system for elimination.

Lymph

This is tissue fluid, which is usually clear and watery, and has the same constituents as plasma. In the presence of infection, foreign proteins are also drained in the lymph from the affected tissue. This stimulates an immunological response, including the formation of specific antibodies and lymphocytes (see Box 13.1 for a definition of lymphoedema).

Organs

Skin

This produces and secretes antimicrobial proteins and immune cells.

Bone marrow

This produces phagocytes, macrophages, and antigen-presenting cells by a process known as haematopoiesis.

Thymus

This lymphoid organ is located in the lower part of the neck. It produces mature T cells from immature thymocytes that have migrated from the bone marrow to be released into the circulation.

Spleen

This lymphoid organ is located in the left upper quadrant region of the abdomen (see ➲ p. 297). It contains B and T lymphocytes, macrophages, natural killer cells, and dendritic cells.

Box 13.1 Lymphoedema

This is defined as an accumulation of lymph in the interstitial space. It occurs as a result of impaired drainage into the lymphatic system.

Pathogens

A pathogen is a disease-causing microorganism (see Box 13.2 for a list of microorganisms).

Box 13.2 Microorganisms

- Prokaryotes (have a non-membrane-bound nucleus):
  - bacteria and mycobacteria.
- Eukaryotes (have a membrane-bound nucleus):
  - viruses
  - fungi
  - protozoa/parasites.

Cells

Granulocytes

These are a type of leucocyte, and include basophils, eosinophils, and neutrophils. Through a process of degranulation, antimicrobial cytotoxic chemicals are released from secretory vesicles (granules). Neutrophils are the most numerous granulocyte, and are also able to engulf microorganisms by phagocytosis.

Mast cells

These cells can mediate allergic reactions by releasing inflammatory chemicals such as histamine.

Monocytes

These cells develop into *macrophages*, which are present in the circulation and in tissues. They coordinate an immune response by signalling to other immune cells and ingesting microorganisms. Macrophages also break down erythrocytes (this occurs without activation of the immune response).

Dendritic cells

These are a type of antigen-presenting cell (APC) located in the lymph nodes, thymus, spleen, and plasma. They are responsible for processing antigens from foreign cells so that they can be recognized by B or T cells in the presence of the major histocompatibility complex (MHC). The latter helps immune cells to distinguish between host and foreign cells.

Natural killer cells

These are responsible for recognizing and killing virus-infected cells or tumour cells. They also contain granules which, when released, can destroy the cell membrane and also coordinate cell apoptosis (programmed cell death). Unlike necrosis, in apoptosis there is no further immune activation.

Antibodies

- These are large protein molecules called immunoglobulins.
- Each immunoglobulin has a unique antigen-binding site that allows the antibody to recognize a matching antigen.
- There are nine classes of human immunoglobulins—IgG (four types), IgA (two types), IgM, IgE, and IgD. Each class has specific functions, including prevention of colonization, allergy response, activation of granulocytes, and antigen receptor.

B cells

- These produce antibodies in response to antigens (proteins) present on the surface of microorganisms.
- The antibodies circulate in the blood and lymph, binding to particular antigens and marking them for destruction by other immune cells (e.g. in the spleen).
- Some antibodies that are bound to antigens activate the complement system to destroy the microorganism.
- Other antibodies block viruses from entering cells.

T cells

- There are two types of T cells.
- T-helper cells (CD4 cells):
  - coordinate immune regulation
  - potentiate the immune response by secreting substances that activate other leucocytes and macrophages
  - signal B cells to make antibodies.
- T-killer cells (CD8 cells):
  - direct the destruction of virus-infected cells, tumour cells, and parasites
  - have an important role in down-regulation of the immune system.

The immunocompromised patient

The immunocompromised patient

The immunocompromised patient exhibits reduced resistance to infection due to an abnormality in the immune system. Causes include:

- malnutrition (reduces T-cell number, depresses antibody response, zinc deficiency can cause lymphoid atrophy)
- previous exposure to vaccination or infection (e.g. HIV)
- autoimmune disorders (e.g. SLE, rheumatoid arthritis)
- medication:
  - H_2 blockers (e.g. ranitidine)
  - antibiotics (e.g. chloramphenicol)
  - cardiovascular drugs (e.g. propranolol)
  - non-steroidal anti-inflammatory drugs (NSAIDs)
  - heparin
  - propofol
  - specific immunosuppressive drugs (e.g. steroids, cytotoxic drugs, monoclonal antibodies)
- major surgery or trauma (suppresses T-cell production and reduces neutrophil chemotaxis)
- hypoxaemia (hypoxia stimulates prostaglandin and tumour necrosis factor production)
- acute or chronic kidney injury (reduced neutrophil activity, inappropriate macrophage activation, impaired macrophage antigen presentation, and defective T-cell function).

Nursing the immunocompromised patient

- Ensure compliance with infection prevention and control measures.
- Consider isolation, preferably with positive, negative, or laminar flow and high-efficiency particulate air (HEPA) (see Box 13.3).
- Direct care equipment (e.g. stethoscopes) should be patient-specific.
- Limit stock to avoid waste.
- Observe for signs of infection at cannulae sites, wounds, and drains, remove within recommended timescales, and conduct microbial screening (e.g. wounds, blood, skin).
- Minimize invasive procedures and monitoring.

Box 13.3 Positive, negative, and laminar flow

Positive air flow maintains a flow of air out of the room to prevent contaminants or pathogens from entering (e.g. use for HIV patient).

Negative air flow maintains a flow of air into the room to prevent contaminants or pathogens from exiting (e.g. use for TB patient).

Laminar flow maintains an even, smooth flow of air that enters the room, flows over the patient, and exits on the other side (e.g. use in theatre).

Human immunodeficiency virus (HIV)

This is a retrovirus (i.e. its genetic material is RNA, not DNA) that causes an autoimmune response in the form of acquired deficiency syndrome (AIDS). Following the initial exposure, viral replication continues with progressive destruction of helper T cells (CD4 lymphocytes). Eventually the rate of production of new CD4 cells cannot match the rate of destruction, and the clinical picture of AIDS develops. Cell-mediated immunity is lost, and the body becomes progressively more susceptible to opportunistic infections.

Admission to the critical care unit

This may be due to:

- co-infections (e.g. hepatitis B, hepatitis C, TB)
- acute respiratory failure (e.g. pneumocytis pneumonia)
- altered conscious level or intractable seizures secondary to neurological manifestations (e.g. CNS toxoplasmosis, CNS lymphoma, cryptococcal meningitis)
- surgical or medical issues unrelated to the HIV infection.

Complications of HIV infection

Respiratory

Table 13.1 lists the causes of acute respiratory failure. The commonest cause is *Pneumocystis carinii*.

- *P. carinii* is a fungus, transmitted through air, that causes upper and lower respiratory tract infection.
- The patient presents with fever, tachycardia, and cough.
- Exertional dyspnoea develops with severe tachypnoea and hypoxia.
- Pneumatocoeles (air-filled cysts) on chest X-ray predispose to pneumothorax.
- Treatment is with antibiotics (e.g. high-dose co-trimoxazole), high-dose steroids and, if needed, ventilatory support.

Neurological

HIV is a neurotrophic virus (i.e. it affects the proteins responsible for growth and maintenance of neurons) that can cause:

- acute myelopathy
- encephalopathy
- meningitis
- cerebral mass lesions
- secondary brain infection, such as toxoplasmosis (a parasitic infection).

Gastrointestinal

- Peritonitis from small bowel or colonic enteritis.
- AIDS cholangiopathy causing biliary sepsis.

AIDS-related malignancies

- Kaposi's sarcoma.
- Lymphomas.
- Cervical carcinomas related to human papilloma virus.
- Hepatitis-B-related carcinomas.
- Non-Hodgkin's lymphoma.

Table 13.1 Causes of acute respiratory failure in HIV disease

Bacterial pneumonia	*Streptococcus pneumoniae* *Staphylococcus aureus* *Haemophilus influenzae* *Pseudomonas* species (e.g. *Serratia marcescens*)
Atypical pneumonia	*Mycobacterium tuberculosis* *Mycoplasma pneumoniae*
Fungal pneumonia	*Pneumocystis carinii* *Cryptococcus neoformans* *Histoplasma capsulatum* *Coccidioides immitis* *Aspergillus fumigatus*
Cytomegalovirus pneumonia	
Lymphocytic interstitial pneumonia	
Toxoplasma gondii pneumonitis	
Non-Hodgkin's lymphoma and pulmonary Kaposi's sarcoma	

Further reading

DeFreitas A et al. Pharmacological considerations in human immunodeficiency virus-infected adults in the intensive care unit. *Critical Care Nurse* 2013; **33**: 46–56.

Prout J and Agarwal B. Anaesthesia and critical care for patients with HIV infection. *Continuing Education in Anaesthesia, Critical Care & Pain* 2005; **5**: 153–6.

Shrosbree J et al. Anesthesia and intensive care in patients with HIV. *Trends in Anaesthesia and Critical Care* 2011; **1**: 153–61.

Systemic lupus erythematosus (SLE)

This is a chronic, potentially fatal autoimmune disease with a high prevalence in young black women. It is termed a connective tissue disorder, and is characterized by the presence of arthritis/arthralgia, vasculitis, and immunological features such as autoantibodies and deposition of immune complex (a network of antigens and antibodies cross-linked to form a large mass that, if trapped in the tissue, can initiate further inflammatory reactions).

Clinical manifestations of SLE

Skin and mucosa

- Photosensitivity with flushing on the face, and rashes and urticaria on sun-exposed parts of the body.
- Alopecia (hair loss).
- Mucosal ulceration conjunctivitis.

Renal

- Lupus nephritis (persistent inflammation of the kidney).

Haematological

- Anaemia, leucopenia, thrombocytopenia.
- Venous or arterial thrombi (causing strokes and pulmonary emboli).
- Prolonged activated partial thromboplastin time.

Cardiac

- Endocarditis, myocarditis, pericarditis.
- Cardiac tamponade from pericardial effusions (rare).
- Chest pain.
- Arrhythmias.

Respiratory

- Pleural effusion.
- Inflammatory pneumonitis.
- Pulmonary hypertension.

Central nervous system

- Isolated nerve palsies.
- Psychosis, personality disorder, dementia.
- Stroke.
- Seizures.

Gastrointestinal

- Peritonitis, pancreatitis.
- Ascites.
- Splenomegaly.

Treatment

- Steroids and/or immunosuppressive drugs (e.g. azathioprine, cyclophosphamide).
- Cessation of drugs that may induce SLE (e.g. procainamide, hydralazine, isoniazid).
- Supportive therapy (e.g. respiratory support, renal replacement therapy).
- Antibiotics for infections.
- Plasma exchange or intravenous immunoglobulin may be useful for pulmonary haemorrhage.
- Long-term anticoagulation (to prevent thrombi and emboli).

Further reading

Demoruelle MK et al. Recent-onset systemic lupus erythematosus complicated by acute respiratory failure. *Arthritis Care & Research* 2013; **65**: 314–23.

Trethewey P. Systemic lupus erythematosus. *Dimensions of Critical Nursing* 2004; **23**: 111–15.

Vasculitic disorders

These are caused by the inflammatory destruction of blood vessels by autoantibodies.

Wegener's granulomatosis/polyarteritis nodosa

This is a necrotizing vasculitis that affects small and medium-sized vessels. Autoantibodies bind to epithelial cells to form immune complexes, which accumulate in the tissues, leading to inflammation of the vessels. Secondary thrombosis and occlusion of the vessels leads to ischaemia and infarction of multiple organs. Small aneurysms develop in weakened tissue walls. Healing can result in fibrosis.

Symptoms

- Cold-like symptoms (fever, weight loss, malaise, myalgia).
- Sinusitis and epistaxis (destruction of nasal cartilage, septal perforation).
- Pulmonary haemorrhage (due to necrotizing capillaries).
- Acute kidney injury (secondary to necrotizing glomerulonephritis).
- Mesenteric artery thrombosis and bowel infarction.
- Myocardial infarction.
- Stroke.

Treatment

- Immunosuppressive drugs (e.g. corticosteroids, cyclophosphamide).
- Renal replacement therapy.
- Balloon dilatation and stent insertion for tracheobronchial stenosis.

Goodpasture's disease

This is caused by antiglomerular basement membrane (anti-GBM) antibodies binding to the glomerulus and alveolus. Patients present with glomerulonephritis and/or pulmonary haemorrhage (particularly if they are smokers).

Treatment

- Immunosuppressive drugs (e.g. corticosteroids, cyclophosphamide).
- Plasma exchange to remove anti-GBM antibodies.

Anaphylactic and anaphylactoid reactions

These are potentially life-threatening, systemic reactions that occur after re-exposure to an antigen, leading to increased vascular permeability and smooth muscle constriction (see Figure 13.1).

Anaphylactic reaction: IgE mediated

There is immediate release of inflammatory mediators (e.g. histamine, kinins, leukotrienes) from tissue mast cells and peripheral basophils.

Anaphylactoid reaction: non-IgE mediated

Tissue mast cells are induced to react following complement activation by immune complexes.

Causes of anaphylactic and anaphylactoid reactions

- Certain foods (e.g. nuts, shellfish, eggs, milk).
- Venom (e.g. bee sting).
- Latex.
- Medication (e.g. vaccine, immunoglobulins, opiates, antibiotics, NSAIDs, dextrans).
- Radiocontrast media.

Symptoms

These can occur within seconds of exposure. However, the extent of the reaction is variable.

- **Cardiovascular symptoms**—vasodilation, myocardial ischaemia, arrhythmias, hypotension, distributive shock.
- **Respiratory symptoms**—nasal congestion, upper airway obstruction, stridor, laryngospasm, bronchospasm, pulmonary oedema.
- **Gastrointestinal symptoms**—nausea, vomiting, abdominal cramps, diarrhoea.
- **Skin symptoms**—flushing, urticaria, pruritus, angio-oedema.

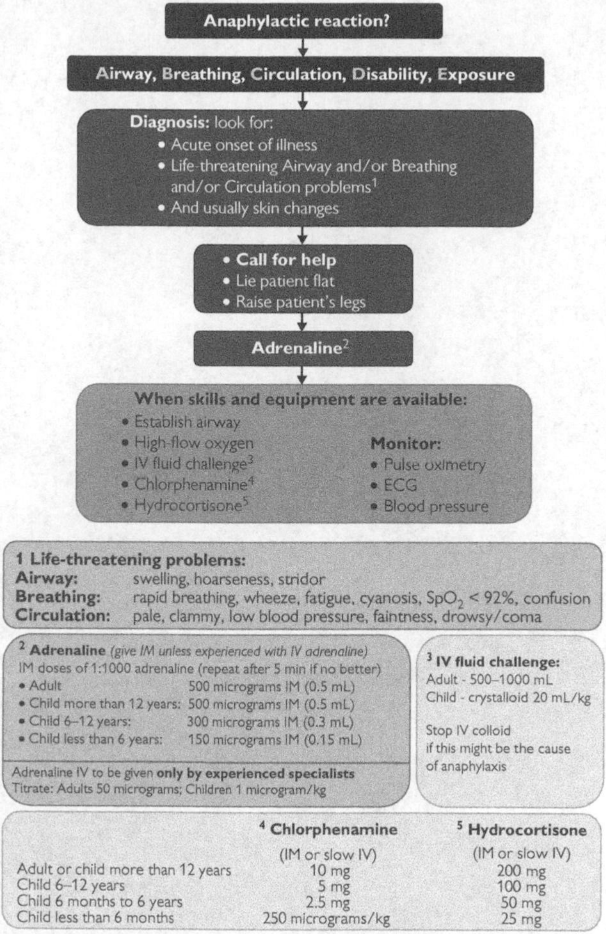

Anaphylactic reaction?
Airway, Breathing, Circulation, Disability, Exposure
Diagnosis: look for:
• Acute onset of illness
• Life-threatening Airway and/or Breathing and/or Circulation problems1
• And usually skin changes
• Call for help
• Lie patient flat
• Raise patient's legs
Adrenaline2
When skills and equipment are available:
• Establish airway
• High-flow oxygen
• IV fluid challenge3
• Chlorphenamine4
• Hydrocortisone5
Monitor:
• Pulse oximetry
• ECG
• Blood pressure
1 Life-threatening problems:
Airway: swelling, hoarseness, stridor
Breathing: rapid breathing, wheeze, fatigue, cyanosis, SpO2 < 92%, confusion
Circulation: pale, clammy, low blood pressure, faintness, drowsy/coma
2 Adrenaline (give IM unless experienced with IV adrenaline)
IM doses of 1:1000 adrenaline (repeat after 5 min if no better)
• Adult 500 micrograms IM (0.5 mL)
• Child more than 12 years: 500 micrograms IM (0.5 mL)
• Child 6–12 years: 300 micrograms IM (0.3 mL)
• Child less than 6 years: 150 micrograms IM (0.15 mL)
Adrenaline IV to be given only by experienced specialists
Titrate: Adults 50 micrograms; Children 1 microgram/kg
3 IV fluid challenge:
Adult - 500–1000 mL
Child - crystalloid 20 mL/kg
Stop IV colloid if this might be the cause of anaphylaxis
4 Chlorphenamine
5 Hydrocortisone
(IM or slow IV)
(IM or slow IV)
Adult or child more than 12 years 10 mg 200 mg
Child 6–12 years 5 mg 100 mg
Child 6 months to 6 years 2.5 mg 50 mg
Child less than 6 months 250 micrograms/kg 25 mg

Figure 13.1 Management of a severe anaphylactic reaction (Resuscitation Council (UK) Anaphylaxis Algorithm). (Reproduced with the kind permission of the Resuscitation Council (UK).)

Chapter 14

Haematology

Erythrocyte disorders

Polycythaemia

This is defined as a red cell count of > 6 × 10^{12}/L or Hb > 180 g/L.

Primary polycythaemia

Blood cell mass (red cells, white cells, and platelets) increases due to excessive bone marrow production. The resultant increase in blood viscosity can cause cardiovascular, neurological, and vascular complications.

Treatment

- Venesection and concurrent volume replacement with crystalloid.
- Aspirin to decrease platelet function and adhesion.
- Cytarabine to reduce platelet production.
- Chemotherapy to depress bone marrow production.

Secondary polycythaemia

Red cell count increases in response to chronic hypoxaemia (e.g. COPD, congenital cyanotic heart disease, adaptation to high altitude).

Sickle-cell anaemia

Sickle-cell haemoglobin (HbS) contains two abnormal beta chains and is inherited as an autosomal-dominant gene. When exposed to low oxygen tensions the red cells become deformed, rigid, and sickle-shaped. The cells aggregate, resulting in the formation of microthrombi in peripheries, causing ischaemia and infarction. Abnormal cells are prematurely destroyed, resulting in a chronic haemolytic anaemia.

Patients with sickle-cell trait (< 50% HbS) are usually symptom-free unless the oxygen tension is very low.

Sickle-cell crisis

Acute haemolytic crises can occur from 6 months of age, and may be precipitated by dehydration and hypoxia. They result in:

- anaemia
- jaundice
- tachycardia
- cardiomegaly
- splenic sequestration—causes the spleen to enlarge, impairs splenic function, and increases the risk of overwhelming infection
- pulmonary sequestration—causes hypoxaemia
- vaso-occlusion—causes tissue infarction (e.g. in bone, spleen, gut, brain, or lung), leading to severe pain.

Management

- Correction or prevention of hypoxaemia:
  - Monitor blood gases, oxygen saturation, and Hb. Aim for steady-state values of Hb and oxygen saturation (i.e. when the patient is clinically well). In the steady state Hb may be only 50–90 g/L and S_pO_2 may be ≥ 90%.
  - Give oxygen therapy, respiratory support, or mechanical ventilation as appropriate.

- Rehydration:
  - Give fluid replacement (this dilutes the blood and decreases agglutination of sickled cells in small vessels).
  - Avoid fluid overload, as this may precipitate heart failure in patients with cardiomyopathy (a common problem in adult sickle-cell patients).
- Analgesia:
  - Oral simple analgesics.
  - Opiate or opioid PCA.
- Infection:
  - Monitor temperature, white cell count, and markers such as CRP.
  - Treat any underlying infection.
  - Patients with splenic dysfunction are prone to infection with encapsulated organisms (e.g. *Pneumococcus, Meningococcus*), and may require long-term prophylactic penicillin.
- Blood transfusion:
  - Give an exchange transfusion (e.g. 4 units can be used to reduce HbS levels during severe crises or before elective surgery).

Further reading

Gladwin M and Sachdev V. Cardiovascular abnormalities in sickle cell disease. *Journal of the American College of Cardiology* 2012; **59**: 1123–33.

Howard J. The role of blood transfusion in sickle cell disease. *International Society of Blood Transfusion Science Series* 2013; **8**: 225–8.

Miller AC and Gladwin MT. Pulmonary complications of sickle cell disease. *American Journal of Respiratory and Critical Care Medicine* 2012; **185**: 1154–65.

Leucocyte disorders

Neutropenia

This is defined as a neutrophil count of $< 2 \times 10^9$/L. The risk of developing life-threatening infection is higher with counts of $< 1 \times 10^9$/L, and such patients are often isolated until the bone marrow recovers. Patients are often asymptomatic until infection develops. Common initial infections include pneumococci, staphylococci, and coliforms. After prolonged immunosuppression and repeated courses of antibiotics, infection with *Pseudomonas*, fungi (*Candida, Aspergillus*), TB, cytomegalovirus, or *Pneumocystis* may occur.

Causes

- Bone marrow failure (leukaemia, myeloma, lymphoma, chemotherapy, radiation).
- Systemic inflammation following severe infection or trauma (causes aggregation of neutrophils in vital organs).
- Infections (typhoid, brucellosis, viral, protozoal).
- Drug related (e.g. carbimazole, sulfonamides).
- Destruction by neutrophil antibodies (e.g. SLE, rheumatoid arthritis).
- Deficiency of vitamin B_{12} or folate (malnutrition).
- Hypersplenism (increased neutrophil destruction).

Management

- Compliance with infection prevention and control, and use of aseptic non-touch technique.
- Discontinuation of implicated drug therapy.
- Protective isolation if neutrophil count is $< 1.0 \times 10^9$/L.
- Avoid uncooked food (e.g. salads).
- Minimize invasive procedures and monitoring.
- Personal hygiene, especially skin, eye, and mouth care. Nystatin mouthwashes for oral thrush, and clotrimazole for fungal skin infections.
- Parenteral antibiotics (broad spectrum if no organism is isolated).
- Regular surveillance for infection, and specific treatment if infection is identified.
- Growth factors, such as granulocyte-colony-stimulating factor (G-CSF), to stimulate the bone marrow.

Leukaemia

This is a neoplastic disorder of the blood-cell-forming tissues (bone marrow, spleen, and lymphatic system), which causes unregulated and prolific accumulation of white cells in the bone marrow, liver, spleen, and lymph nodes, and invasion of the gastrointestinal tract, meninges, skin, and/or kidneys.

Types

Leukaemia is classified according to the site involved as either acute or chronic. Therapy aims to induce remission by the use of cytotoxic drugs, irradiation, and transplant.

Acute lymphatic leukaemia (ALL)

This is common in children. It is a severe disease in which the lymph nodes, bone, and nervous tissue become infiltrated. Around 50% of children aged 2–11 years survive for 5 years.

Chronic lymphatic leukaemia (CLL)

This occurs mainly in adults aged > 50 years. Patients are often symptom-free. Pleural or peritoneal effusions may develop. No treatment is needed if the patient is asymptomatic. Around 50% survive for 5 years.

Acute myeloid leukaemia (AML)

Any age group may be affected, but AML is more common in adults. Around 30–50% of cases survive long term.

Chronic myeloid leukaemia (CML)

This most commonly occurs in the 30–50 years age group. It has an insidious onset with fever and weight loss. Splenomegaly, hepatomegaly, and thrombocytopenia develop later, with a high white cell count. Survival with chemotherapy is about 3 years. With allogenic bone marrow transplantation, around 50% of patients may survive for more than 5 years.

Further reading

Azoulay É and Darmon M. Acute respiratory distress syndrome during neutropenia recovery. *Critical Care* 2010; **14**: 114.

Dowling M, Meenaghan T and Kelly M. Treating chronic myeloid leukaemia: NICE guidance. *British Journal of Nursing* 2012; **21**: S16–17.

Lee Y and Lockwood C. Prognostic factors for risk stratification of adult cancer patients with chemotherapy-induced febrile neutropenia: a systematic review and meta-analysis. *International Journal of Nursing Practice* 2013; **19**: 557–76.

Thrombocyte disorders

Thrombocytopenia

This is defined as a platelet count of $< 150 \times 10^9$/L. Bleeding is unlikely to occur unless the count falls to $< 50 \times 10^9$/L, unless generalized infection is present. Thrombocytopenia is caused by increased destruction, increased consumption, and/or decreased production of platelets.

Causes of increased destruction or consumption of platelets

- Idiopathic thrombocytopenic purpura (ITP).
- Thrombotic thrombocytopenic purpura (TTP).
- Disseminated intravascular coagulation (DIC).
- Heparin-induced thrombocytopenia (HIT) syndrome.
- Sepsis.
- Haemorrhage.
- Autoimmune disorders (e.g. AIDS, malaria).
- Extracorporeal circulation (e.g. dialysis).
- Hypersplenism.

Causes of decreased platelet production

- Drugs (e.g. chemotherapy).
- Uraemia.
- Megaloblastic anaemia.
- Marrow infiltration (e.g. leukaemia, carcinoma, lymphoma).

Idiopathic thrombocytopenic purpura (ITP)

This is an autoimmune disorder in which autoantibodies are directed against platelets, considerably shortening their lifespan. It is more common in young adults, particularly following respiratory or gastrointestinal viral infections, and may be acute or chronic.

Clinical manifestations include:

- petechiae, multiple bruising, and epistaxis
- prolonged bleeding time but normal coagulation times.

Treatment

There is no definitive treatment.

- In the acute form of ITP, steroids tend not to increase the platelet count, but may reduce the incidence of bleeding.
- Platelet and red cell transfusions are generally avoided unless severe bleeding occurs.
- In the chronic form of ITP, steroids may cause a rise in platelet count.
- Intravenous immunoglobulin.
- Rituximab (an anti-CD20 monoclonal antibody that depletes B cells).
- Splenectomy, if the patient is unresponsive to medical management.

Thrombotic thrombcytopenic purpura (TTP)

This disorder is characterized by fever, thrombotic microangiopathy (TMA), haemolytic anaemia, neurological symptoms (including drowsiness, transient or permanent strokes, and blindness), and renal dysfunction. TTP has many clinical similarities to haemolytic uraemic syndrome (HUS). However, HUS predominantly affects the kidneys and usually follows a diarrhoeal illness, whereas TTP more frequently affects the brain in adults.

Symptoms

- Abdominal pain.
- Purpura (the appearance of red or purple discolouration on the skin that does not blanch when pressure is applied).
- Fever.
- Hypertension.
- Neurological signs.
- Haematuria (may progress to acute kidney injury).

Treatment

- Plasma exchange (using FFP).
- Steroids.
- Intravenous immunoglobulin.
- Rituximab (anti-CD20 monoclonal antibody that depletes B cells).
- Avoidance of platelet transfusion unless there is severe bleeding.

Drug-induced thrombocytopenia

Causes

Numerous drugs can cause thrombocytopenia, including:

- heparin
- quinine
- antituberculous drugs
- thiazide diuretics
- penicillins
- sulfonamides
- anticonvulsants
- chemotherapy.

Heparin-induced thrombocytopenia (HIT) syndrome

Antibodies generated during exposure to heparin affect platelet activation and cause endothelial dysfunction. This occurs with all heparins, including low-molecular-weight heparin (LMWH), which forms antibodies against platelets. Most patients who are affected do not suffer clinical consequences. HIT syndrome rarely occurs with transient exposure to heparinoids, typically appearing after 7–10 days of use.

Treatment

Treatment of drug-induced thrombocytopenia is supportive, and includes discontinuation of heparin. Platelet transfusions may be needed for active bleeding or if platelet levels are very low. For HIT syndrome there should be total avoidance of heparin administration (including the small amounts used in arterial flush solutions). As up to 50% of patients will develop a thromboembolic event if taken off heparin and not continued on another anticoagulant, alternative anticoagulation therapy should be commenced promptly.

Further reading

Barbani F et al. Heparin-induced thrombocytopenia incidence in the ICU: preliminary results. *Critical Care* 2010; 14 (Suppl. 1): P637.

Davies J, Patel P and Zoumot Z. Diagnosing heparin induced thrombocytopenia in critically ill patients. *Intensive Care Medicine* 2010; **36**: 1447–8.

Hunt BJ. Bleeding and coagulopathies in critical care. *New England Journal of Medicine* 2014; **370**: 847–59.

Urden L, Stacy K and Lough M. *Critical Care Nursing: diagnosis and management*, 7th edn. Mosby: St Louis, MO, 2014.

Watson H, Davidson S and Keeling D. Guidelines on the diagnosis and management of heparin-induced thrombocytopenia: second edition. *British Journal of Haematology* 2012; **159**: 528–40.

Anticoagulation therapy

This is used alone to prevent the intravascular formation of thrombi [illegible] [illegible] haemorrhage [illegible] therefore patients must be observed closely for signs of bleeding:

- Observe and report any signs of haematuria.
- Observe and test faeces and gastric aspirate for blood.
- Observe cannula sites, wounds, and drains for bleeding.
- Observe the skin for purpura and bruising.
- Perform regular laboratory investigations of clotting.
- Avoid invasive procedures and intramuscular injections.
- Hard lines and [illegible] [illegible]

Anticoagulants

Heparin

[illegible] low molecular weight heparin (LMWH) [illegible]

[illegible]

- [illegible]
- VTE and pulmonary embolus
- acute coronary syndromes.

[illegible]

Warfarin

Warfarin is a vitamin K antagonist [illegible]

[illegible]

Reversal

- For non-major bleeding give vitamin K (1–3 mg IV).
- For major bleeding give vitamin K (5 mg IV) and prothrombin complex concentrate (PCC) 25–50 U/kg.

Anticoagulation therapy

This is used either to prevent thrombus formation or to prevent extension of an existing thrombus. Haemorrhage is a potential complication. Therefore patients must be observed closely for signs of bleeding:

- Observe and test urine daily for haematuria.
- Observe and test tracheal and nasogastric aspirate for blood.
- Observe cannulae sites, wounds, and drains for bleeding.
- Observe the skin for purpura and bruising.
- Perform regular laboratory coagulation screens.
- Avoid vigorous endotracheal or nasogastric tube suction.
- Place lines and tubes either after cessation of anticoagulant therapy or after correction of coagulopathy.

Anticoagulants

Heparin

Unfractionated heparin inhibits FXa and thrombin, and has a half-life of 45–90 min. LMWH (fractionated heparin) derived from unfractionated heparin inhibits FXa and thrombin, is more predictable, and no monitoring is required (an antiXa test can be used). Its half-life is 4 h. Reversal is with protamine sulfate 1 mg per 80–100 units up to a maximum of 50 mg. Consider rFVIIa if there is active bleeding.

Given intravenously, heparin has a rapid onset of action, with a half-life of 90 min. Overdose can be reversed with protamine sulfate (1 mg neutralizes 100 IU of heparin). Unfractionated heparin given by continuous infusion is recommended for patients with renal failure and for anticoagulation of extracorporeal circuits (e.g. haemofiltration, cardiopulmonary bypass). The dosage is monitored by the activated partial thromboplastin time (APTT).

Low-molecular-weight heparin (e.g. enoxaparin, dalteparin) is now the treatment of choice for:

- thromboprophylaxis
- VTE and pulmonary embolus
- acute coronary syndromes.

Fixed dosages are given and no laboratory monitoring is necessary.

Warfarin

Warfarin inhibits vitamin K to stop production of factors II, VII, IX, and X and anticoagulant proteins C and S.

Given orally, it takes at least 3–5 days of loading to achieve full anticoagulation. Therefore heparin cover should be provided for 72 h when warfarin is commenced. Interactions which may lead to under- or over-anticoagulation (e.g. levels of free warfarin) rise with some drugs (e.g. aspirin, amiodarone). Dosage is controlled using the international normalized ratio (INR), and a ratio of 2:3 is usually targeted for adequate anticoagulation. Excess levels are treated by reducing or temporarily discontinuing warfarin.

Reversal

- For non-major bleeding give vitamin K (1–3 mg IV).
- For major bleeding give vitamin K (5 mg IV) and prothrombin complex concentrate (PCC), 25–50 U/kg.

- If INR is > 5 but there is no bleeding, withhold or reduce the warfarin dose and investigate the causes of elevated INR.
- If INR is > 8 but there is no bleeding, give vitamin K (5 mg orally).
- For surgery that can be delayed for 6–12 h, correct with IV vitamin K.
- For surgery that cannot be delayed, correct with PCC and IV vitamin K. PCC should not be used to enable elective or non-urgent surgery.

Fresh frozen plasma should not be used for warfarin reversal except with haematology approval.

Indications

- Long-term thromboprophylaxis (e.g. metal heart valves, atrial fibrillation) (see NICE guidance[1]).
- Long-term anticoagulation for thrombosis or emboli.

Factor Xa inhibitors (FXaIs) (e.g. rivaroxaban, apixaban)

FXaIs bind with the section of factor Xa that catalyses the activation of factor II (prothrombin), so that no thrombin is present. Direct FXaIs can inhibit free factor Xa, clot-bound factor Xa, and factor Xa bound to the prothrombinase complex. They are indicated for the prevention of thromboembolism in patients with atrial fibrillation, and for the prevention of VTE and pulmonary embolism in patients undergoing major orthopaedic surgery.

There is no specific reversal agent, but the short half-life means that discontinuation of the drug is sufficient to correct most bleeding problems caused by its use. The most effective monitor of the anticoagulant effect is an anti-factor Xa assay. However, no routine laboratory test monitoring of coagulation should be required except possibly in special circumstances, such as renal failure, obesity, or severely underweight patients.

Fondaparinux

Fondaparinux is a synthetic pentasaccharide with indirect anti-Xa activity. Its half-life is 17 h, and there is no specific reversal agent. Consider recombinant factor VIIa if there is active bleeding.

Clopidogrel

Clopidogrel is metabolized by CYP450 enzymes to produce the active metabolite that inhibits platelet aggregation. This action is irreversible, so platelets that are exposed to the active metabolite of clopidogrel will be affected for the rest of their lifespan (about 7–10 days). Routine blood monitoring is not required. The platelet count will be unaffected. However, the function of the platelets will be impaired.

Indications

- Single antiplatelet therapy for the prevention of atherothrombotic events in patients with myocardial infarction, ischaemic stroke, or established peripheral arterial disease.
- Or in combination with aspirin in patients suffering from acute coronary syndrome (ACS) or patients undergoing a stent placement following percutaneous coronary intervention (PCI).

Prostacyclin/epoprostenol (PGI_2) or prostin (PGE_1)
These drugs inhibit platelet aggregation. The effect stops within 30 min of discontinuation. The main side effect is vasodilation, which can cause flushing, hypotension, and tachycardia.

Indications
- As an alternative to heparin in renal replacement therapy.
- Pulmonary hypertension.
- Poor gas exchange in ARDS (nebulized).
- Digital ischaemia (e.g. severe sepsis, autoimmune disease).

Thrombolytic agents (e.g. streptokinase, tissue plasminogen activator (tPA))
These drugs are used to break down a thrombus that has already formed. Allergic reactions can occur, and are more likely with streptokinase. tPA and newer related agents (e.g. reteplase, tenecteplase) are easier to administer, but need to be given with heparin. Bleeding may be a major complication, and should be corrected with the antifibrinolytic agent tranexamic acid, plus FFP, cryoprecipitate, and red cell transfusion as necessary.

Indications
- Acute myocardial infarction.
- Stroke.
- Pulmonary embolism.
- Distal emboli (e.g. in the leg).

Direct thrombin inhibitors (e.g. lepirudin, argatroban, dabigatran)
Lepirudin is a recombinant form of hirudin (extracted from leeches), whereas argatroban is derived from arginine. Both form an irreversible complex with thrombin. These drugs are unrelated to and not affected by heparin. Antibody formation occurs in approximately 40% of patients treated with lepirudin for > 6 days. These drugs have long half-lives and there are no antidotes, so they are contraindicated in patients with active haemorrhage. Bivalirudin is related to hirudin but is reversible, with a short half-life of only 25 min.

Danaparoid
This is a heparinoid given intravenously that has therapeutic similarities to heparin. Its use is generally restricted to treatment of HIT syndrome and VTE prophylaxis, although there is a 10–20% risk of cross-reactivity. No antidote is available.

Reference

1 National Institute for Health and Care Excellence (NICE). *Atrial Fibrillation: the management of atrial fibrillation*. CG180. NICE: London, 2014. www.nice.org.uk/guidance/cg180

Further reading

Makris M et al. Guideline on the management of bleeding in patients on antithrombotic agents. *British Journal of Haematology* 2012; **160**: 35–46.

Soff G. A new generation of oral direct anticoagulants. *Arteriosclerosis, Thrombosis, and Vascular Biology* 2012; **32**: 569–74.

Clotting disorders

Disseminated intravascular coagulation (DIC)

DIC is an excessive, dysfunctional activation of the clotting cascade, which [illegible] deposition of fibrin in small vessels with the [illegible] ischaemia and consumption of clotting factors and platelets. The resulting depletion of clotting factors can lead to haemorrhage that may be relatively mild (e.g. oozing from venepuncture sites) or severe (e.g. frank [illegible]). DIC often arises as a poor prognostic indicator of an underlying [illegible] dysfunction.

Conditions that may trigger DIC

- [illegible] (acute, chronic, or metastatic)
- Obstetric disorders (e.g. septic abortion, placental abruption, amniotic fluid embolism, intrauterine fetal death)
- Liver disorders (e.g. cirrhosis, acute hepatic necrosis)
- Malignant disease (e.g. [illegible] leukaemia)
- Trauma (e.g. crush injuries, burns)
- Hypotension/shock
- Pulmonary embolism or fat embolism
- Graft rejection
- Blood transfusion reactions
- Extracorporeal circulatory bypass
- Heat stroke.

Symptoms

- Haemorrhage
- [illegible] (e.g. haemoptysis, haematuria, gastrointestinal haemorrhage)
- Acute kidney injury due to [illegible]
- Cerebral ischaemia [illegible]
- Symptoms of [illegible]
- Small bowel [illegible]
- Skin [illegible], bruising, and [illegible] purpura [illegible].

Management

- Adequate [illegible] treatment and [illegible] (tissue perfusion)
- Treatment of the underlying cause (e.g. infection)
- Careful monitoring of [illegible] and arterial blood gases
- [illegible] should be [illegible] be used
- [illegible] for [illegible]
- [illegible] (including fibrinogen, [illegible] time, and D-dimers)
- [illegible] and blood components [illegible] platelets.

Laboratory values in DIC

- Prolonged prothrombin time (> 12–13 s)
- Prolonged partial thromboplastin time (> 40–50 s)
- Prolonged thrombin time (> 15–20 s)

Clotting disorders

Disseminated intravascular coagulation (DIC)

DIC is an excessive systematic activation of the coagulation cascade, which causes the generation of thrombin and fibrin within circulating blood, resulting in the formation of microthrombi. The resulting depletion of clotting factors can lead to haemorrhage that may be relatively mild (e.g. into skin, haematuria, or around catheter and drain sites) or severe (e.g. major gastrointestinal bleed). It often arises as a secondary complication of an underlying condition.

Disorders that may trigger DIC

- Infection (bacterial, viral, or parasitic).
- Obstetric disorders (e.g. septic abortion, eclampsia, amniotic fluid embolism, placental abruption).
- Liver disorders (e.g. cirrhosis, cholestasis, acute hepatic necrosis).
- Malignant disease (e.g. carcinoma, leukaemia).
- Trauma (e.g. crush injuries, burns).
- Hypovolaemic shock.
- Pulmonary embolism or fat embolism.
- Organ transplant rejection.
- Blood transfusion reaction.
- Extracorporeal circulatory bypass.
- Acute pancreatitis.

Symptoms

- Haemorrhage.
- Respiratory failure due to haemorrhage, haemothorax, or embolism.
- Acute kidney injury due to microemboli or hypovolaemia.
- Cerebral ischaemia or infarction due to haemorrhage or thrombus.
- Gastrointestinal haemorrhage.
- Small bowel infarction due to mesenteric embolus.
- Skin petechiae, purpura, bruising, and necrosis resulting from decreased capillary refill and/or infarction.

Management

- Adequate fluid replacement and restoration of tissue perfusion.
- Treatment of the underlying cause (e.g. sepsis).
- Careful monitoring of haemodynamics and arterial blood gases.
- Observation of endotracheal and nasogastric aspirate, urine, and stool for blood.
- Observation of the skin and extremities for ischaemia.
- Regular blood tests, particularly clotting screen, including fibrinogen, thrombin time, and D-dimers.
- Heparin is not usually given, and blood component transfusions are avoided if there is no active bleeding.

Laboratory values in DIC

- Prolonged prothrombin time (> 15 s).
- Prolonged partial thromboplastin time (> 60–90 s).
- Prolonged thrombin time (> 15–20 s).

- Low fibrinogen levels (< 75–100 mg/dL).
- Low platelet count (< 20–75 × 10^9/L).
- High levels of fibrin degradation products (> 100 mg/mL).
- Raised levels of D-dimers.

Note: not all of the results will necessarily be abnormal.

Haemophilia

This is a genetic disorder which can cause severe bleeding from minor trauma, and disabling muscle and joint haemorrhages.

- Haemophilia A is caused by deficiency of factor VIII.
- Haemophilia B is caused by deficiency of factor IX.

Treatment

- Administer factor VIII or IX concentrate (give prophylactically prior to surgery or dental extraction).
- Aim to raise the factor to above 30% of normal.
- Repeat infusions every 8–10 h as necessary.
- Never give aspirin, as this impairs platelet function.
- Avoid the use of intramuscular injections.

Further reading

Levi M et al. Guidelines for the diagnosis and management of disseminated intravascular coagulation. *British Journal of Haematology* 2009; **145**: 24–33.

Richards M et al. Guideline on the use of prophylactic Factor VIII concentrate in children and adults with severe haemophilia A. *British Journal of Haematology* 2008; **149**: 498-507.

Blood components for transfusion

Packed red blood cells

- Leucocyte depleted as standard.
- CMV-negative and irradiated on request.
- Cross-matching is required.
- Stored at 2–6°C in a dedicated blood fridge.
- Once removed from the fridge, administer within 30 min or return to storage.
- Transfuse using a dedicated transfusion giving set, finishing the transfusion within 4 h of removal of the unit from the fridge.
- Red blood cell transfusion contains no therapeutic amounts of clotting factors or platelets.
- Transfusion of 1 unit should raise the Hb concentration by 10 g/L.

Packed red blood cells are used in anaemic patients with:

- chronic, persistent blood loss
- bone marrow failure
- major haemorrhage (see ➔ p. 470).

Platelets

- Leucocyte depleted as standard.
- CMV-negative and irradiated on request.
- Adult therapeutic dose is pooled from four separate donors or one single apheresis donor.
- Cross-matching is required.
- Stored at 22°C under gentle agitation in dedicated storage.
- Transfuse using a dedicated transfusion giving set within 60 min of out-of-storage time.

Platelets are used in thrombocytopenic patients with:

- chronic, persistent low platelet counts
- bone marrow failure
- immune thrombocytopenia
- acute DIC (see ➔ p. 396)
- major haemorrhage (see ➔ p. 470)
- uraemia.

Fresh frozen plasma (FFP)

- Leucocyte depleted as standard.
- Methylene blue on request.
- Cross-matching is not required.
- Dose is 12–15 mL/kg.
- Stored frozen, and once thawed has a shelf life of 24 h.
- Transfuse full dose using a dedicated transfusion giving set within 4 h.

FFP is used for:

- replacement of coagulation factor deficiencies where there is no specific factor concentrate available
- immediate reversal of warfarin in the presence of life-threatening bleeding

- acute DIC (see ➲ p. 396)
- thrombotic thrombocytopenic purpura
- plasma exchange
- advanced liver disease (see ➲ p. 312)
- major haemorrhage (see ➲ p. 470).

Cryoprecipitate

- Leucocyte depleted as standard.
- Cross-matching is not required.
- Contains factor VIII, fibronectin, and fibrinogen.

Cryoprecipitate is used to provide replacement factors in patients with:

- haemophilia or von Willebrand's disease
- major bleeding associated with hypofibrinogenaemia (< 1 g/L) or uraemia
- acute DIC (see ➲ p. 396)
- advanced liver disease (see ➲ p. 312)
- bleeding associated with thrombolytic therapy
- major haemorrhage (see ➲ p. 470).

Further reading

www.transfusionguidelines.org.uk

Blood transfusion complications

Transfusion reactions due to allergens, bacteria, or incompatible blood usually occur within 10–15 min of starting the transfusion. Monitoring (including haemodynamics and temperature) is essential throughout this period. Correct identification of the patient at the sampling and administration stage will prevent significant errors and harm to the patient.

Febrile non-haemolytic reactions

Causes

- Incompatibility of donor red cells, white cells, platelets, or plasma proteins.
- Anti-HLA (human lymphocyte antibodies), granulocyte-specific, and platelet-specific antibodies in the recipient as a result of sensitization during pregnancy or previous transfusions.

Symptoms

- Pyrexia.
- Urticaria.
- Pruritus.

Management

- Antipyretics (aspirin, paracetamol).
- Antihistamines (e.g. chlorphenamine).
- Hydrocortisone.
- Continue the transfusion slowly if there is only a mild reaction.
- Stop the transfusion if rigors or fever > 38°C occur.
- Send the implicated unit to the laboratory for examination.

Acute haemolytic reactions

Causes

- Incompatible ABO blood group.
- Incorrectly stored blood.
- Out-of-date blood.
- Overheated blood.
- Infected blood.
- Mechanical destruction of the red cells due to administering the infusion under pressure.
- Mixing of blood with hypotonic infusion fluids.

Symptoms

- Pain at the infusion site.
- Pyrexia, facial flushing, rigors, nausea, and vomiting.
- Dyspnoea.
- Headache, chest, abdominal, and loin pain.
- Tachycardia and hypotension leading to circulatory collapse.
- Oliguria and renal failure.
- DIC.

Management

- Stop the blood transfusion immediately.
- Retain the unit and return it to the laboratory with samples to check the blood group, FBC, coagulation screen, fibrinogen, U&E, and direct antiglobulin test.
- Take blood cultures if sepsis is suspected.
- Take a urine sample for haemoglobinuria.
- Resuscitative measures, including mechanical ventilation.
- Continuous cardiovascular monitoring.
- 12-lead ECG.
- Maintain urine output at > 1 mL/kg/h.
- If DIC develops, clotting factor replacement may be required.
- Provide renal support if acute kidney injury develops.

Circulatory overload

Patients are less able to tolerate the fluid load associated with blood transfusion, and can develop pulmonary oedema and heart failure. The evidence suggests that overload can occur with transfusion volumes of as little as 1 unit (median volume of transfusion is 2 units).

Symptoms

- Dyspnoea or tachypnoea.
- Hypertension.
- Elevated jugular venous pressure.
- Tachycardia.

Management

- Continuous cardiovascular monitoring.
- Diuretics.
- Respiratory support, including non-invasive ventilation.
- Avoid circulatory overload by administering diuretic at the beginning of the transfusion.

Transfusion-related acute lung injury (TRALI)

This is associated with leucocyte antibodies present in donor blood reacting with recipient white blood cells. Clinical features typically occur within 1–2 h of transfusion, and include chills, fever, non-productive cough, dyspnoea, cyanosis, hypotension that is unresponsive to fluid challenge (10–15%), or hypertension (15%). Radiological signs include bilateral pulmonary infiltrates and scattered opacities.

Transfusion-associated graft versus host disease

This condition is rare, but usually fatal. It is caused by engraftment of viable T lymphocytes, which cause widespread tissue damage. It can occur in immunosuppressed patients (e.g. bone marrow transplant recipients). It can be prevented by irradiating blood products (red cells, platelets, and white cells) prior to transfusion.

Blood transfusion hazards

Bacterial contamination

Contamination of blood is rare, but may be lethal. Contaminants from the donor's skin can enter the blood during donation. Gram-negative bacteria grow slowly at 4°C, but their growth accelerates at room temperature. Onset of pyrexia and circulatory collapse can be rapid. Failure to maintain aseptic technique in the setting up of the transfusion is another contamination hazard.

Transmission of disease

Donor selection criteria and testing of donor blood for infectious agents have decreased transmission of disease, but have not completely eradicated it.

Diseases that may potentially be transmitted include:

- hepatitis B and C
- cytomegalovirus (CMV)
- malaria
- HIV.

Hazards of massive blood transfusion

Massive blood transfusion is defined as the transfusion of the patient's own volume of blood within a 24-h period.

Hypothermia

- Transfused red cells can rapidly cool the patient. Use a thermostatically controlled blood warmer if giving more than several units of blood to a normothermic patient.
- Hypothermia increases the risk of cardiac arrhythmias, reduces the rate of metabolism, and shifts the oxygen dissociation curve to the left.
- Citrate toxicity is more likely to occur if the patient is hypothermic.

Acid–base and electrolyte disturbances

- Stored blood is acidic (pH 6.6–6.8) due to the citric acid that is used as an anticoagulant and the lactic acid that is generated during storage. Both are metabolized by the liver in the well-perfused patient, but may cause a metabolic acidosis in the hypoperfused patient or the patient with liver failure. Monitor with regular acid–base measurements.
- The sodium content of FFP is higher than that of normal blood due to the sodium citrate anticoagulant. Monitor Na^+ levels (particularly in patients with renal failure and hypernatraemia).

Hypocalcaemia

- Stored red cells contain anticoagulants such as citrate that can cause calcium depletion. Monitor ionized calcium levels and give supplements as necessary.
- Observe the patient for tetany, muscle tremors, cardiac dysfunction, and prolonged QT interval on ECG.

Further reading

Contreras M (ed.). *ABC of Transfusion*, 4th edn. Wiley-Blackwell: Chichester, 2009.
McClelland D. *Handbook of Transfusion Medicine*. 5th edn. TSO: London, 2013.
Serious Hazards of Transfusion (SHOT). ↗ www.shotuk.org
↗ www.transfusionguidelines.org.uk/

Chapter 15

Managing emergencies

Cardiac arrest and advanced life support

Cardiac arrest is defined as the absence or severe reduction of cardiac output, resulting in inadequate perfusion of vital organs.

Cardiac arrests are rarely unforeseen, and the evidence suggests that patients normally exhibit one or more signs of physiological deterioration in the hours prior to arrest.[1] Clinical indicators of potential deterioration are listed in Box 15.1, and it is important that the critical care nurse is responsive to these.

The incidence of cardiac arrest in critical care is increased because of the acuity levels of this patient group. There are many factors that can cause a sudden deterioration in the patient's condition. The causes of cardiac arrest are manifold, and the common causes are listed in Table 15.1.

Box 15.1 Indicators of potential deterioration

- Threatened airway
- Increased or decreased respiratory rate
- Saturations of < 90%
- Heart rate < 40 beats/min or > 130 beats/min
- Systolic blood pressure < 90 mmHg
- Urine output < 50 mL in 4 h
- Acute mental status change

Table 15.1 Common causes of cardiac arrest

System	Potential causes
Cardiac	Myocardial infarction
	Heart failure
	Dysrhythmia
	Coronary artery spasms
	Cardiac tamponade
Respiratory	Respiratory failure
	Respiratory depression
	Airway obstruction
	Impaired gaseous exchange
Haematological	Hyperkalaemia
	Hypokalaemia
	Hypomagnesaemia
	Hypercalcaemia
	Hypocalcaemia
Treatment causes	Pulmonary artery catheterization
	Cardiac catheterization
	Surgery
	Side effects of medications

Cardiac arrest is associated with the following dysrhythmias:

- ventricular fibrillation (VF)
- ventricular tachycardia (VT)
- pulseless electrical activity (PEA)
- asystole.

The Resuscitation Council (UK) publishes guidelines pertaining to CPR recommendations, which are available on its website.[2] It is essential that critical care nurses regularly update their knowledge of these, as recommendations change in line with additions to the current evidence base.

The advanced life support (ALS) guidelines[3] note the following:

- the need to maintain minimally interrupted chest compressions
- reduced importance given to the role of the precordial thump
- delivery of drugs via the endotracheal route is no longer recommended
- changes in timing of the first dose of adrenaline when treating VF/VT
- atropine is no longer recommended for routine use in asystole or PEA
- capnography is recommended to confirm and monitor endotracheal tube (ETT) placement and to monitor the effectiveness of CPR
- recommendations for post-resuscitation care are also provided.

The ALS algorithm (see Figure 15.1) highlights the need to:

- summon immediate help
- begin CPR as early as possible in a ratio of 30:2
- minimize interruptions to chest compression.

Two different pathways are identified for ALS:

- a pathway for shockable rhythms (VT and VF)
- a pathway for non-shockable rhythms (asystole and PEA).

Potentially reversible causes

It is useful to consider causes or aggravating factors during cardiac arrest. As an aid to memory these have been divided into two groups of four.

4 H's

- **Hypoxia**—check air entry, provide 100% oxygen, check that ETT is not misplaced.
- **Hypovolaemia**—check for signs of haemorrhage, restore intravascular volume, determine the cause of hypovolaemia if present, consider surgical intervention.
- **Hyperkalaemia, hypokalaemia, hypocalcaemia, acidaemia, and other metabolic disorders**—check blood results , review patient history for causes of electrolyte imbalance.
- **Hypothermia**—suspect if near drowning, check with low-reading thermometer, consider rewarming.

4 T's

- **Tension pneumothorax**—diagnosis is normally made by clinical examination and ultrasound. It requires decompression with needle thoracocentesis followed by chest drain insertion.
- **Tamponade**—consider causes (e.g. trauma, recent cardiac surgery). Tamponade may be present if distended neck veins are present. It requires an ECG, and thoracotomy may be necessary.

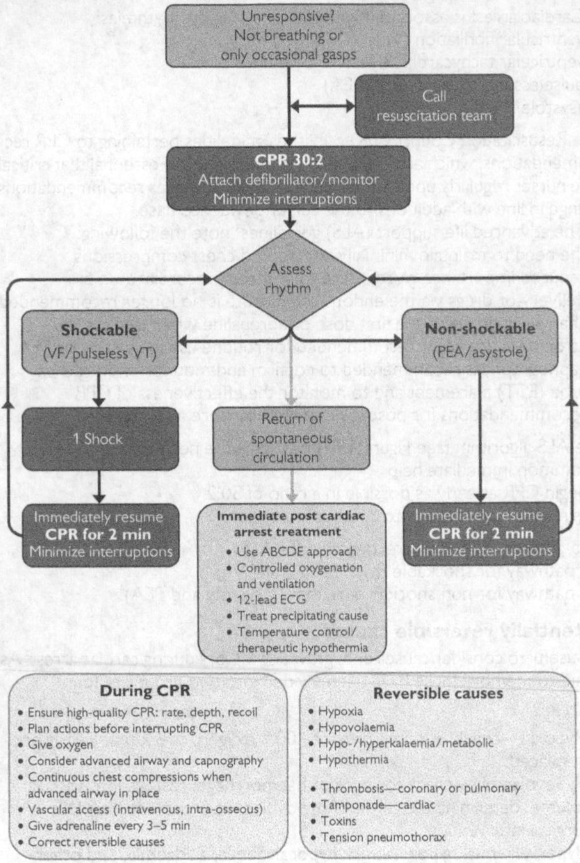

Figure 15.1 Adult advanced life support (ALS) guidelines for resuscitation.[3] VF, ventricular fibrillation; VT, ventricular tachycardia; PEA, pulseless electrical activity. (Reproduced with the kind permission of the Resuscitation Council (UK).)

- **Toxic substances**—consider the likelihood of accidental or deliberate ingestion of toxins. A drug screen is required. Consider antidotes if appropriate.
- **Thromboembolism**—most commonly massive pulmonary embolism. Consider the need for thrombolysis.

Drugs that may be administered

Adrenaline

This should be administered after the third shock in shockable rhythms and repeated every 3–5 min. In non-shockable rhythms, adrenaline should be administered once access is gained, and given every 3–5 min thereafter. CPR should not be stopped to allow the administration of drugs.

Anti-arrhythmic medication

There is little evidence to support their effectiveness, but medical staff may use various anti-arrhythmic medications for the management of arrhythmias in cardiac arrest.

Amiodarone

This may be used for persistent VF or VT. The usual dose is 300 mg by a bolus injection. An infusion may follow the bolus. Consideration may also be given to the use of lidocaine, but *not* if the patient has already had amiodarone.

Magnesium

This may be administered for refractory VF if hypomagnesaemia is suspected. It is also useful in torsades de pointes or if digoxin toxicity is suspected.

Bicarbonate

This is not recommended routinely. Acidosis is better corrected by restoration of circulation. However, bicarbonate may be used if arrest is associated with hyperkalaemia or tricyclic antidepressant overdose.

Calcium

This is recommended only if specifically indicated (e.g. in arrests caused by hyperkalaemia, hypocalcaemia, or overdose of calcium-channel-blocking medications).

Use of mechanical CPR aids

Prolonged cardiac compression can be extremely tiring, and rescuer fatigue can reduce the effectiveness of CPR. There are several ongoing trials exploring mechanical resuscitation aids. However, the Resuscitation Council (UK) has highlighted the need for further research before firm recommendations are made about their use.

Post-resuscitation care

Following successful resuscitation, correct management of post-resuscitation complications (post-cardiac arrest syndrome) is needed to enable complete recovery from cardiac arrest.

Post-cardiac arrest syndrome includes:

- brain injury
- myocardial dysfunction
- ischaemia or reperfusion response
- persistence of existing pathology.

Various recommendations have been made for improving the outcome of patients after cardiac arrest. These include the following:

- **Effective oxygenation.** Maintenance of normal O_2 and CO_2 levels is recommended. The use of end-tidal CO_2 monitoring is encouraged.
- **Effective circulatory support.** Early PCI is recommended if cardiac arrest is related to STEMI. Otherwise supportive measures to maintain cardiac output (fluids and vasoactive drugs) are needed. An intra-aortic balloon pump may be required if conservative measures do not work.
- **Control of seizures.** Seizures will occur in 5–15% of patients. These should be controlled with anticonvulsant drugs or barbiturates. There is no direct recommendation that prophylactic anticonvulsants should be used.
- **Glucose control.** Hypoglycaemia should be avoided. Current recommendations are to maintain the glucose level at 10 mmol/L, but tight glycaemic control is *not* recommended after cardiac arrest because of the risk of hypoglycaemia.
- **Temperature control.** Pyrexia should be avoided, and treatment of post-arrest hyperpyrexia may require antipyretics or active cooling measures.

Therapeutic hypothermia

The evidence suggests that therapeutic hypothermia may be beneficial post cardiac arrest, as it decreases the cerebral oxygen requirement and may inhibit the release of excitory amino acids and free radicals. It may also have a role in reducing the post-arrest inflammatory response.

Therapeutic hypothermia consists of three basic stages:

- **Induction.** This involves cooling the patient using cooled fluid infusions, cooling blankets, gel pads, or a bypass machine. The body temperature is usually lowered to 32–34°C.
- **Maintenance.** Fluctuation of temperature is best avoided during this stage, so it is suggested that cooling devices that measure and regulate temperature are best suited to this stage.
- **Rewarming.** This should be achieved slowly, and current recommendations are to increase body temperature by 0.25–0.5°C per hour.

It is important to remember that hypothermia has associated risks (e.g. cardiac arrhythmia, coagulopathies, etc.). Therefore careful monitoring for side effects of hypothermia is required.

References

1 Morton PG and Fontaine DK. *Critical Care Nursing: a holistic approach*, 10th edn. Lippincott Williams & Wilkins: Philadelphia, PA, 2012.
2 Resuscitation Council (UK). www.resus.org.uk
3 Resuscitation Council (UK). *Resuscitation Guidelines*. www.resus.org.uk/pages/Guide.htm

Anaphylaxis

Anaphylaxis is a life-threatening [illegible] generalized hypersensitivity reaction [illegible]. It is characterized by life-threatening [illegible] problems in the airway, breathing and circulation. Symptoms may include the following:

Airway:

- Airway obstruction
- Pharyngeal or laryngeal oedema
- Hoarseness of voice
- Stridor

Breathing:

- [illegible] for breathing
- Shortness of breath
- Wheeze
- [illegible] and [illegible]
- Hypoxia
- Cyanosis

Circulation:

- Cardiac arrest
- Signs of shock
- Tachycardia
- Hypotension

The Resuscitation Council (UK) and NICE [illegible] that [illegible] anaphylaxis [illegible] likely diagnosis if the patient presents with:

- sudden onset and rapid progression of symptoms
- life-threatening airway, breathing, and/or circulation problems
- skin and/or mucosal changes (flushing, urticaria, angioedema).

However, it is important to note that skin or mucosal changes may not be present, and [illegible] may have severe reactions without mucosal or skin changes. In addition, some patients may present with gastrointestinal symptoms (e.g. vomiting, abdominal pain, incontinence).

Anaphylaxis can be immunologically mediated or non-immunologically mediated [illegible]:

- IgE-mediated reactions occur as a result of a previous exposure to an allergen. The immune system [illegible] antibodies [illegible] of [illegible] that lead to anaphylaxis.
- Non-IgE mediated reactions occur when [illegible] without [illegible] IgE [illegible].
- Idiopathic reactions [illegible] and the cause of the reaction is not ever determined.

Anaphylaxis

Anaphylaxis is defined as a severe, life-threatening, generalized hypersensitivity reaction.[4] It is characterized by life-threatening changes in the airway, breathing, and circulation, which may include the following:

Airway
- Airway obstruction.
- Pharyngeal and laryngeal oedema.
- Hoarseness of voice.
- Stridor.

Breathing
- Cessation of breathing.
- Shortness of breath.
- Wheeze.
- Increased tiredness and workload of breathing.
- Hypoxia.
- Cyanosis.

Circulation
- Cardiac arrest.
- Signs of shock.
- Tachycardia.
- Hypotension.

The Resuscitation Council (UK)[5] and NICE[4] have both highlighted difficulties in diagnosing anaphylaxis correctly, and suggest that anaphylaxis is a likely diagnosis if the patient presents with:
- a sudden onset and rapid progression of symptoms
- life-threatening airway, breathing, and/or circulatory problems
- skin and mucosal changes (flushing, urticarial rash, erythema, angioedema).

However, it is important to note that in some patients changes may not be overt, and they may simply have severe hypotension without mucosal or skin changes. In addition, some patients may also present with abdominal symptoms (e.g. vomiting, abdominal pain, incontinence).

Anaphylaxis can be immunoglobulin E mediated, non-immunoglobulin E mediated (anaphylactoid), or idiopathic.
- **IgE-mediated reactions** occur as a result of a previous exposure to an antigen. The immune system develops a immune response to that antigen that triggers the release of the chemical mediators that initiate anaphylaxis.
- **Non-IgE-mediated reactions** occur without the presence of IgE antibodies, and can occur *the first time that the patient is exposed to the antigen.*
- **Idiopathic reactions**—a large proportion of reactions can present as anaphylaxis, and the cause of the reaction is never determined.

Box 15.2 Common triggers of anaphylaxis

- Insect stings
- Nuts
- Other food
- Antibiotics
- Anaesthetic drugs
- Other drugs and medicinal products
- Contrast medium

Triggers of anaphylaxis

There are a plethora of causative factors. The evidence suggests that these vary with age. Generally, younger patients are more likely to have food allergies, whereas older patients may be more likely to react to medication. Virtually any food, medicine, or medicinal product can trigger an allergic reaction. Common allergens noted by the Resuscitation Council (UK)[5] are listed in Box 15.2.

Management of the patient with anaphylaxis

Where possible the trigger should be removed. If the patient is receiving IV medications or IV infusions that may cause a reaction, these should be stopped immediately. Vomiting should *not* be induced if the allergy is thought to be a food allergy.

Other treatment should focus on assessing and managing the patient systematically. See Chapter 13 (➔ p. 381) for a summary algorithm of the management of a severe anaphylactic reaction.

Airway

- The patient should be assessed for signs of complete or partial airway obstruction. This requires immediate intervention, and specialist help should be sought.
- The patient may require an artificial airway, and early intubation is recommended.
- Emergency tracheostomy may be required if normal endotracheal intubation is not possible.

Breathing

- Respiratory function should be assessed.
- If the patient is not breathing, ALS guidelines should be followed.
- If the patient is breathing, they should be positioned in an upright position.
- High-flow oxygen should be provided.
- Nebulizers may be needed if the patient has bronchoconstriction.

Circulation

- Cardiovascular assessment should be undertaken.
- If the patient has no cardiac output, ALS guidelines should be followed.
- The patient's position may need to be changed if they are hypotensive, so long as this does not affect respiratory function. A flat position with the legs elevated is recommended for hypotension.
- IV access should be secured, preferably with a wide-bore cannula.
- IV fluid challenge should be given (500–1000 mL of crystalloid is recommended).

Disability

- Neurological function should be assessed using the AVPU or GCS score.
- Pupil reactions should be assessed.
- Blood glucose levels should be monitored.

Exposure

- Skin should be assessed for flushing, urticarial rash, and erythema.
- The patient should be observed for signs of angio-oedema.

Medication for anaphylaxis

Several medications may be required. These include the following:

Adrenaline

This is normally administered intramuscularly. Adrenaline may be administered intravenously (reduced dose), but only by specialist experienced medical staff. It is important to note that IV adrenaline in a patient with cardiac output can cause life-threatening cardiac arrhythmias, life-threatening hypertension, and severe myocardial ischaemia.

Antihistamine

This can be given after the initial resuscitation. It may be administered intravenously or intramuscularly. Chlorpheniramine is normally the drug of choice.

Steroids

These are given after the initial resuscitation. The drug normally given is hydrocortisone, and it may be administered intravenously or intramuscularly.

Bronchodilators

These may be given for bronchoconstriction. They can be administered by nebulizer (e.g. salbutamol, ipratropium) or they may be administered intravenously (e.g. aminophylline, magnesium). Note that magnesium is a vasodilator, so it may worsen hypotension.

Cardiac drugs

Adrenaline is the main cardiac drug administered, but other vasopressors, such as noradrenaline, may be needed, especially if the patient requires critical care admission. Glucagon can be useful if administered to patients who are receiving beta blockers. Some patients develop profound bradycardia, and atropine may be useful in the treatment of this.

Aftercare

Close monitoring of the patient is essential following management of a severe allergic reaction, as they may require transfer to critical care. In addition to monitoring, the patient may require:

- timed blood tests (mast-cell tryptase may be helpful for confirming the diagnosis of anaphylaxis; it usually peaks 1–2 h after the onset of symptoms)
- referral to an allergy specialist for testing.

References

4 National Institute for Health and Care Excellence (NICE). *Anaphylaxis: assessment to confirm an anaphylactic episode and the decision to refer after emergency treatment for a suspected anaphylactic episode*. CG134. NICE: London, 2011. www.nice.org.uk/guidance/cg134

5 Working Group of the Resuscitation Council (UK). *Emergency Treatment of Anaphylactic Reactions: guidelines for healthcare providers*. Resuscitation Council (UK): London, 2008.

Massive haemorrhage

Definition

Massive haemorrhage is defined as a situation in which a patient is bleeding uncontrollably and requires more than 10 units of red blood cells in a 24-h period. It is argued that this definition is difficult to apply in practice, so more specific definitions identify the following as signs of massive haemorrhage:

- blood loss of > 150 mL/min
- haemodynamic instability.

Massive haemorrhage may be associated with:

- trauma (see ➲ p. 470)
- obstetric emergencies (see ➲ p. 432)
- gastrointestinal bleeds (see ➲ p. 318).

The mortality rate in this group of patients is as high as 50%, and therefore the early recognition of massive haemorrhage and correct management are important.

The use of massive transfusion protocols has been recommended for the correct management of this patient group. The UK blood transfusion and tissue transplantation services have published such protocols,[6] and it is recommended that these are followed to enable timely and effective management of this patient group.

An ABC approach

Early involvement of the haematology department and/or consultant haematologist is recommended to ensure adequate provision of blood and blood products, rapid haematological blood results, and timely expert advice. This will need to be coordinated by a senior nurse or a doctor.

Treatment of the patient requires systematic assessment and management.

Airway

- The patient's ability to maintain an airway should be assessed.
- If necessary, intubation should be considered.

Breathing

- High-flow oxygen should be administered if the patient is self-ventilating.
- If the patient is being ventilated, normal blood gases should be maintained by adjustment of ventilation if necessary.
- Respiratory assessment should be performed to assess the adequacy of ventilation.

Circulation

- The effects of blood loss should be monitored.
- The target systolic blood pressure is 90–100 mmHg, or higher if clinically indicated (e.g. if trauma involves neurological damage).
- Additional monitoring may be required.
- Wide-bore cannulas should be inserted to facilitate the rapid administration of blood products as needed.
- Bleeding should be arrested as soon as possible. This may require early surgical, radiological, or endoscopic intervention.

- A tourniquet or pressure dressing should be used if external bleeding is apparent.
- Resuscitation with fluids and blood should occur until haemostasis is secured. Blood and FFP should be transfused in accordance with massive haemorrhage guidelines, and 10 mL of blood products per kg is recommended. The timing will be dependent upon the severity of blood loss. See ➔ p. 470 for principles of damage-control resuscitation with traumatic haemorrhage.
- Cell salvage can be considered if appropriate.
- Drugs to arrest bleeding should be administered following the manufacturer's guidelines as clinically indicated (see Box 15.3).
- Consideration may be given to the transfusion of other blood products, such as platelets, cryoprecipitate, and clotting factors.
- Blood samples should be sent to the laboratory on initial presentation and throughout the resuscitation period to monitor the effects. The blood tests that are required are listed in Box 15.4.
- Body temperature should be closely monitored and appropriate steps taken to avoid hypothermia (warming of replacement fluid, warming blankets, etc.).
- Close monitoring for signs of adverse blood transfusion reactions is required.
- Close monitoring of renal function and urine output is needed.
- An accurate input/output fluid chart should be maintained.

Box 15.3 Drugs required during massive transfusion

It is recommended that tranexamic acid is given to all patients within 1 h of the onset of massive haemorrhage.

Other drugs may include:

- vitamin K
- prothrombin complex
- other reversal agents following discussion with a consultant haematologist

Box 15.4 Essential blood tests

- Emergency cross-matching
- Full blood count
- Clotting studies to include prothrombin time (PT), activated partial thromboplastin time (APTT), and fibrinogen
- Urea and electrolytes
- Calcium
- Blood gases
- Thromboelastography

Other considerations

Adverse complications of massive transfusion should be monitored for and treated promptly. Problems associated with massive haemorrhage are normally linked to fluid resuscitation attempts and the components of or chemicals used in stored blood. They include:

- dilutional coagulopathies and DIC (see ➲ p. 396)
- hypothermia
- electrolyte disturbances:
  - potassium
  - calcium
  - magnesium
- transfusion reactions (see ➲ p. 400):
  - allergic
  - haemolytic
  - non-haemolytic
- immunological reactions:
  - acute lung injury
  - immunosuppression
  - transfusion-related purpura
- acidosis/alkalosis
- air embolism.

Later problems include:

- transfusion-related acute lung injury (see ➲ p. 401)
- non-cardiogenic pulmonary oedema
- infection
- multi-organ failure
- death.

Reference

6 Joint United Kingdom Blood Transfusion and Tissue Transplantation Services Professional Advisory Committee (JPAC). Transfusion management of major haemorrhage. http://www.transfusionguidelines.org.uk/transfusion-handbook/7-effective-transfusion-in-surgery-and-critical-care/7-3-transfusion-management-of-major-haemorrhage

Further reading

Bird J. Massive blood transfusion for trauma patients. *Emergency Nurse* 2012; **20**: 18–20.

Pham HP and Shaz BH. Update on massive transfusion. *British Journal of Anaesthesia* 2013; **111** (Suppl. 1): i71–82.

Preparing for health emergencies

[illegible] Social Care [illegible] legal responsibility [illegible] sustainable response to emergency situations. This [illegible] have [illegible] to ensure [illegible] preparedness, resilience and response [illegible].

A wide range of events can cause [illegible] emergencies [illegible] appropriate planning. These may include:

- natural disasters
- major accidents
- outbreaks of disease
- terrorist incidents.

The Department of Health has developed guidelines for [illegible] of [illegible] Critical Care [illegible] of [illegible] services [illegible] units [illegible] and patients who require [illegible] support.

This document [illegible] increasing demand for [illegible] platelets [illegible] that [illegible] should [illegible] likely [illegible] massive haemorrhage [illegible].

The key aims of [illegible] are:

- to [illegible] due to [illegible] being [illegible]
- [illegible]
- [illegible] available resources are being utilized
- [illegible] collections
- [illegible] practicable
- [illegible] all patients
- [illegible] hospital.

[illegible] (such as those triggered by a major [illegible] incident) [illegible] will be [illegible]:

- [illegible] 10 [illegible]
- [illegible] network [illegible]
- [illegible]
- [illegible] demand.

Preparing for health emergencies

The reorganization of healthcare provision following the Health and Social Care Act (2013) saw a contractual responsibility for NHS trusts to ensure robust and sustainable responses to emergency situations. NHS trusts therefore have a requirement to ensure appropriate Emergency Preparedness, Resilience and Response (EPRR).

A wide range of events can cause health emergencies and require the need for appropriate planning. These may include:

- natural hazards
- major accidents
- outbreaks of disease
- terrorist attacks.

The Department of Health has developed guidelines for responding to emergency situations for each part of the health sector.

Critical care units are guided by the NHS England document, *Management of Surge and Escalation in Critical Care Services: standard operating procedure for adult critical care.*[7] (Separate guidance has been issued for critical care units that specialize in burns, paediatrics, and patients who require ECMO support.)

This document identifies changes that are required during periods of increasing demand for critical care beds, and includes provision for increasing demand during a 'major incident.' It emphasizes that during an emergency surge in demand for critical care beds, critical care units should act as a network, as it is unlikely that one unit would be able to offer sufficient beds to meet a rapid increase in demand.

The key aims of the guidance are:

- to prevent mortality due to patients not being able to access critical care beds when these are required
- to maximize capacity in a range of scenarios
- to maximize capacity until all available resources are being utilized.

The guidance highlights the need for:

- maintaining normal critical care services for as long as is reasonably practicable
- equity of access and treatment for all patients
- management of critical care resources across a network rather than one hospital.

During emergency surges in demand (such as those triggered by a major incident), critical care units will be expected to:

- collectively deliver a 100% increase in Adult Level 3 Critical Care bed capacity (in response to either a 'big bang' or a 'slow burn' scenario)
- assist other critical care units in the network to facilitate coping with the increase in demand for beds
- identify non-critical-care-trained nursing staff to care for patients during an emergency surge in demand
- increase capacity using a stepped approach as demand increases
- be coordinated by local Critical Care Networks and by NHS England during a wider surge in demand

- ensure that difficult decisions relating to access to critical care are made in conjunction with local critical care network policies rather than patient assessment criteria.

The guidelines highlight the need to continue to maintain 'normal critical care services' for as long as possible. However, in emergency situations they identify the need to potentially cancel elective critical care admissions. It is suggested that suspension of elective activity should occur in three stages:

- Stage 1—cancellation of all elective, non-life-threatening, non-oncology surgery that requires critical care admission.
- Stage 2—as for Stage 1, but also including cancellation of all non-life-threatening cardiac and general surgery that requires critical care admission.
- Stage 3—as for Stages 1 and 2, but also including cancellation of all cardiac and oncology surgery.

Each NHS trust and critical care network should have local guidelines with regard to emergency preparedness, and it is important that these are available to the critical care team and that local training is provided.

If the incident is local in nature (e.g. a major road incident) it is likely to be managed by the critical care network. More widespread emergencies (e.g. an influenza pandemic) may require regional or national management.

In the event of an emergency situation it is likely that local guidelines will identify a coordinator to manage the emergency situation.

Critical care nurses will need to consider a number of practical points. These could include:

- patient acuity levels of all patients in critical care beds within the critical care network
- potential transfer of level 2 patients to another area (step down, HDU, etc.)
- review of staff levels and staff skill mix
- use of non-critical-care-trained nurses within the unit
- availability of equipment
- availability of pharmaceuticals
- availability of support staff
- availability of other consumables (e.g. sterile supplies).

Reference

7 NHS England. *Management of Surge and Escalation in Critical Care Services: standard operating procedure for adult critical care*. NHS England: London, 2013.

Chapter 16

Obstetric emergencies

The pregnant patient in critical care

Admission to critical care

Pregnant women may be admitted to critical care units for a variety of reasons. Admission may be triggered by complications of pregnancy or pre-existing medical conditions. Common causes of critical care admission during pregnancy include:

- pre-eclampsia or eclampsia
- postpartum haemorrhage
- placental abruption
- amniotic fluid embolism
- infection
- cardiac complications
- severe gestational diabetes
- stroke.

The effect of critical care on the pregnant mother and fetus will depend upon the severity of the illness. It is important to remember that because care interventions may have a profound impact on both mother and fetus, they must be carefully considered by the critical care team in order to minimize complications.

Additional considerations

The maintenance of fetal oxygenation is an important consideration. Therefore careful attention must be paid to:

- adequate maternal blood pressure and cardiac output
- adequate oxygenation
- adequate perfusion to the fetus
- appropriate monitoring.

Early involvement of the midwifery and obstetric team is essential, and the decision may be made to monitor the fetus while the mother is critically ill. Fetal monitoring and interpretation of the monitoring remain the responsibility of the midwifery/obstetric team. However, some important issues that critical care staff should be aware of include:

- normal fetal heart rate (110–160 beats/min)
- decelerations from baseline may indicate fetal distress
- abnormal fetal heart rates or tracings require prompt intervention.

Close liaison between critical care staff and the obstetric/midwifery team is vital, and any concerns about the mother or fetus should be escalated immediately, as interventions such as early Caesarean section may be required.

Indications for early Caesarean section

Caesarean section may be indicated for the following reasons:

- critical deterioration in maternal health
- death of the mother (in which case it needs to be performed within 4 min of cessation of maternal circulation)
- instability of the fetus
- the decision by the team that Caesarean section is safest for mother and fetus.

Caesarean section can normally be considered as an option once the fetus has reached 24 weeks, as it is then considered viable.

In addition to the indications listed on ➔ p. 424, Caesarean section may be performed to assist with maternal resuscitation in maternal collapse from 20 weeks' gestation (see ➔ p. 438).[1]

Equipment for emergency Caesarean section should be available whenever there is a pregnant patient in the critical care area.

Reference

1 Royal College of Obstetricians and Gynaecologists. *Maternal Collapse in Pregnancy and the Puerperium (Green-top Guideline No. 56)*. RCOG: London, 2011.

Pre-eclampsia and eclampsia

Definition

Pre-eclampsia is defined by NICE as new hypertension presenting after 20 weeks' gestation with significant proteinuria.[2] (Significant proteinuria is diagnosed if the urinary protein:creatinine ratio is higher than 30 mg/mmol or a validated 24-h urine collection result shows more than 300 mg protein.)

It is a relatively common occurrence in pregnancy, affecting 2–8% of all pregnancies. It has associated mortality and morbidity risks to the patient, and is one of the leading causes of maternal death in the UK. The risk to the mother is relatively small if pre-eclampsia occurs after 36 weeks' gestation, but it increases significantly if it occurs before 33 weeks' gestation. Complications of pre-eclampsia include:

- pulmonary oedema
- seizures (i.e. eclampsia)
- intracerebral haemorrhage.

Risk factors for the development of pre-eclampsia include:

- primigravidae
- multiple pregnancies
- obesity
- age > 40 years
- previous history of pre-eclampsia
- family history of pre-eclampsia
- pregnancy interval of more than 10 years
- diabetes mellitus.

Eclampsia is typically defined as a complication of severe pre-eclampsia, resulting in new onset of grand mal seizure activity and/or unexplained coma during pregnancy or postpartum in a woman with signs or symptoms of pre-eclampsia.

Urgent diagnosis and intervention are required for pre-eclampsia and eclampsia.

Assessment

Assessment of the mother should follow a systematic ABCDE approach (see ➲ p. 18). Two cardinal signs should be present to confirm severe pre-eclampsia requiring admission to a higher level of care. These are:

- systolic blood pressure > 140 mmHg systolic or 90 mmHg diastolic
- protein urea > 300 mg in 24 h.

Additional assessment findings may include changes to renal, neurological, abdominal, and haematological function, and may cause:

- oliguria
- elevated serum creatinine levels
- elevated LFTs
- pulmonary oedema or decreased saturations
- severe headache
- visual disturbances

- seizures
- epigastric or upper right quadrant pain
- thrombocytopenia.

NICE[3] highlights the need for transfer to higher levels of care if the patient requires:

- stabilization of blood pressure
- support of failing systems (haematological, respiratory, or cardiovascular)
- assessment following neurological changes
- mechanical ventilation.

Management

Management of pre-eclampsia is based on continuous assessment of the mother and fetus and associated:

- management of hypertension
- accurate fluid balance
- management of complications
- preparedness for early fetal delivery.

Management of hypertension

NICE[3] highlights the need for continuous blood pressure assessment and control of blood pressure using oral or intravenous medication. This may include:

- labetalol
- nifedipine
- hydralazine.

Responses to antihypertensive treatment should be closely monitored, as should adverse complications of treatment for the mother and fetus.

Strict fluid balance

- Accurate intake and output are essential, and urinary catheterization may be required.
- Fluid resuscitation may be required if the mother's blood pressure falls in response to antihypertensive medication (this is especially likely when administering hydralazine).
- Limit IV fluid to 80 mL/h unless there are ongoing fluid losses or hypotension.

Management of complications

- The risks and manifestation of ongoing complications should be assessed.
- Severe hypertension (160/110 mmHg) may require the administration of IV magnesium sulfate, as does the presence of eclamptic convulsions.[3]

Preparedness for early delivery

- Steroids should be administered if early delivery is likely to occur at 24–35 weeks' gestation.
- Normal delivery can be considered if blood pressure is controlled.
- Mothers with uncontrolled blood pressure despite medication may require operative delivery.

Eclampsia and pre-eclampsia normally begin to resolve after the removal of the placenta, but it is necessary to continuing monitoring for pre-eclampsia and eclampsia after delivery, as complications can occur and continue for 48–72 h after delivery.

References

2 National Institute for Health and Care Excellence (NICE). *Hypertension in Pregnancy: the management of hypertensive disorders during pregnancy*. CG107. NICE: London, 2010. www.nice.org.uk/guidance/cg107

3 National Institute for Health and Care Excellence (NICE). *Severe Hypertension, Severe Pre-Eclampsia and Eclampsia in Critical Care*. NICE: London, 2011. https://pathways.nice.org.uk/pathways/hypertension-in-pregnancy/severe-hypertension-severe-pre-eclampsia-and-eclampsia-in-critical-care

Further reading

European Society of Intensive Care Medicine. *Obstetric Critical Care: clinical problems*. http://pact.esicm.org/media/Obstetric%20critical%20care%2030%20April%202013%20final.pdf

Royal College of Obstetricians. https://www.rcog.org.uk/

HELLP syndrome

Definition

[illegible]

Assessment

[illegible]

Management

[illegible]

HELLP syndrome

Definition

HELLP is an acronym that stands for Haemolysis, Elevated Liver Enzymes and Low Platelets. It is considered to be a varying presentation of severe pre-eclampsia. It can arise either in the antenatal period or shortly after delivery. Mortality and morbidity rates are high. The pathophysiology relating to HELLP is unclear. It may occur without hypertension and other signs of pre-eclampsia.

Assessment

Some of the signs and symptoms are related to vasospasm of the hepatic vessels. They include:
- nausea
- vomiting
- abdominal pain (typically epigastric or right upper quadrant pain)
- generalized oedema
- malaise.

Laboratory investigations may indicate:
- reduced haematocrit
- elevated bilirubin
- reduced platelet count
- elevated AST/ALT and APT.

Complications include:
- DIC (see ➲ p. 396)
- pulmonary oedema
- hepatic dysfunction
- hepatic rupture and infarction.

Management

Some of the management is similar to that of pre-eclampsia. Treatment should focus on:
- control of symptoms
- stabilization of the patient
- observing for signs of haemorrhage (see ➲ p. 416)
- management of bleeding or transfusion of blood products (see ➲ p. 398)
- urgent Caesarean section.

Postpartum haemorrhage

Definition

Postpartum haemorrhage (PPH) may be primary or secondary. Primary PPH is the loss of 500 mL or more of blood from the genital tract within 24 h of the birth of the baby. According to the Royal College of Obstetricians and Gynaecologists, PPH can be minor (500–1000 mL) or major (> 1000 mL). Secondary PPH is defined as abnormal or excessive bleeding from the birth canal between 24 h and 12 weeks postnatally.[4]

PPH is the leading cause of maternal death worldwide, and accounts for 30% of maternal deaths. Around 1% of deliveries are associated with PPH.

Risk factors include:

- previous PPH
- increased BMI
- four or more previous babies
- antepartum haemorrhage
- over-distended uterus
- uterine abnormalities
- low-lying placenta
- women over 35 years of age.

Labour risks include:

- induction
- prolonged stages of labour
- use of oxytocin
- operative birth.

Causes of PPH include:

- tone—uterine atony (inability to contract)
- trauma—tear of uterus, cervix, or vaginal wall
- tissue—retained placenta
- thrombin—coagulation deficits.

Assessment

Assessment of the mother should follow a systematic ABCDE approach (see ➔ p. 18). Particular attention must be focused on assessment of signs of hypovolaemic shock or massive haemorrhage. This will include:

- obvious signs of haemorrhage (see ➔ p. 416)
- hypotension
- tachycardia
- tachypnoea
- increased capillary refill time
- decreased urine output
- increased SVR
- decreased level of consciousness.

Management

Management is based on accurate assessment, fluid resuscitation, stabilization of the patient, intervention to stop further bleeding, and monitoring for complications arising from PPH. Note that accurate assessment of blood loss in PPH is difficult, as blood loss may be concealed and other fluids such as amniotic fluid may also be present.

Assessment of the patient

Timely and accurate assessment using an ABC approach is required to determine the consequences of PPH for the mother.

Fluid resuscitation

Massive fluid resuscitation may be required, using blood products, colloids, and crystalloid.

- Guidelines relating to massive haemorrhage should be followed (see ➲ p. 416).
- Two wide-bore peripheral cannulae should be inserted.
- Central line insertion may also be required.
- FBC and coagulation tests will be needed.
- Techniques to increase uterine contraction may be required.

Stabilization of the patient

Interventions and/or medications may be needed to stabilize the patient. These may include:

- high-flow oxygen in self-ventilating patients
- mechanical ventilation if the patient's condition is poor
- vasopressors to maintain appropriate cardiac output and blood pressure
- invasive blood pressure monitoring (see ➲ p. 218)
- measurement of cardiac output (see ➲ p. 226).

Intervention to stop further bleeding

If bleeding is not stopped by conservative measures, administration of haemostatic agents may be recommended.

If this fails, surgical or radiological intervention may be needed. This may include:

- manual removal of the placenta if it has not already been delivered
- uterine tamponade
- haemostatic brace suturing (e.g. B-Lynch suture)
- surgical ligation of uterine and/or internal iliac arteries
- radiological embolization
- hysterectomy.

Monitoring for complications

There are several potential complications of PPH. Some of these relate to massive blood transfusion, while others are directly linked to the PPH. It is important that the critical care nurse closely monitors the patient for these complications. They include:

- acute lung injury
- electrolyte imbalance
- coagulopathies
- increased risk of thrombosis
- increased risk of acute kidney injury
- Sheehan's syndrome (damage to the anterior lobe of the pituitary gland, which inhibits lactation).

Reference

4 Royal College of Obstetricians and Gynecologists (RCOG). *Postpartum Haemorrhage, Prevention and Management (Green-top Guideline No. 52)*. RCOG: London, 2011.

Further reading

Pollock W and Fitzpatrick C. Pregnancy and postpartum considerations. In: D Elliott, L Aitken and W Chaboyer (eds) *ACCN's Critical Care Nursing*, 2nd edn. Elsevier Australia: Chatswood, NSW, 2012. pp. 710–45.

Amniotic fluid embolism

Definition

[illegible]

Risk factors include: [illegible]

- [illegible]
- [illegible]
- [illegible] delivery
- [illegible]
- Cervical lacerations
- Eclampsia

Assessment

[illegible]

- The initial phase [illegible]
- The second stage [illegible] cardiac failure
- [illegible]

The patient is likely to present with:

- [illegible]

Management

[illegible]

- [illegible]
- [illegible]
- [illegible]
- [illegible]
- Fluid resuscitation should follow massive haemorrhage protocols (see [illegible]).

Amniotic fluid embolism

Definition

Amniotic fluid embolism (AFE) is a rare and potentially catastrophic complication of pregnancy. Its incidence is about 8–10 per 100 000 pregnancies. It predominantly occurs as a result of labour, but can occur throughout pregnancy. Its aetiology is not known, but it is suggested that exposure of amniotic fluid to the maternal circulation is the catalyst for AFE. Recent discussions relating to AFE have likened its consequences to a severe anaphylactoid response, and the term 'anaphylactoid syndrome of prègnancy (ASP)' has been suggested. Regardless of the mechanism involved, mothers with AFE/ASP will deteriorate rapidly, and require urgent medical intervention.

Risk factors include:

- induction of labour
- forceful uterine contractions
- Caesarean section or instrumental delivery
- placenta praevia and abruptio placentae
- cervical lacerations
- eclampsia.

Assessment

A thorough assessment of the mother with AFE is essential, and it should follow a systematic ABCDE approach (see ➔ p. 18). The symptoms are likely to present in phases.

- The initial phase is characterized by disturbances in respiratory function and severe pulmonary oedema.
- The second stage is characterized by cardiovascular changes secondary to left-sided cardiac failure.
- Finally, haemorrhagic complications may follow, causing DIC (see ➔ p. 396).

The patient is likely to present with:

- acute dyspnoea
- severe hypoxaemia
- pulmonary oedema
- ARDS
- hypotension
- coagulopathies
- severe haemorrhage (see ➔ p. 416).

Management

Management is mostly supportive in nature and directed towards failing systems.

- Intubation is likely to be needed, due to respiratory failure.
- Mechanical ventilation may be required, and it may be necessary to use high concentrations of oxygen to correct the hypoxaemia.
- In severe cases, nitric oxide therapy or ECMO may be needed.
- Haemodynamic monitoring and restoration of blood pressure are required.
- Fluid resuscitation should follow massive haemorrhage protocols (see ➔ p. 416).

- Strict fluid assessment is required.
- Support of failing cardiovascular status with inotropes and vasopressors may be necessary.
- DIC is a likely consequence, so blood, blood components, and clotting factors will be required to reduce the effects of DIC (➔ p. 396).
- Delivery of the fetus should be expedited if AFE occurs antepartum.

Further reading

European Society of Intensive Care Medicine. *Obstetric Critical Care: clinical problems*. http://pact.esicm.org/media/Obstetric%20critical%20care%2030%20April%202013%20final.pdf

Pollock W and Fitzpatrick C. Pregnancy and postpartum considerations. In: D Elliott, L Aitken and W Chaboyer (eds) *ACCN's Critical Care Nursing*, 2nd edn. Elsevier Australia: Chatswood, NSW, 2012. pp. 710–45.

Cardiac arrest in pregnancy

Special precautions

Significant physiological changes in cardiac output, oxygenation, and circulatory volume occur in pregnancy, and these need to be considered in the event of a maternal cardiac arrest. In addition, the impact of the uterus in the later stages of pregnancy can adversely affect cardiac output.

Although cardiac arrest in pregnancy is relatively rare (1 in 300 000 deliveries), common causes have been identified. These include:

- cardiac disease
- pulmonary embolus
- severe hypertension
- haemorrhage
- severe infection
- AFE/ASP
- ectopic pregnancy.

Resuscitation following cardiac arrest will largely follow the guidelines for general resuscitation (see ➲ p. 406). However, there are some important modifications of this that should be considered.

- When summoning immediate assistance it is important to contact an obstetrician as well as the cardiac arrest team.
- CPR should commence as soon as possible, and the evidence suggests that good-quality cardiac compressions increase the likelihood of success.
- After 20 weeks' gestation, care should be taken with maternal positioning. The gravid uterus may compress the inferior vena cava and decrease venous return and preload. The mother should therefore be positioned to avoid this. The uterus should be manually displaced, and once this has been done the mother should be placed in a position that provides a left lateral tilt (with pillows and/or specially designed wedges). The tilt should be approximately 15–30° and should facilitate Caesarean delivery if this is deemed necessary.
- Equipment should be available for an emergency Caesarean section if this is deemed appropriate by the medical team.
- If there is no response to correctly performed CPR within 4 min of maternal collapse, or if resuscitation is continued beyond this in women beyond 20 weeks' gestation, delivery should be undertaken to assist maternal resuscitation. This should be achieved within 5 min of the collapse.[5]
- As there is an increased risk of pulmonary aspiration, early tracheal intubation is recommended.

Reference

5 Royal College of Obstetricians and Gynaecologists (RCOG). *Maternal Collapse in Pregnancy and the Puerperium (Green-top Guideline No. 56)*. RCOG: London, 2011.

Further reading

Resuscitation Council (UK). *Cardiac Arrest in Special Circumstances*. ℜ https://lms.resus.org.uk/modules/m10-v2-cardiac-arrest/10346/resources/chapter_12.pdf

Chapter 17

Poisoning

Assessment of poisoning

Poisoning caused by a harmful substance can be acute or chronic, and may be intentional or accidental. It can result from:

- ingestion
- injection
- inhalation
- exposure of body surfaces (skin, eyes, mucous membranes)
- venomous stings or bites.

The National Poisons Information Service provides expert advice to healthcare professionals on chronic and acute poisoning:

- TOXBASE® (www.toxbase.org)—a continually updated online database that provides guidance on individual poisons
- a 24-hour telephone helpline to provide specific advice for healthcare professionals about complex poisoning situations.

The consequences of poisoning depend on:

- the patient's age, size, and general health
- the medication(s) or other substance(s) taken
- the route and quantity of these
- onset or period of exposure
- other substances taken at the same time (e.g. alcohol).

Focused health history

Subjective information about the patient's symptoms and the known or suspected drug or substance can be obtained from:

- evidence such as empty bottles, syringes, drugs, or suicide note
- the patient, their relatives, ambulance personnel, friends, or GP
- the patient's medical history, including mental illness and previous overdose attempts
- supervisors and co-workers from the same workplace order to ascertain the use of or exposure to any industrial chemicals or gases

Consider prescribed and illicit drugs, 'legal highs', complementary therapies, the use of herbs, plants, and mushrooms, and recent travel.

Focused physical assessment

Signs may be suggestive of particular substances. For example:

- toxidromes—a collection of characteristic signs and symptoms that are elicited by a particular substance when it is taken in excess (see ➔ p. 444)
- breath odour:
  - cyanide—bitter almonds odour
  - phenol, salicylates, isopropyl alcohol—acetone odour
  - heavy metals, organophosphates—garlic odour
- needle tracks or venepuncture marks from recreational drug use
- colour of the skin and mucous membranes (jaundice, cherry red, cyanosed)
- pupil size (e.g. opioids cause pinpoint pupils, anticholinergics cause dilated pupils)
- presence of rashes, blisters, or other lesions.

In patients presenting with an altered conscious level, other causes of neurological dysfunction must be considered (e.g. meningoencephalitis, head injury, stroke, hypoglycaemia, hepatic encephalopathy).

Laboratory investigations

Guidance on investigations to be carried out should be obtained from the National Poisons Information Service's TOXBASE®, and typically includes:

- specific tests to confirm the presence of known or suspected poison(s) (e.g. in blood, urine, gastric aspirate, or vomitus)
- blood glucose levels
- urea, creatinine, and electrolytes
- FBC
- clotting screen
- osmolality
- LFTs
- urinalysis
- arterial blood gas (if carbon monoxide poisoning is suspected, use a co-oximeter to measure oxygen saturation, as it can identify the concentration of carboxyhaemoglobin)
- 12-lead ECG
- chest X-ray if indicated (aspiration is common, and pulmonary oedema may occur with salicylate and heroin poisoning).

Conditions that require admission to the critical care unit

- Hypotension and hypertension.
- Potential or actual cardiac arrhythmias and other ECG abnormalities (e.g. prolonged QT or QRS segments).
- Heart failure.
- Reduced conscious level (e.g. GCS score ≤ 8 or continuing to fall).
- Repeated or prolonged seizures.
- Need for endotracheal intubation with or without mechanical ventilation.
- Need for specialist support (e.g. haemo(dia)filtration, haemoperfusion, temporary pacing).
- Management of bleeding (e.g. from warfarin overdose).

Further reading

Boyle JS, Bechtel LK and Holstege CP. Management of the critically poisoned patient. *Scandinavian Journal of Trauma, Resuscitation and Emergency Medicine* 2009; **17**: 29.

Ghannoum M and Gosselin S. Enhanced poison elimination in critical care. *Advances in Chronic Kidney Disease* 2013; **20**: 94–101.

Patel SR. Toxicological emergencies in the intensive care unit: managing reversal agents and antidotes. *Critical Care Nursing Quarterly* 2013; **36**: 335–44.

Pettie J and Dow M. Management of poisoning in adults. *Nursing Standard* 2013; **27**: 43–9.

Management of poisoning

Initial management

- Maintain a patent airway—if the patient is comatose, or there is no cough or gag reflex, endotracheal intubation and mechanical ventilation will be required.
- Monitor heart rate, blood pressure, O_2 saturation, and respiratory rate.
- Give O_2 therapy to maintain O_2 saturations at ≥ 94%.
  - The exception to this is carbon monoxide poisoning, in which case give 100% O_2 because O_2 saturation monitoring is unreliable (see ➔ p. 453).
- Continuous ECG monitoring and regular rechecking of 12-lead ECG.
- Haemodynamic monitoring.
- Establish IV access, correct hypovolaemia, and treat excessively high or low blood pressures.
- Recognize and promptly manage seizures.
- Monitor core temperature and treat hyper- or hypothermia.
- Monitor blood glucose levels and treat hypo- or hyperglycaemia.
- Monitor renal function and electrolytes and treat accordingly.
- Perform a thorough neurological assessment and institute regular neuromonitoring with GCS scoring.
- Monitor liver function.
- Check the limbs, buttocks, and back for evidence of compartment syndrome, and the blood and urine for rhabdomyolysis.
- Examine the skin for signs of injury, blisters, or venepuncture marks.
- Regularly reassess the patient.
- Review the TOXBASE® guidelines if the poison is known or a particular poison is suspected.
- Educate the patient and their family as appropriate.

Minimizing further absorption of poison

Gastric lavage and emesis are rarely used, due to doubts about their efficacy and also the risk of serious complications.

Activated charcoal

- This prevents absorption from the stomach.
- Give 1 g/kg charcoal orally or via nasogastric tube.
- Ideally give it as early as possible after ingestion of the substance, although it can be effective up to 24 h after ingestion.
- It is effective for benzodiazepines, anticonvulsants, antihistamines, phenothiazines, tricyclics, and theophylline, but not for heavy metals (e.g. iron).
- The airway must be protected, as there is a risk of aspiration.
- Do not give charcoal to patients with an ileus.

Whole bowel irrigation

- A solution of polyethylene glycol is given orally or via nasogastric tube at a rate of 2 L/h until the rectal effluent runs clear.
- This procedure is used for substances such as enteric-coated preparations, those for which activated charcoal is ineffective, and for intact elimination of packets of cocaine or heroin.
- Do not use in patients with an unprotected airway, ileus, bowel obstruction, or perforation.

Increasing excretion of poison

Forced diuresis

Large volumes of IV fluid are infused with diuretics to promote urinary excretion. Forced diuresis is contraindicated in patients with renal dysfunction or heart failure.

- Maintain urine output at > 200 mL/h.
- Avoid excess positive fluid balance.
- Monitor blood electrolytes and magnesium levels.
- For forced alkaline diuresis (used for acid poisons such as aspirin), infuse aliquots of 8.4% sodium bicarbonate to maintain urinary pH at > 7. If the pH is > 7.5, alternate with 0.9% saline or 5% glucose.
- For forced acid diuresis (used for soluble alkaline drugs), use 5% glucose with added ammonium chloride to maintain urinary pH close to 6.5.

Extracorporeal elimination

- This involves the use of haemodialysis, haemofiltration/diafiltration, or haemoperfusion.
- It is effective for removal of small-molecule poisons with limited protein binding (e.g. methanol, ethylene glycol, lithium, theophylline).

Antidotes and alteration of drug metabolism

Specific antidotes can be given for certain poisons (e.g. naloxone for opiates, flumazenil for benzodiazepines, ethanol for methanol, acetylcysteine for paracetamol).

Mental health assessment

An assessment of the patient's mental health should be undertaken if clinically appropriate (i.e. if the patient is able to speak or communicate well using aids). This is particularly important if the poisoning was an intentional overdose. For a systematic approach to assessment of mental health, see ➲ p. 28. Consideration should be given to whether there is a need for referral to mental health services both while the patient remains in the critical care setting and upon discharge.

Further reading

Brooks DE et al. Toxicology in the ICU: Part 2: specific toxins. *Chest* 2011; **140**: 1172–85.

Levine M et al. Toxicology in the ICU: Part 1: general overview and approach to treatment. *Chest* 2011; **140**: 795–806.

Levine M et al. Toxicology in the ICU: Part 3: natural toxins. *Chest* 2011; **140**: 1357–70.

Toxidromes

A toxidrome is a collection of characteristic signs and symptoms elicited by a particular substance when taken in excess, and based on the pharmacology and physiological effects of the substance. Recognizing a toxidrome helps to guide treatment without specific knowledge of the substance. Table 17.1 provides a list of common toxidromes and their corresponding signs and symptoms.

Table 17.1 Common toxidromes

Toxidrome	Signs and symptoms	Examples of drugs
Anticholinergic	Hypertension Tachycardia Dilated pupils Hyperthermia Delirium Dry, flushed skin Urinary retention Seizures Coma Psychosis	Atropine Antihistamines Psychoactive drugs
Cholinergic	Bradycardia Hypotension Tachypnoea Confusion Seizures Sweating Vomiting Lacrimation Defaecation Fasciculations Dilated pupils	Organophosphates Nerve agents (e.g. sarin) Common pesticides
Sedative/hypnotic	Respiratory depression Slurred speech Depressed mental state Ataxia	Barbiturates Ethanol Anticonvulsants Benzodiazepines Some antidepressants
Opioid	Respiratory depression Depressed mental state Bradycardia Hypotension Pinpoint pupils	Morphine Heroin Fentanyl Codeine

Paracetamol poisoning

Definition

[illegible]

Assessment findings

[illegible]

- [illegible]
- hypoglycaemia
- hypotension
- lactic acidosis
- coagulopathy
- acute liver failure (on day 2–7)
- acute kidney injury (on day 2–3)

Investigations

- [illegible]
- ECG
- Arterial blood gas
- [illegible]

Management

- Consider activated charcoal [illegible]
- [illegible]
- [illegible]

Paracetamol poisoning

Definition

Hepatic glucuronide and sulphate are depleted following a paracetamol overdose, with a consequent increase in P450-catalysed oxidation. This leads to increased production of a reactive arylating metabolite, N-acetyl-p-benzoquinone imine (NAPQI). NAPQI is usually rendered non-toxic by conjugation with glutathione, but this is reduced following overdose. NAPQI causes cellular damage and hepatic necrosis.

Toxic effects are serious or fatal at 150 mg/kg in adults, or around 75 mg/kg in those with impaired hepatic metabolism. For example:

- malnutrition—decreases glutathione stores
- alcoholism—decreases glutathione stores
- HIV infection—decreases glutathione stores
- chronic disease—decreases glutathione stores
- enzyme-inducing drugs (e.g. rifampicin, barbiturates, carbamazepine, ethanol, phenytoin)—increase P450 activity.

Assessment findings

Patients are often asymptomatic for the first 24 h, or experience non-specific abdominal pain, nausea, and vomiting. After 24 h, hepatic necrosis develops, causing elevated transaminase activity, jaundice, and right upper quadrant pain. This can progress to:

- encephalopathy
- oliguria
- hypoglycaemia
- hypotension
- lactic acidosis
- coagulopathy
- acute liver failure (on day 2–7)
- acute kidney injury (on about day 3).

Investigations

- Serum paracetamol levels—take the first sample as soon as possible after 4 h post ingestion.
- Urea, creatinine, and electrolytes—if needed, repeat 12-hourly.
- LFTs—if needed, repeat 12-hourly (ALT > 1000 IU/L indicates severe liver damage).
- Clotting screen—monitor INR (perform 12-hourly if needed).
- FBC.
- Arterial blood gas.
- Regular monitoring of blood glucose levels.

Management

- Consider activated charcoal (50 mg) if more than 150 mg/kg paracetamol or 12 g, whichever is the smaller, has been ingested, and if it can be given within 1 h of the overdose.
- Monitor urine output.
- Take hourly blood glucose measurements—treat hypoglycaemia.
- Provide renal support for acute kidney injury.

- Acetylcysteine:
  - acts as a precursor for glutathione, promoting normal conjugation of the remaining paracetamol
  - its protective effect is greatest within 12 h of ingestion, but can decrease mortality in late-presenting patients up to 36 h
  - protection is most effective if given within 8 h of ingestion.
- Start acetylcysteine infusion if:
  - the paracetamol level exceeds the treatment line on the paracetamol treatment graph (see Figure 17.1)
  - > 150 mg/kg paracetamol has been ingested within the past 8–24 h
  - the overdose was staggered or the time of ingestion is uncertain
  - the patient is a late presenter (> 24 h) with detectable paracetamol levels or elevated transaminase levels
  - there is evidence of severe toxicity regardless of time of overdose
  - consider its use for high-risk patients with depleted glutathione levels or on enzyme-depleting drugs.

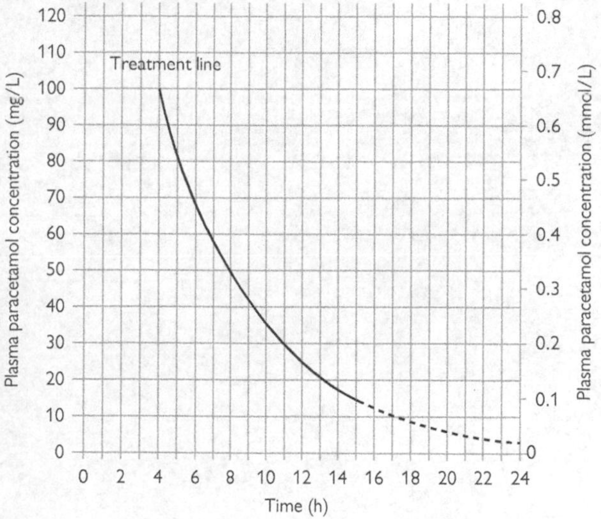

Figure 17.1 Paracetamol treatment graph. (Reproduced from Singer and Webb (2005) with permission from Oxford University Press.)

- **Liver transplantation**—contact the Regional Liver Centre. Consider liver transplantation if:
  - arterial pH is < 7.3 or arterial lactate level is > 3.0 mmol/L after fluid resuscitation
  - creatinine concentration is > 300 µmol/L
  - prothrombin time is > 100 s
  - INR is > 6.5
  - there is grade III/IV encephalopathy in a 24-h period.
- Provide psychosocial support for the patient and their family, and refer the patient to mental health services as appropriate.

Further reading

Singer M and Webb AR. *Oxford Handbook of Critical Care*, 3rd edn. Oxford University Press: Oxford, 2009.

Salicylate poisoning

Definition

[illegible]

Investigations

[illegible]

Salicylate poisoning

Definition

The most common cause of salicylate poisoning is ingestion of aspirin, and it is less commonly caused by ingestion of oil of wintergreen (used in liniments) or methyl salicylate. The toxic blood level is > 150 mg/kg.

Salicylates impair cellular respiration by uncoupling oxidative phosphorylation, stimulating the respiratory centre in the medulla, and interfering with lipid, amino acid, and carbohydrate metabolism. They may also cause gastrointestinal erosions, bleeding, ulceration, and (rarely) perforation, as well as renal or liver failure.

Assessment findings

Mild to moderate poisoning (150–300 mg/kg)

- Vertigo.
- Tinnitus.
- Diarrhoea.
- Vomiting.
- Headache.
- Confusion.
- Tachycardia.
- Hyperventilation.

Severe poisoning (300–500 mg/kg)

- Altered mental state (delirium, hallucinations, coma).
- Acid–base disturbances (respiratory alkalosis due to central stimulation, followed by metabolic acidosis due to the acidic nature of the drug and increased metabolic rate).
- Pulmonary oedema.
- Seizures.
- Gastrointestinal bleeding.
- Liver failure.
- Acute kidney injury.
- Respiratory failure.
- Rhabdomyolysis.
- Hypoglycaemia.
- Hyperthermia.
- Dehydration and electrolyte imbalance (renal Na^+, K^+, and water loss is increased).

Investigations

- Serum salicylate levels (serial levels are needed to determine whether absorption is continuing).
- Arterial blood gases.
- Blood glucose levels.
- Coagulation studies (including INR).
- Urea, creatinine, and electrolytes.
- LFTs.
- Serum creatine kinase and urinary myoglobin if rhabdomyolysis is suspected.

Management

- Give activated charcoal to prevent absorption (give as soon as possible after acute ingestion).
- Urinary alkalinization increases elimination—aim for a urinary pH in the range 7.5–8.0.
- Forced diuresis—aim for a urine output of 2–3 mL/kg/h, although the evidence for any benefit over urinary alkalinization is weak.
- Correct dehydration.
- Avoid fluid overload, particularly in the elderly or those with cardiac or renal disease.
- Monitor electrolytes—give K^+ supplements as required.
- Monitor blood glucose levels—treat hypoglycaemia.
- Observe for seizures—treat with benzodiazepines.
- Monitor core temperature—active cooling is needed if the patient is hyperthermic.
- Haemodialysis is required for significant acute kidney injury, refractory acidosis, coma, seizures, pulmonary oedema, or serum salicylate level > 6.2 mmol/L.

Carbon monoxide poisoning

Definition

Carbon monoxide (CO) is a colourless, odourless gas produced by the incomplete burning of organic compounds. Haemoglobin has a greater affinity for CO than for O_2, forming carboxyhaemoglobin, which then prevents the uptake of O_2 on to the Hb. The oxyhaemoglobin (OxyHb) dissociation curve is shifted to the left, decreasing release of O_2 at the tissues. CO also binds to myoglobin, which has an even greater affinity for it than does Hb, further exacerbating tissue hypoxia.

The elimination half-life of CO from blood is:

- 4.5 h in room air
- 1.5 h in 100% O_2
- 15–23 min in 2.5 atm hyperbaric O_2.

CO also competes with O_2 for binding to the haem moiety within cytochrome oxidase, the last part of the mitochondrial electron transport chain responsible for generating most of the body's ATP. As mitochondrial pO_2 levels are much lower than arterial levels, the CO is harder to displace—hence the rationale for hyperbaric treatment.

Assessment findings

- Headache.
- Nausea.
- Vomiting.
- Tiredness and weakness.
- Confusion, memory disturbance, and amnesia.
- Abdominal pain.
- Coordination problems.
- Angina (if there is pre-existing heart disease).
- Dyspnoea.
- Loss of consciousness.
- Coma.
- Seizures.
- The classic cherry-red appearance of the skin and mucosa rarely occurs—usually there is pallor.
- Tachycardia.
- Hypotension or hypertension.
- Hyperglycaemia.
- Hypokalaemia.
- Hyperthermia.
- Bright red retinal veins.
- Papilloedema.
- Retinal haemorrhages.
- Non-cardiogenic pulmonary oedema.

Complications

- Myocardial depression, ischaemia, or infarction.
- Cardiac arrhythmias secondary to hypoxia or myocardial injury.
- Non-traumatic rhabdomyolysis.
- Renal failure (secondary to myoglobinuria from rhabdomyolysis).
- Cerebral oedema.
- White matter demyelination.
- Permanent brain damage or long-term neuropsychiatric sequelae.

Investigations

Do not rely on O_2 saturation monitoring by pulse oximetry (PaO_2) or from the arterial blood gas analysis (SaO_2). Machines are unable to tell the difference between carboxyhaemoglobin (COHb) and oxyhaemoglobin (OxyHb), and may give falsely high and inaccurate O_2 saturation results.

- COHb levels—measure on a co-oximeter.
- Arterial blood gases—metabolic acidosis may be present secondary to lactic acidosis.
- Troponin.
- Creatinine kinase and urine myoglobin.
- FBC, U&Es, LFTs, and glucose.
- 12-lead ECG.
- Urinalysis—this is positive for albumin and glucose in chronic intoxication.
- Chest X-ray.
- CT of the head if the patient is comatose or has unresolving CNS symptoms.

Management

- Give 100% O_2 (do not rely on pulse oximetry to guide O_2 therapy).
- Continue 100% oxygen until COHb levels are < 10%.
- Give ventilatory support as required.
- Give hyperbaric oxygen (if feasible) if COHb levels are > 25%. Benefits have been shown for long-term cognition.
- Continuous haemodynamic monitoring.
- Serial neurological assessments.
- Monitoring of electrolytes—correct hypokalaemia.
- Monitoring of blood glucose levels.

Tricyclic antidepressant poisoning

Definition

Tricyclic antidepressants are rapidly absorbed and then metabolized in the liver. Conjugates are subsequently excreted renally, and impaired renal function may prolong toxicity. They have long elimination half-lives (often > 24 h).

Assessment findings

Toxic effects are related to the following:

- Anticholinergic effects:
  - dry mouth and blurred vision
  - urinary retention
  - agitation and hallucinations
  - depressed mental state
  - pyrexia
  - delayed gastric emptying.
- Direct alpha blockade—vasodilation causing profound hypotension.
- Inhibition of noradrenaline (norepinephrine) and serotonin reuptake—hypokalaemia.
- Blockade of fast sodium channels in myocardial cells, causing depression of myocardial contractility and arrhythmias.

Cardiovascular effects

- Prolonged PR and QT interval, and widened QRS.
- Unstable ventricular arrhythmias or asystole.
- Atrioventricular block.
- Sinus tachycardia.
- Hypotension.

Neurological effects

- Drowsiness or coma.
- Rigidity.
- Extrapyramidal signs.
- Ophthalmoplegia.
- Respiratory depression (causing hypoxia).
- Delirium.
- Seizures.

Investigations

- U&Es.
- LFTs.
- Arterial blood gases.
- Toxicology screen is not particularly helpful, as serum tricylic antidepressant levels do not correlate with toxic effects. The high degree of protein binding and their lipophilic nature mean that tissue levels are often much higher than serum levels of free drug.
- 12-lead ECG.
- Chest X-ray.

Management

- Give activated charcoal to reduce absorption.
- Provide respiratory support:
  - monitor respiratory rate
  - give O_2 therapy
  - intubate to protect the airway if the patient is obtunded or comatose
  - use mechanical ventilation for severe respiratory depression.
- Continuous haemodynamic monitoring—treat hypotension with fluid with or without inotropes (use agents with α-adrenergic effects).
- Continuous ECG monitoring—observe for arrhythmias. Correct hypotension, hypoxia, and acidosis, and consider magnesium therapy before using anti-arrhythmic drugs, as these may potentially worsen myocardial depression (e.g. beta blockers) and/or further prolong the QT interval (e.g. amiodarone), increasing the risk of serious ventricular arrhythmias. Monitoring should continue for 24 h after the patient is symptom-free.
- Serum alkalinization is required, using sodium bicarbonate to achieve a blood pH in the range 7.45–7.55. This increases protein binding, decreases QRS width, stabilizes arrhythmias, and can raise blood pressure. Administer sodium bicarbonate as an initial slow bolus of 1–2 mEq/kg body weight (70–140 mL of 8.4% solution for a 70 kg adult) through a central venous catheter, followed by an infusion.
- Observe for seizures—treat with benzodiazepines if necessary.
- Use a urinary catheter to relieve retention and monitor output.

Illicit drug overdose

Street drugs are often 'cut' with various contaminants. Purity, and hence dosage, is therefore difficult to determine. Allergic reactions to the cutting agents (e.g. quinine) can also occur.

Assessment and management

- **Respiratory**—monitor respiratory rate. Endotracheal intubation may be required for airway protection with or without mechanical ventilation.
- **Neurological**—assess conscious level, and observe for and treat seizures.
- **Cardiovascular**—provide continuous cardiac monitoring, and treat hypertension and hypotension.
- **Renal**—monitor urine output, and provide renal support if necessary.
- **Active cooling if patient is hyperthermic**—dantrolene may be considered if the core temperature exceeds 40°C.
- **Specific antidotes**—these are available for some of these agents (e.g. naloxone for opiates, flumazenil for benzodiazepines). Short-term reversal may be useful for diagnostic purposes or in life-threatening situations where respiratory support is not immediately available. The half-lives of these drugs are short, so the patient may deteriorate within minutes. Longer-term infusions are very expensive, and in general such patients are intubated and may also be ventilated until the airway, respiratory, and neurological depressant effects of the overdose have worn off. Sudden reversal of the neurological depression with flumazenil or naloxone may precipitate seizures, so these drugs should generally be avoided if the patient has a history of epilepsy or presents with seizure activity.

Illicit drugs

Cocaine

This is a potent CNS stimulant. Crack cocaine is made from cocaine 'cooked' with ammonia or sodium bicarbonate to create 'rocks' that can be smoked.

Symptoms

- Hyperthermia, hypertension, cerebral haemorrhage.
- Myocardial infarction or cardiomyopathy, leading to heart failure.
- Seizures, tremors, delirium.
- Acute kidney injury.

Ecstasy (methylenedioxymethamphetamine, or MDMA)

This is a stimulant and hallucinogenic drug. Adverse effects are more likely to occur with exercise in hot environments (e.g. dancing in nightclubs). Encouragement to drink large volumes of water has led to cases of death from severe hyponatraemia.

Symptoms

- Tachycardia, hypertension, heart failure.
- Hyperthermia and dehydration (sometimes severe).
- Loss of consciousness, seizures, stroke, DIC.
- Muscle cramps.
- Rhabdomyolysis leading to compartment syndrome and acute kidney failure.
- Permanent neurological damage (e.g. impaired thinking and memory).

Heroin (diamorphine)

This is an opiate synthesized from morphine.

Symptoms

- Slow, shallow, and laboured breathing, respiratory arrest.
- Hypotension.
- Disorientation, delirium, drowsiness, coma.
- Pinpoint pupils, and cold, clammy skin.
- Muscle cramps, gastrointestinal spasms.

Specific treatment

- Naloxone.

Benzodiazepines

These include short-acting (e.g. midazolam), medium-acting (e.g. lorazepam), and long-acting (e.g. diazepam) agents.

Symptoms

- Respiratory depression.
- Confusion, drowsiness, coma.
- Blurred vision, slurred speech.

Specific treatment

- Flumazenil.

Gamma-hydroxybutyrate (GHB)

This is a synthetic depressant, which can be snorted, smoked, or mixed into drinks.

Symptoms

- Nausea, dizziness, amnesia.
- Drowsiness, visual disturbances.
- Respiratory distress.
- Seizures, coma.

Amphetamines

These potent psychostimulants cause release of the neurotransmitters dopamine and noradrenaline (norepinephrine).

Symptoms

- Tachypnoea, tachycardia.
- Confusion, hallucinations, psychosis.
- Arrhythmias, hypertension.
- Hyperthermia.
- Stroke, seizures, coma.

Specific treatment

- Acidification of the urine can increase excretion.
- IV phentolamine for severe hypertension.

Barbiturates

These depress the activity of the CNS, respiratory, and cardiovascular systems.

Symptoms

- Severe weakness.
- Confusion, extreme drowsiness.
- Shortness of breath.
- Bradycardia.
- Hypotension.

Specific management

Alkalinization of the urine increases the elimination of phenobarbital.

Chapter 18

Trauma

Introduction

Trauma is the leading cause of death in children and in adults under 44 years of age, and results in significant long-term physical and psychological effects for those surviving from major injuries.[1,2] The assessment and management of trauma patients are complex due to the following:

- the individual nature of each patient's injuries, including internal injuries which may initially be missed
- the potential for rapid deterioration due to either life-threatening injuries or secondary clinical problems
- the potential for various types of shock to develop, such as hypovolaemic, distributive, or traumatic shock (see ➲ p. 174), each of which requires a different type of approach to the clinical management
- the need for involvement of a variety of different types of healthcare professionals while the patient is in critical care which, depending on the type of injury, may include specific surgical teams, physiotherapists, occupational therapists, psychological counsellors, and specialist trauma practitioners.

Trauma assessment and management

In order to immediately identify and treat life-threatening problems while following up ongoing clinical issues, a systematic and structured approach to the assessment and management of the patient with trauma should be adopted. The assessment and management stages are typically undertaken simultaneously, and may involve a variety of healthcare professionals. This chapter will provide an overview of the trauma primary survey (see ➲ p. 462), secondary survey (see ➲ p. 463), tertiary survey (see ➲ p. 468), and a trauma-focused nursing assessment (see ➲ p. 464).

While assessing and caring for a patient with trauma, it is useful to consider the underpinning nature of any injuries, including the following:

Type of injury

- Unintentional.
- Self-inflicted.
- Assault.

Mechanism of injury

- Road traffic accident—car, motorcycle, bicycle, or pedestrian.
- Fall—consider the height and how the patient landed.
- Penetrating (e.g. stabbing, gunshot, other objects).
- Blunt force trauma.
- Blast injuries.
- Other types of injury (e.g. shearing, crushing, compression, chemical, thermal, electric).

Areas of the body affected

- Head.
- Spine.
- Chest.
- Abdomen.
- Pelvis.
- Limbs.
- Internal organs.

References

1 National Confidential Enquiry into Patient Outcome and Death (NCEPOD). *Trauma: who cares?(2007)*. ✈ www.ncepod.org.uk/2007t.htm

2 Trauma Audit and Research Network (TARN). *Trauma Care*. ✈ www.tarn.ac.uk

Further reading

Alzghoul MM. The experience of nurses working with trauma patients in critical care and emergency settings: a qualitative study from Scottish nurses' perspective. *International Journal of Orthopaedic and Trauma Nursing* 2014; **18**: 13–22.

Christie RJ. Therapeutic positioning of the multiply-injured trauma patient in ICU. *British Journal of Nursing* 2008; **17**: 638–42.

Smith J, Greaves I and Porter K (eds). *Oxford Desk Reference: major trauma*. Oxford University Press: Oxford, 2011.

Tisherman SA and Forsythe RM. *Trauma Intensive Care*. Oxford University Press: New York, 2013.

Trauma.Org ✈ www.trauma.org/index.php

Initial management

The primary survey is conducted at the scene of the trauma by pre-hospital staff, and then continues in the Emergency Department. It is concerned with the identification and management of life-threatening injuries using an ABCDE approach. For trauma patients with serious injuries, each section of the ABCDE model should be assessed simultaneously in an efficient manner, which can be achieved by a trauma team whose members have pre-determined roles. Box 18.1 summarizes the key immediate actions to be taken while resuscitating a patient during the primary survey.

Primary survey

Airway maintenance and cervical spine control

- Establish a patent airway by chin-lift or jaw-thrust manoeuvres.
- Remove debris, blood clots, and loose-fitting false teeth.
- Use airway adjuncts or suction.
- Use endotracheal intubation, cricothyroidotomy, or tracheostomy as required.
- Consider cervical spine injuries—do not hyperextend the neck.

Breathing and ventilation

- Give manual ventilation as required (apnoea, reduced respiratory rate).
- Give high-concentration oxygen therapy and monitor SpO_2.
- Expose the chest to assess respiratory movements (look, listen, and feel).
- Consider the possibility of tension or open pneumothorax, or flail chest with pulmonary contusions.

Circulation and haemorrhage control

- Assess haemodynamic status (ECG, blood pressure, heart rate, temperature, capillary refill time, skin colour).
- Control external haemorrhage by direct pressure or pneumatic splints.

Disability and dysfunction

- Assess neurological status (GCS, AVPU, pupillary reaction).
- Consider potential reversible causes of abnormal neurological findings (hypoxia, hypoglycaemia, toxins).

Exposure and environmental control

- Undress the patient so that a rapid assessment can be made of injuries to the trunk and limbs.

Box 18.1 Resuscitation phase

The management of shock is initiated by replacement of lost intravascular volume (see ➲ p. 470), oxygenation reassessment, and haemorrhage control re-evaluation. If not contraindicated, a urinary catheter is inserted. Life-threatening conditions identified during the primary survey are constantly reassessed as management continues.

Secondary survey

This begins after life-threatening conditions have been identified and treated and shock therapy has begun. It involves a thorough head-to-toe assessment in which each region of the body is examined in detail. Laboratory studies, X-rays, scans, and special investigations (e.g. peritoneal lavage) are undertaken.

Definitive care phase

All injuries are managed comprehensively. Fractures are stabilized, and the patient is transferred to the operating theatre if immediate surgery is necessary, or stabilized in preparation for transfer to the critical care unit or other specialist area.

Arrival on the critical care unit

Equipment should be prepared and tested prior to the patient's arrival. Depending on the patient's injuries, an appropriate bed or pressure-relieving mattress may be required (e.g. Stryker frame for spinal injuries). Ensure that any traction can be affixed to the particular bed used.

Checklist for equipment preparation

- Humidified oxygen mask and delivery system/ventilator.
- Rebreathing circuit/Ambu bag.
- Suctioning equipment.
- Volumetric pumps and syringe drivers.
- Pressure bags for rapid IV infusion.
- Stethoscope.
- Continual monitoring equipment—ECG, temperature, pulse oximeter.
- Non-invasive blood-pressure-measuring device.
- Primed transducers for invasive monitoring.
- Trolley for central venous/arterial cannulation.
- Nasogastric tube.
- Blood- and body-warming devices.
- Chest drain sets.
- Ensure that alarm limits are set on monitoring equipment.

Immediate assessment

- Temperature, pulse, respiratory rate, blood pressure.
- If the patient is intubated, mechanical ventilator settings and monitoring.
- ECG rhythm.
- Central venous pressure.
- Neurological status.
- Drainage volumes (urine, wound, chest).
- Chest drain checks—unclamped, patent, and appropriate position.
- Infusion checks—ensure the correct rate for all IV fluids and drugs.
- Patient positioning—ensure that this is appropriate, depending upon injuries.
- Ensure that fractured limbs are supported and traction is fitted properly.

If the patient is stable at this stage, a full trauma-focused nursing assessment (see ➜ p. 464) should be carried out. If the patient is haemodynamically unstable, ventilatory support is inadequate, or the patient is in pain, these aspects must be corrected first.

Trauma-focused nursing assessment

Respiratory assessment

- Airway assessment (patient should be intubated if GCS score is < 8).
- Assess respiratory rate, rhythm, depth, effort, SpO_2, and ABG.
- Particular patterns are characteristic of head injuries in spontaneously breathing patients. Cheyne–Stokes respiration (irregular breathing of fast, deep breaths alternated with slower, shallow breaths and periods of apnea) is seen in bilateral cerebral hemisphere damage, hyperventilation in midbrain injuries, apneustic respiration (prolonged inspiration) in pontine injuries, and ataxic (random) respiration in medullary injuries.
- Observe whether the chest is moving symmetrically with each respiration, and auscultate breath sounds to all lung regions.
- If chest movement is unilateral, the trachea is displaced, or the breath sounds are diminished in any region, consider intraluminal obstruction (e.g. blood clot, tooth), malposition of the endotracheal tube (if intubated), pneumothorax, haemothorax, rupture of a bronchus, or pulmonary contusions.
- If the patient has multiple rib fractures or a flail segment, this will impede movement of the chest wall, and (if the patient is breathing spontaneously) paradoxical chest wall movement may be evident over the flail segment.
- For chest drains, note the type (blood, haemoserous fluid, air) and amounts of drainage, and observe whether the drains swing with respiration or are bubbling.
- Consider underlying respiratory disease, such as asthma or COPD.

Cardiovascular assessment

- Use continuous ECG monitoring and 12-lead ECG.
- Assess trends with regard to vital signs—blood pressure, heart rate, respiratory rate, O_2 saturations, and temperature.
- The frequency of blood pressure recording will depend on the extent of the injuries.
  - Continuous blood pressure monitoring allows blood pressure changes to be detected immediately—this is essential in shocked patients and those with multiple injury .
  - Changes in blood pressure should not be considered in isolation but related to other changes, such as those in heart rate, CVP, and stroke volume.
  - Consider the effects of drug therapy (e.g. sedation, analgesia) as a potential cause of blood pressure changes.
- If haemodynamic monitoring is being used, assess for trends in cardiac output, systemic vascular resistance, stroke volume, etc.
- Assess the presence and strength of central pulses and rhythm.
- Assess for cardiac tamponade (Beck's triad—lowered blood pressure, distended jugular veins, and muffled heart sounds).

Neurological assessment

- A full neurological assessment must be made to provide a baseline for sequential appraisal and detection of deterioration (see ➲ p. 242).
- The frequency of recordings will depend on the patient's injuries, and the presence of or potential for head injury.
- The scalp should be examined for lacerations, bruising, and obvious deformity. Bruising behind the ears may indicate bleeding into the mastoid space, which is a late sign of basal skull fracture. Otorrhoea, rhinorrhoea, and bilateral black eyes (panda/raccoon) are also suggestive of basal skull fracture.

Skin

- Examine the skin for bruising, lacerations, and abrasions, and consider whether any of these may indicate underlying injuries (e.g. seat-belt marks).
- Feel for subcutaneous emphysema, which may arise from external (e.g. stab wound) or from internal (e.g. rib fractures lacerating the underlying lung) injuries.
- Observe for cyanosis, which can occur if there is rapid deterioration (e.g. due to a tension pneumothorax).

Limbs

- Note any bruising, lacerations, swelling, or compartment syndrome.
- Assess skin colour, warmth, and capillary refill time in each limb.
- Check the strength of distal pulses and ensure that dressings, splints, plaster casts, or traction on limbs are not impeding circulation.
- Ensure that pressure is not exerted on healthy skin by plaster casts or traction devices (observe for tissue swelling and breaks in the skin).

Renal assessment

- Use a urethral urinary catheter to monitor urine output.
- If there is trauma to the urethra, a suprapubic catheter is used.
- Perform routine urinalysis—observe for frank haematuria, myoglobinuria (black urine), debris, and clots.
- Examine the genitalia for bruising, lacerations, and oedema.
- Raised blood creatine kinase levels increase the risk of AKI.

Gastrointestinal assessment

- All ventilated patients should have a nasogastric tube inserted unless contraindicated (e.g. due to nasal or basal skull injuries, in which case an orogastric tube should be inserted). The tube should be left to drain freely and aspirated regularly—observe and test for blood.
- Examine the abdomen for bruising and lacerations, rigidity, pain on palpation, distension, and raised intra-abdominal pressure.
- Note any rectal bleeding.

Pain

- Determine whether there is pain or tenderness over a particular area of the chest, or on inspiration, which may limit chest movement.
- Assess for pain or discomfort in any other areas of the body.

Investigations

- FBC, LFTs, clotting, U&E, lactate, glucose, creatine kinase.
- Review radiology reports.

Psychosocial assessment

- Assess the impact of the trauma on the patient's mental well-being, and provide reassurance and support.
- Provide the family with reassurance and support as required.
- Refer the patient to other relevant services (e.g. specialist trauma team, critical care outreach, social services, mental health services).

Tertiary survey

The primary and secondary surveys for trauma patients focus on [illegible] the identification and management of life-threatening injuries, and lesser injuries may be missed. In addition to the primary and secondary surveys, the tertiary survey aims to address [illegible]. The purpose of the tertiary survey is to review all of the clinical information to ensure that all injuries and potential complications are addressed and appropriate care is planned for ongoing rehabilitation.

Missed injuries

- Factors that increase the risk of missed injuries include a high injury severity score, severe traumatic brain injury, emergency surgical interventions, and [illegible].
- [illegible] commonly missed injuries [illegible] extremities, spine, abdomen, [illegible] and pelvis.

Timing of the tertiary survey

The tertiary survey of [illegible] patients [illegible] may be performed by a doctor or [illegible] practitioner. Although [illegible] nurses [illegible] the [illegible] their [illegible] survey. [illegible] the [illegible] survey will depend on how long [illegible] the patient [illegible] and the [illegible] in which the patient [illegible]. Suggested times [illegible] to perform the tertiary survey include:

- [illegible] admission [illegible]
- within 24h of [illegible] patient [illegible]
- once the patient is awake [illegible]
- [illegible] when the survey [illegible] completed.

The tertiary survey should be repeated if the patient [illegible], or [illegible] concerns [illegible] the [illegible] survey [illegible].

Tertiary survey process

- Confirm the mechanism of injury and the patient's [illegible] history.
- Confirm the assessment findings, including [illegible] primary and secondary survey.
- Perform a thorough head-to-toe physical assessment.
- Review [illegible] radiology [illegible] and [illegible].
- [illegible]

Further reading

[illegible]

Tertiary survey

The primary and secondary surveys for trauma patients focus on the initial identification and management of life-threatening injuries, and less serious injuries may be missed. In addition, the primary and secondary surveys may be interrupted to address critical abnormalities. The purpose of the tertiary survey is to review all of the clinical information to ensure that all injuries and potential complications are addressed and a holistic plan of care can be planned for ongoing rehabilitation.

Missed injuries

- Factors that increase the risk of missed injuries include a high Injury Severity Score, severe traumatic brain injury, emergency interventions, and primary intensive care unit admission.
- Body areas to consider for a missed injury are the head and neck, extremities, chest, spine, abdomen, soft tissues, and pelvis.

Timing of the tertiary survey

The tertiary survey of a trauma patient in the critical care setting may be performed by a doctor or an advanced nurse practitioner, although the bedside nurses can also contribute valuable clinical information based on their ongoing assessment while nursing the patient. The timing of the tertiary survey will depend on how long it takes to manage any life-threatening injuries, and the clinical context in which the patient is managed. Suggestions as to when to undertake the tertiary survey include the following:

- after the patient has been stabilized
- within 24 h of the patient's admission to critical care
- once the patient is awake, extubated, and/or ambulatory
- prior to discharging the patient from critical care if the survey has not yet been completed.

The tertiary survey should be repeated for patients who previously had a reduced level of consciousness or who were not fully mobilizing when the initial tertiary survey was undertaken.

Tertiary survey process

- Confirm the mechanism of injury and the patient's background history.
- Confirm the assessment findings and diagnoses from primary and secondary surveys.
- Conduct a comprehensive, full head-to-toe physical assessment.
- Review reports from all laboratory and radiology investigations.
- Review reports from all medical and surgical interventions.

Further reading

Giannakopoulos GF et al. Missed injuries during the initial assessment in a cohort of 1124 level-1 trauma patients. *Injury* 2012; **43**: 1517–21.

Mirhadi S, Ashwood N and Karagkevrekis B. A review of tertiary survey and its impact. *Trauma* 2014; **16**: 79–86.

Traumatic brain injury

Patients with suspected traumatic brain injury should have a CT scan of the head performed and be referred to specialist neurological services as needed (for the assessment and management of trauma patients with brain injury, see ➲ p. 256).

Traumatic haemorrhage

Uncontrolled haemorrhage with trauma shock can cause a deadly combination of coagulopathy, hypothermia, and acidosis, with each of these exacerbating the others (see Figure 18.1). The influence of inflammation and fibrinolysis, which are both triggered after trauma, also enhances the tissue hypoxia and acidosis from shock, leading to even further coagulopathy. Resuscitation of trauma patients requires the addressing of all three aspects of the lethal triad (see Table 18.1).

Principles of damage-control resuscitation

- Permissive hypotension aiming for a systolic blood pressure of 90 mmHg:
  - prevents renewed bleeding in damaged blood vessels which have just clotted as part of the repair process.
- Minimal crystalloids:
  - prevents dilution coagulopathy.
- Haemostatic resuscitation:
  - transfusion of blood products aiming to resemble whole blood
  - fresh frozen plasma, packed red blood cells, and platelets given in a ratio of 1:1:1
  - recombinant factor VIIa, cryoprecipitate, and tranexamic acid may also be considered
  - for further information on massive blood transfusions, see ➲ pp. 416 and 402.
- Warm the patient to correct hypothermia.
- Damage-control surgery should be postponed until hypothermia, acidosis, and coagulopathy have been resolved.

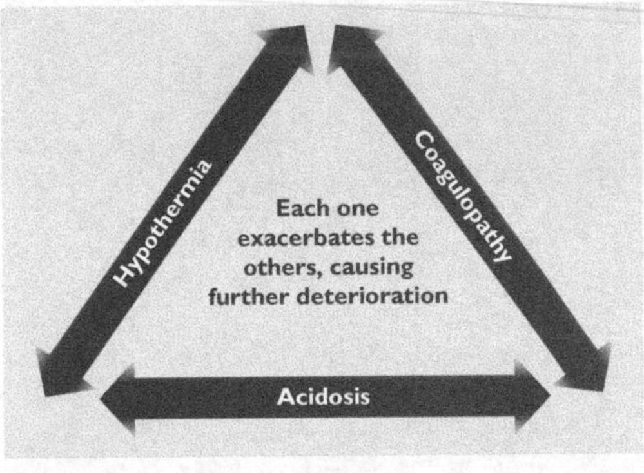

Figure 18.1 The lethal triad of trauma.

Table 18.1 Traumatic haemorrhage pathway checklist

Initial assessment and management	Extent of traumatic haemorrhage assessed
	Patient in shock with identified source of bleeding treated immediately
	Patient in shock with unidentified source of bleeding sent for further investigation
	Coagulation, haematocrit, serum lactate levels, and base deficit assessed
	Antifibrinolytic treatment initiated
	Patient history of anticoagulant therapy assessed (vitamin K antagonists, antiplatelet agents, oral anticoagulants)
Resuscitation	Systolic blood pressure of 80–100 mmHg achieved in absence of traumatic brain injury
	Measures to achieve normothermia implemented
	Target Hb level of 7–9 g/dL achieved
Surgical interventions	Abdominal bleeding controlled
	Pelvic ring closed and stabilized
	Peritoneal packing, angiographic embolization, or surgical bleeding control completed in haemodynamically unstable patient
	Damage-control surgery performed in haemodynamically unstable patient
	Local haemostatic measures applied
	Thromboprophylactic therapy recommended
Coagulation management	Coagulation, haematocrit, serum lactate levels, base deficit, and calcium levels reassessed
	Target fibrinogen level of 1.5–2 g/L achieved
	Target platelet level achieved
	Prothrombin complex concentrate administered if indicated due to vitamin K antagonist or viscoelastic monitoring

Source: Spahn DR et al. Management of bleeding and coagulopathy following major trauma: an updated European guideline. *Critical Care* 2013; 17: R76. (Reproduced with permission from BioMed Central.)

Further reading

Jansen JO et al. Damage control resuscitation for patients with major trauma. *British Medical Journal* 2009; **338**: b1778.

Pearson JD, Round JA and Ingram M. Management of shock in trauma. *Anaesthesia and Intensive Care Medicine* 2011; **12**: 387–9.

Sweeney J. Mass transfusion to combat trauma's lethal triad. *Journal of Emergency Nursing* 2013; **39**: 37–9.

Spinal cord injuries

Spinal cord injuries are often associated with other injuries, particularly to the head and chest. Any unconscious, multiply injured patient must be assumed to have spinal injuries until these have been excluded by expert opinion. The management of the airway, breathing, and circulation must take priority, although precautions should also be taken to prevent exacerbation of any neurological damage.

Airway maintenance with cervical spine control

- In high cervical spine injuries, intubation may be required to protect the airway and/or provide a means of ventilatory support. Vertebral fractures above C5 lead to loss of diaphragmatic function, and those above C8 cause loss of intercostal function.
- A difficult intubation should be anticipated. Endotracheal intubation should be performed by an experienced anaesthetist with an assistant responsible for controlling the head and neck and minimizing spinal movement.
- A fibre-optic laryngoscope or bronchoscope should be available.
- Pharyngeal stimulation may provoke a vagal reflex, causing severe bradycardia (this can be prevented by administering atropine or glycopyrronium bromide prior to the procedure).
- The neck must be stabilized at all times using a rigid collar of appropriate size with sand bags on each side of the head.
- Stabilization of the neck must be continued throughout all procedures (e.g. X-rays, CVP line insertion).
- If X-rays confirm spinal damage, more definitive stabilization may be considered (e.g. skull tongs, halo-pelvic traction, spinal fusion).

Breathing

- Careful observation is required in a patient with a spinal injury who is breathing spontaneously. Ascending oedema of the traumatized cervical cord may lead to deterioration in respiratory status.
- Equipment for manual ventilation must be at the bedside at all times.
- Arterial blood gas analysis and pulse oximetry should be used to identify hypoxaemia as early as possible.
- Vital capacity should be monitored, particularly in patients with fractures above C8 (a forced vital capacity of < 10–15 mL/kg body weight may indicate the need for ventilatory support).
- The patient should be nursed on a bed capable of lateral tilting and longitudinal elevation, while keeping the spine straight.
- Keep the head tilted up and the feet down at 30° if possible to increase functional capacity and help to prevent atelectasis.
- Regular physiotherapy and assisted coughing (supporting the diaphragm) is essential to help to remove chest secretions.

Circulation

- **Neurogenic shock**—reduced sympathetic outflow between T1 and T12 may cause hypotension and bradycardia (see ➔ p. 177).
- Neurogenic shock must be distinguished from hypovolaemic shock (hypotension and tachycardia), as aggressive fluid replacement is detrimental and may precipitate pulmonary oedema.

- Atropine or glycopyrronium bromide may be needed if the heart rate is < 50 beats/min with associated hypotension (< 80 mmHg systolic).
- Fluid challenges may be needed if the patient is hypotensive and bradycardic, but with careful ongoing assessment to avoid over-resuscitation.
- Hypotension and inadequate tissue perfusion may lead to irreversible neurological damage, and frequent monitoring of vital signs is required—noradrenaline may be needed to maintain sufficient MAP.
- ECG monitoring is required due to the increased risk of arrhythmias.
- Temperature may be fluctuating due to loss of sympathetic control.
- Abdominal or other occult trauma may not be recognized because the abdominal wall is anaesthetized and flaccid. Signs of visceral perforation and haemorrhage may not be readily apparent.
- Peritoneal lavage, ultrasound, and X-ray procedures may be necessary if abdominal trauma is suspected.
- Prophylaxis of venous thromboembolism is required.
- **Autonomic dysreflexia**—excessive uncontrolled sympathetic output is triggered by a stimulus (e.g. full bladder or bowel) and results in extremely severe hypertension. It is treated by removing the stimulus and administering an antihypertensive drug as necessary to prevent stroke or cerebral haemorrhage.
- **Spinal shock**—this is loss of reflexes, sensation, and movement below the level of the spinal cord injury due to swelling (it can last from hours to several weeks, and resolves once the swelling around the injury subsides).

Specific nursing management

- Cervical spine immobilization and log rolling until the cervical spine is cleared.
- Nasogastric tube insertion (unless contraindicated) and regular aspiration. Paralytic ileus and gastric dilatation are common in spinal cord trauma. The patient should be nil by mouth for 48 h.
- Urethral catheter (unless contraindicated), as urinary retention may develop. Urine output should be monitored regularly.
- Regular urinalysis should be performed (and the colour observed) and body temperature recorded to detect urinary tract infections.
- Regular administration of laxative and enemas as per unit protocol.
- Prevention of pressure sores and limb deformities by correct positioning of limbs and joints.
- Physiotherapy and passive limb movements to preserve joint motion and stimulate the circulation.
- Adequate nutrition to prevent hypoalbuminaemia.
- Psychosocial care for the patient and their family.

Further reading

Jia X et al. Critical care of traumatic spinal cord injury. *Journal of Intensive Care Medicine* 2013; 28: 12–23.
Pellatt GC. Spinal surgery for acute traumatic spinal cord injury: implications for nursing. *British Journal of Neuroscience Nursing* 2010; 6: 271–5.

Chest injuries

Airway and breathing

- A patent airway must be secured—endotracheal intubation or tracheostomy may be required.
- Chest X-ray is needed to identify the specific location of injuries.
- Mechanical ventilation, CPAP, non-invasive ventilation, or oxygen therapy should be instituted according to the patient's condition.
- Any pneumothorax must be identified and drained.
- Continuous pulse oximetry and regular arterial blood gas analysis should be performed in conjunction with respiratory observations to monitor respiratory function.
- The self-ventilating patient requires careful and continuous observation in order to detect respiratory distress and the need for further intervention.

Circulation

- Continuous ECG and monitoring of vital signs are essential.
- Observe for signs of hypovolaemia (tachycardia, hypotension) and frank blood loss via drains and wounds.
- Monitor haemoglobin levels.
- Myocardial contusions may give rise to tachyarrhythmias and conduction abnormalities.
- Large blood losses may result from tearing of thoracic vessels and haemothoraces.
- Major cardiac or vascular lacerations may have had haemorrhage arrested by a tamponade effect. Rapid transfusion and the subsequent rise in arterial pressure may result in uncontrollable bleeding.

Specific chest injuries

Pulmonary contusions

Shearing and crushing forces within the thoracic cage cause disruption of the microcirculation. Extravasation of red cells and plasma occurs, and these fluids fill the alveoli. Interstitial haemorrhage and alveolar collapse result, impairing gas exchange. Perfusion is maintained in the unventilated lung segments, causing intrapulmonary shunting and hypoxaemia. Management involves treating hypoxia (with mechanical ventilation, non-invasive ventilation, or O_2 therapy), ensuring that there is adequate pain control, and providing physiotherapy.

Rib fractures

Sharp edges of fractured rib may lacerate the underlying lung or blood vessels. If several ribs are fractured in more than one place, or the broken ribs are combined with fracture dislocation of the costochondrial junctions or sternum, a flail segment can move independently of the rib cage. Management is the same as for pulmonary contusions.

Pneumo/haemothoraces

- **Simple pneumothorax**—air in the pleural cavity is caused by damage to lung tissue.
- **Open pneumothorax**—air enters the pleural cavity from a penetrating injury.

- **Tension pneumothorax**—air enters the pleural cavity and increases with each respiration. The affected lung is compressed and collapses, pushing the mediastinal structures to the unaffected side. Cardiovascular collapse will ensue unless immediate decompression is undertaken.
- **Haemothorax**—blood is present in the pleural cavity.
- Pneumo/haemothoraces impair ventilation and may result in hypoxaemia. A chest drain is usually inserted, particularly if mechanical ventilation is necessary, as the likelihood of tension pneumothorax is greatly increased.

Pericardial tamponade

Penetrating or blunt trauma causes the pericardium to fill with blood. This condition is characterized by:

- Beck's triad—lowered blood pressure, jugular venous distension, and muffled heart sounds
- tachycardia
- increased CVP
- reduced cardiac output and other signs of obstructive shock (see ➔ p. 178)
- pulsus paradoxus (a fall in blood pressure during inspiration)
- ST-segment changes and low-voltage QRS complexes on ECG
- arrhythmias.

Treatment is by pericardiocentesis.

Myocardial contusions

These are caused by blunt trauma to the chest or by deceleration trauma. They are characterized by:

- non-specific ST-segment and T-wave changes on ECG
- arrhythmias
- elevated cardiac enzymes.

Diaphragmatic rupture

This is caused by blunt or penetrating injuries. The abdominal contents may be pushed through the laceration. Surgical repair is usually necessary.

Aortic rupture

This is characterized by persistent or recurrent hypovolaemia despite fluid replacement. It is frequently fatal.

Major airway injuries

These are characterized by:

- surgical emphysema
- stridor
- aphonia
- haemoptysis
- respiratory distress.

They are often accompanied by injuries to the oesophagus, carotid artery, and jugular vein, and may be associated with pneumo/haemothoraces.

Abdominal injuries

Initial priorities are the maintenance of airway, breathing, and circulation. Specific treatment of abdominal injury should not delay correction of hypoxaemia and tissue hypoperfusion. Urgent laparotomy may be indicated if hypovolaemia persists after adequate fluid replacement and the cause cannot be attributed to other injuries.

Blunt abdominal trauma can result in significant internal injuries without obvious external physical signs, and abdominal organs may rupture and/or haemorrhage several hours or days after the traumatic incident. Causes of blunt abdominal trauma include road traffic accidents (including seat-belt injuries), falls, physical fights, and sports injuries. Penetrating abdominal injuries may be due to gunshots, knives, or stabbing with any other type of object inserted into the abdomen.

Assessment

- ABCDE assessment, observing for signs of hypovolaemic shock (see ➔ p. 175).
- Presence of increasing abdominal pain, rigidity, or distension.
- Presence of bruising, lesions, or wounds to the abdomen or flanks (see Table 18.2).
- For penetrating trauma, check the groin, buttocks, and armpits.
- Urine output, volume, and colour, and presence of blood in the urine.
- Abdominal pressure (for the assessment and management of intra-abdominal hypertension, see ➔ pp. 300 and 322).
- Haemoglobin and coagulation profile to assess whether these indicate ongoing internal bleeding.
- LFTs, U&E, and glucose levels to assess liver and kidney function.

Specific nursing management

- Closely monitor vital signs and haemoglobin levels.
- Provide IV fluids and/or blood products as required.
- Insert a nasogastric tube (unless contraindicated) in order to:
  - decompress the stomach
  - reduce the risk of aspiration pneumonia
  - detect the presence of upper gastrointestinal injury (indicated by blood in the nasogastric aspirate).
- Closely monitor temperature, peritonism (see Table 18.3), and purulent discharge from wounds or drains.
  - Patients with abdominal injuries are particularly at risk of local infection, septicaemia, and multi-organ dysfunction syndrome (MODS), so must be regularly monitored for potential infection.
  - If the spleen has been removed, there is an increased risk of overwhelming bacterial sepsis due to reduced humoral immunity.

Table 18.2 Abdominal signs

Name	Assessment	Causes
Grey Turner's sign	Bruising to lower abdomen and back	Acute pancreatitis, retroperitoneal bleeding, ruptured abdominal aortic aneurysm, ruptured ectopic pregnancy
Cullen's sign	Bruising and oedema near the umbilical area	Acute pancreatitis, retroperitoneal bleeding, ruptured abdominal aortic aneurysm, ruptured ectopic pregnancy
Ballance's sign	Left upper quadrant percussion—dullness Right upper quadrant percussion—shifting dullness	Splenic rupture or injury (coagulated blood around splenic area and free blood in peritoneum)
Kehr's sign	Acute pain in shoulder tip, which increases while lying down with feet up	Referred pain from diaphragmatic irritation due to intraperitoneal blood, clots, or air (e.g. splenic injury, ruptured ectopic pregnancy)

Table 18.3 Peritonism*

Peritoneal sign	Assessment
Acute abdominal pain	Pain to the abdomen increases with movement of the peritoneum (e.g. ask patient to cough, flex and rotate hip, lie on their side and hyperextend hip)
Guarding	Voluntary contraction of abdominal muscle upon palpation (may decrease if the patient is reassured or distracted)
Rigidity	Involuntary reflex in which abdominal muscles contract upon palpation; it persists on repeat examinations
Rebound tenderness	Increased pain when the fingers are quickly withdrawn after firmly palpating into the abdomen

*Peritonism refers to an acute abdomen which is probably due to peritonitis and presents with the peritoneal signs listed above.

Pelvic fractures

Causes of a fractured pelvis include falls from standing (patients with osteoporosis are particularly at risk), falls from a considerable height, road traffic accidents, and crush injuries. The following are specific examples of different types of pelvic injuries:

- lateral compression fracture (see Figure 18.2)
- anterior–posterior compression fracture (open book) (see Figure 18.3)
- vertical sheer fracture (see Figure 18.4).

Injury to the pelvis can result in severe and uncontrollable haemorrhage. Therefore continuous recording of vital signs is essential, and fluid resuscitation should be given as necessary. Immobilization and external fixation can help to control bleeding, but surgical repair of torn vessels or angiography and embolization may be required.

Care of pressure areas may pose particular problems, and clear instructions must be given by the surgeon as to the degree of mobility the patient is allowed. A pressure-relieving mattress is essential, as movement remains limited even after external/internal fixation.

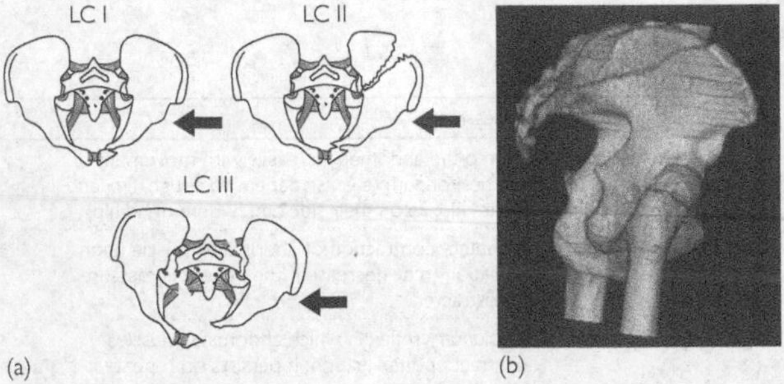

Figure 18.2 Pelvic injury: lateral compression (LC) fracture. (Reproduced from Bulstrode C et al., *Oxford Textbook of Trauma and Orthopaedics*, 2011. By permission from Oxford University Press.)

Further reading

Bodden J. Treatment options in the hemodynamically unstable patient with a pelvic fracture. *Orthopedic Nursing* 2009; **28**: 109–16.

McMaster J. Pelvic ring fractures: assessment, associated injuries, and acute management. In: C Bulstrode et al. (eds) *Oxford Textbook of Trauma and Orthopaedics*, 2nd edn. Oxford University Press: Oxford, 2011. pp. 1253–64.

Walker J. Pelvic factures: classification and nursing management. *Nursing Standard* 2011; **26**: 49–58.

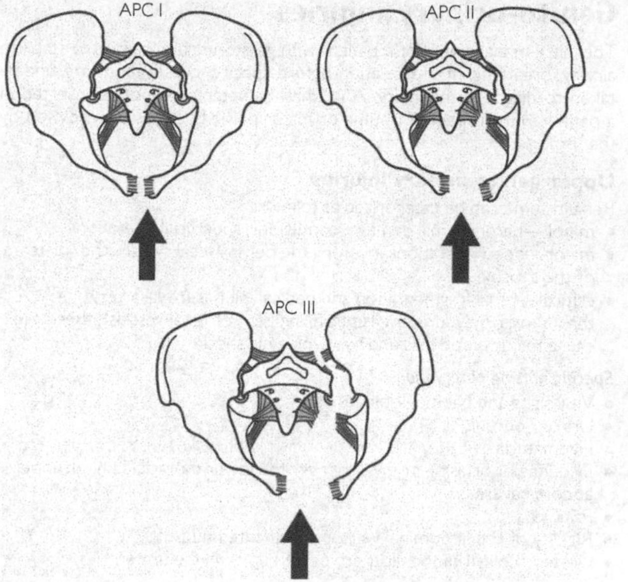

Figure 18.3 Pelvic injury: anterior–posterior compression (APC) fracture (open book). (Reproduced from Bulstrode C et al., *Oxford Textbook of Trauma and Orthopaedics*, 2011. By permission from Oxford University Press.)

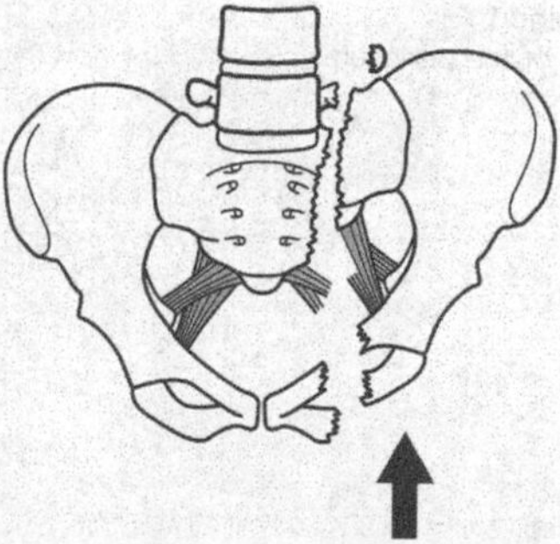

Figure 18.4 Pelvic injury: vertical sheer fracture. (Reproduced from Bulstrode C et al., *Oxford Textbook of Trauma and Orthopaedics*, 2011. By permission from Oxford University Press.)

Genito-urinary injuries

The initial management of a patient with genito-urinary injury is to stabilize airway, breathing, and circulation before specific investigations are undertaken to diagnose the injury. A urethral catheter must not be inserted in a patient with suspected trauma or major pelvic fractures until advised by the urologist.

Upper genito-urinary injuries

Renal trauma can be categorized as follows:

- **minor**—parenchymal damage, contusions, superficial lacerations
- **major**—deep lacerations involving the pelvicalyceal system and/or tears of the capsule
- **critical**—renal fragmentation and pedical injuries (renal artery thrombosis, pelvi-ureteric rupture, avulsion of renal vessels); these can cause major blood loss and hypovolaemic shock.

Specific nursing observations

- Vital signs and haemoglobin levels.
- Urinary output.
- Haematuria.
- Evidence of bruising or swelling over the lower thoracic, loin, or upper abdominal areas.
- Pain.
- Rigidity of the abdominal wall on the affected side.
- Ureteric colic if blood clots are passed through the ureter.

Lower genito-urinary injuries

Specific nursing observations

- Vital signs and haemoglobin levels.
- Urinary output.
- Haematuria.
- Inspect the urethral meatus for blood.
- Evidence of bruising, particularly of the perineum.
- Abdominal pain or rigidity.

Musculoskeletal injuries

Management is standard [illegible] (see [illegible] airway, breathing, and circulation [illegible] [illegible] injuries.

- [illegible] amputations
- [illegible] the point and [illegible]
- [illegible] fractures
- [illegible]
- [illegible]
- [illegible] (see [illegible] pp. [illegible] and [illegible]), which [illegible] and [illegible] the [illegible]

Specific observations of limbs

- [illegible]
- Colour
- [illegible]
- Pulses
- [illegible]
- [illegible]

Specific nursing management

[illegible] (see [illegible] pp. [illegible])

Traction

- [illegible] pressure areas
- [illegible] clean and dry
- [illegible]
- [illegible]
- [illegible]

Plaster cast

- [illegible] (see [illegible] p. [illegible])
- Check [illegible]
- Check for pain [illegible] the plaster cast
- Check [illegible]
- [illegible]

Potential complications

- Haemorrhage [illegible] levels [illegible]
- [illegible]
- Compartment syndrome [illegible] the [illegible]
- [illegible]
- [illegible]
- [illegible]
- [illegible]

Musculoskeletal injuries

Management is secondary to resuscitation and control of the airway, breathing, and circulation. Life-threatening conditions include:

- traumatic amputations
- severe crush injuries to the pelvis and abdomen
- multiple long bone fractures
- vascular injuries
- open fractures
- haemorrhagic shock (see ➲ pp. 175 and 416), which must be identified and treated before definitive treatment of the injury.

Specific observation of limbs

- Temperature.
- Colour.
- Capillary refill time.
- Pulses.
- Sensation and pain.
- Local compression (plaster of Paris, splints, bandages).

Specific nursing management

This depends on the extent of the injuries and degree of immobility.

Traction

- Frequent and meticulous attention to pressure areas, and use of a pressure-relieving mattress.
- Inspect pin sites, and keep them clean and dry.
- Passive/active limb exercises for non-immobilized joints.
- Traction weights should hang free, with the knots secure.
- Retain traction when moving the patient, and support the weights.

Plaster cast

- For a description of specific observation of limbs, see ➲ p. 482.
- Check for constriction due to swelling.
- Check for pain under the plaster cast.
- Check skin integrity around the plaster edge.
- Elevate the limb to alleviate swelling.

Potential complications

- **Haemorrhage**—monitor vital signs and haemoglobin levels, and observe wounds and drains.
- **Compartment syndrome**—monitor the area affected by trauma for swelling and signs of poor perfusion (report suspected compartment syndrome to the doctor immediately because of the need for urgent surgical intervention).
- **Infection**—monitor temperature, and observe wounds, cannulae, and pin sites.
- **Deep vein thrombosis**—inspect the calves for swelling and pain, and consider anti-embolic stockings/prophylactic anticoagulation.

- Rhabdomyolysis—monitor creatine kinase and renal function.
- Fat embolism syndrome:
  - This is associated with fractures to the long bones and pelvis, polytrauma, and after orthopaedic surgery
  - Fat macroglobules released from the bone damage the endothelium, leading to respiratory failure, cerebral dysfunction, and skin petechiae (although the patient may be asymptomatic).
  - It is difficult to diagnose (so is often diagnosed by exclusion of other causes), and management includes respiratory support and fluid resuscitation.

Flaps

Free or pedical flaps are used to correct an anatomical defect. Post- operative survival of the flap depends on adequate perfusion. Close and frequent observation of the flap is essential in order to detect changes as soon as possible. Assess and document the flap condition according to local protocol, and report any changes immediately. Factors that are detrimental to flap survival include:

- hypotension
- vasopressors
- hypovolaemia
- poor positioning.

Specific flap observations

- Temperature—core, peripheral, and flap.
- Colour.
- Capillary refill time.
- Turgidity.
- Pulse.

Specific flap management to maintain core–flap temperature difference of < 1.5°C

- Keep the flap warm—use a body-warming device if necessary.
- Keep the vessels dilated—use IV glyceryl trinitrate.
- Keep Hb < 10 g/dL to reduce blood viscosity.
- Maintain blood pressure and CVP within set parameters.

Blast injuries

Victims of blast injuries experience trauma from a number of sources. The initial source of trauma is the blast wave (primary injury), and this is often accompanied by blunt or penetrating trauma associated with projectile debris from the explosive device or the surrounding area (secondary injury). Further injury can be caused by being thrown against stationary objects, or by building collapse (tertiary injury). There may also be exposure to toxic or radioactive substances (quaternary injury).

The predominant injuries seen after bomb blasts are pulmonary, abdominal, orthopaedic (including soft tissue), neurological, and ontological.

Blast wave or primary injury

Injuries are caused by the slamming impact of the high-pressure energy wave on the body. This causes injuries to hollow organs, such as the ears, respiratory tract, and abdominal viscera. These injuries may manifest little in the way of external evidence of trauma, so patients require careful assessment for any clinical manifestations (see Table 18.4).

Blast-wave-related traumatic brain injury is also frequent, and has the hallmark of diffuse brain injury. This is thought to be related to transfer of the kinetic energy of the blast pressure to the central nervous system.

Secondary injuries

These are commonly multiple, involving shrapnel wounds, traumatic amputations, fractures, and internal injuries. Victims may also receive extensive burns from the blast energy and blast-related fire. These injuries can rapidly lead to haemorrhagic shock and a severe systemic inflammatory response syndrome, and require immediate and effective treatment.

Management of blast injuries

- Immediate management will follow the ABCDE priorities of any acute trauma. A primary assessment is needed to ensure that airway, breathing, and circulation are supported, followed by a thorough secondary assessment.
- **Airway**—should be secured by endotracheal intubation if there are signs of compromise, upper airway burns or smoke inhalation, or impending respiratory failure.
- **Breathing**—adequate arterial oxygen saturations should be maintained with additional inspired oxygen plus mechanical ventilation. If there are concerns about pulmonary blast injury, care should be taken not to deliver too much fluid during resuscitation.
- **Circulation**—an adequate circulating intravascular volume and organ perfusion should be maintained by filling against markers such as blood pressure, CVP, urine output, and metabolic acidosis. Hypotension usually requires correction with whole blood, clear fluids (colloid/crystalloid), and blood products to maintain haemostasis.

Table 18.4 Impact of blast injuries

Pathology	Clinical signs
Blast lung (alveolar rupture, pneumothorax, pulmonary contusion, and haemorrhage)	Tachypnoea
	Hypoxaemia
	Cyanosis
	Wheezing
	Decreased breath sounds
	Haemoptysis
	Cough
	Chest pain
	Dyspnoea
	Haemodynamic instability
Tympanic membrane rupture and damage	Deafness
	Bleeding from the ear
Abdominal haemorrhage and perforation	Abdominal pain and rectal bleeding
	Liver or spleen lacerations
	Rebound tenderness
	Guarding
	Absent bowel sounds
	Signs of hypovolaemia
	Nausea and vomiting
Traumatic brain injury	Loss of consciousness
	Headache
	Fatigue
	Poor concentration
	Lethargy
	Amnesia

Major burns

Expert advice for patients with major burn injuries should be sought from a specialist burns unit or centre. While the patient is waiting to be transferred to a specialist unit, protective isolation in an environment with humidity and temperature control should be provided if possible. Initial history taking and rapid assessment should identify the causative factor (e.g. flame, electrical, chemical, explosion, radiation, or cold), and the depth, size, and location of the burn.

Airway

- Early intubation may be needed before laryngeal oedema and facial swelling increase over time.
- Do not cut the oral endotracheal tube (OETT) prior to intubation. Do assess the tie tapes frequently because of facial swelling.

Breathing

- Give humidified O_2 and mechanical respiratory assistance as required.
- Mechanical ventilation should follow protective lung strategies (see ➲ p. 157) due to the high risk of ARDS.
- Use regular suctioning and nebulizers—bronchial lavage may also be required to clear secretions.
- Monitor ABG, lactate, and carboxyhaemoglobin levels.

Smoke inhalation

- Chemicals in smoke cause inflammation and damage to the airway and lungs, leading to mucosal dysfunction, airway coagulopathy, laryngospasm, bronchospasm, pulmonary oedema, and ARDS.
- There is an increased risk with fire in a confined space or prolonged exposure to smoke—bronchoscopy is required to confirm the diagnosis.
- Do not rely on O_2 saturation readings (see ➲ p. 452 for an overview of the effects of carboxyhaemoglobin on pulse oximetry).
- Use nebulized agents according to local protocol (e.g. normal saline, salbutamol, bicarbonate, acetylcysteine, anticoagulant).

Circulation

Burn shock

- Poor tissue perfusion results from combined hypovolaemic, distributive, and cardiogenic shock due to a reduced effective circulating blood volume, SIRS, and decreased myocardial contractility.

Fluid resuscitation

- Massive intravascular fluid deficit can occur due to direct fluid loss at the burn site and third spacing (fluids shift to the interstitial space as a result of decreased albumin and increased capillary permeability).
- Formulae exist for IV fluid replacement regimes, but should be used as a guide only—seek expert advice from the specialist burns unit and use end points of resuscitation goals (e.g. heart rate, blood pressure, urinary output, haemoglobin, lactate, and base deficit) to prevent under- or over-resuscitation.
  - Fluid creep—fluid overload from over-resuscitation with excessive administration of IV fluids.

- Inotropes and/or vasoconstrictor may be required if low blood pressure and low cardiac output persist despite fluid resuscitation.
- Close monitoring of blood electrolytes, clotting, and full blood count is required.
- Blood components (e.g. packed red blood cells, fresh frozen plasma) should be given as required.

Renal monitoring

- Close monitoring of urine output is needed, aiming for 0.5 mL/kg/h.
- Acute kidney injury may result from:
  - lowered blood pressure due to decreased intravascular volume and/or vasodilation
  - myohaemoglobinuria, which occurs with electrical burns or deep dermal/full-thickness burns and causes rhabdomyolysis—use a urine output goal of 1–2 mL/kg/h to flush out the kidneys.

Hypothermia

- Prolonged SIRS and hypermetabolism that occur with major burns result in the body resetting its 'normal' baseline temperature to 38°C. A temperature of 36–38°C is considered to be relative hypothermia.
- Warm the room, and provide inspired air, blankets, and IV fluids as needed.

Infection

- Raised temperature can persist for several days, but may be due to SIRS and not necessarily caused by infection.
- Scrupulous attention to infection prevention and control is essential.
- Observe wounds and discharge for signs of infection.
- Appropriate antibiotics should be given if indicated.

Disability

- Monitor neurological status, sedation level, and pain.
- Provide analgesia, particularly before and during dressing changes.
- Provide blood glucose control according to local protocol.

Exposure

- Liaise with the specialist burns unit with regard to wound management.
- Monitor the abdomen and limbs for signs of compartment syndrome.

Other considerations

- Avoid suxamethonium from 5 to 150 days post-burn, as there is a risk of rapid and severe hyperkalaemia.
- Early enteral nutrition should follow specific guidance from a dietitian.
- A bowel management system should be used if burns affect the buttocks or upper legs.
- Physiotherapy and occupational therapy referral should be arranged.
- Psychological support should be provided for the patient, their family, and staff members.

Further reading

Bishop S and Maguire S. Anaesthesia and intensive care for major burns. *Continuing Education in Anaesthesia, Critical Care & Pain* 2012; 12: 118–22.

Miller AC, Elamin EM and Suffredini AF. Inhaled anticoagulation regimens for the treatment of smoke inhalation-associated acute lung injury: a systematic review. *Critical Care Medicine* 2014; 42: 413–19.

Maxillofacial injuries

Many patients with severe maxillofacial injuries will have other associated injuries, and cervical spine trauma must always be suspected. Extreme care is needed while stabilizing the neck when the airway is being secured. Injuries to the face and neck can be life-threatening because they may compromise the airway and cause major haemorrhage.

Specific fractures

- **Mandible**—may cause airway obstruction if it is a bilateral fracture. Often causes haematoma and swelling of the neck and floor of the mouth. Treatment is by internal wiring or plating.
- **Maxilla**—Le Fort I, II, or III. Le Fort II and III fractures are associated with basal skull fracture and may lead to CSF leakage. Nasal intubation must never be performed. Treatment involves internal wiring and plating and intermaxillary fixation. External fixation is often required.
- **Zygoma and orbit**—fracture and displacement of the zygoma can disrupt the lateral wall and floor of the orbit. Subconjunctival ecchymosis and peri-orbital swelling may be present. Unstable fractures require internal or external fixation, whereas stable fractures can be surgically reduced. Fractures of the orbital walls may tear or compress the optic nerve, and blindness is immediate and permanent. Avoid supra-orbital pressure during neurological assessment of patients with suspected facial fracture.
- **Nasal**—haemorrhage may be severe and may require nasal packing. Closed reduction and external splinting may be required.
- **Larynx**—fracture may severely compromise the airway and necessitate immediate tracheostomy. Surgical exploration and repair are usually necessary.

Specific management

Airway and breathing

- Soft tissue swelling and oedema can increase insidiously.
- A patient without tracheal intubation is at risk of developing airway problems.
- Ensure that oxygen face masks are not tight-fitting if the patient has facial injuries.
- Never use nasal cannulae if there is evidence of rhinorrhoea.
- Observe for increasing difficulty in breathing, stridor, and oedema of the face, neck, and mouth.
- Keep the head of the bed elevated if possible to encourage drainage of blood, saliva, and CSF away from the airway and reduce venous pressure.

Circulation

Significant haemorrhage can occur from closed fractures to the maxilla, nose, and ethmoids, and can cause profound swelling.

- Obtain clear guidelines from the medical staff with regard to specific wound management.
- Check all wounds for foreign bodies such as glass.
- Observe for haemorrhage, haematoma, and infection.
- Ensure that pin sites of external fixation are kept clean and dry.

Mouth

- Mouth care can be difficult, but is essential in patients who have had major oral surgery and have sutures or skin grafts within the oral cavity, have their jaws wired together, or cannot take oral fluids.
- A pair of wire cutters must be available at the bedside if the patient's jaws are wired (in order to cut the wires if the patient vomits and the airway is compromised).
- Regular anti-emetics should be given if the patient is experiencing nausea, as vomiting must be prevented.

Eyes

- Observe for peri-orbital swelling and subconjunctival haemorrhage.
- Pooling of tears may indicate damage to the lacrimal apparatus.
- Proptosis or exophthalmos (bulging of the eye) suggests haemorrhage within the orbital walls.
- Foreign bodies (grit or glass) can penetrate the eye and cause pyrogenic infection.

Nose

- Observe for bleeding.
- Rhinorrhoea suggests a cribriform plate fracture. Do not pass a nasogastric tube in this case or the cranial cavity may be intubated.

Ears

- Observe for bleeding or otorrhoea.
- Look behind the ears for bruising over the mastoid process (Battle's sign), which can indicate a basal skull fracture.

Drowning

Definition

The International Liaison Committee on Resuscitation defines drowning as a 'process resulting in primary respiratory impairment from submersion/immersion in a liquid medium. Implicit in this definition is that a liquid–air interface is present at the entrance of the victim's airway, preventing the victim from breathing air. The victim may live or die after this process, but whatever the outcome, he or she has been involved in a drowning incident.'[3] Hypothermia usually accompanies a drowning incident, and although it has a protective effect against organ damage, it causes loss of consciousness and haemodynamic changes.

Causes

Traditionally, freshwater drowning was thought to lead to rapid absorption of water into the circulation, causing haemolysis, hypo-osmolality, and electrolyte disturbances, whereas inhalation of salt water was believed to cause mucosal injury and osmotic pulmonary oedema. In practice there is little difference between them, as both cause loss of surfactant and severe inflammatory disruption of the alveolar–capillary membrane, leading to ARDS.

Assessment findings

- Hypoxia.
- ARDS.
- Multi-organ dysfunction syndrome.
- Sepsis.
- Pneumonia.
- Circulatory failure.
- Electrolyte imbalance.
- Dysrhythmias.
- Acute kidney injury.
- Neurological damage.
- Gastric dilatation.
- Metabolic acidosis.

Management

- Cardiopulmonary resuscitation is often required initially.
- Airway management and high-concentration O_2 by mask if self-ventilating, or intubation and mechanical ventilation as needed. Early CPAP/PEEP is useful, and high inflation pressures may be required.
- Nebulized β-agonists if bronchospasm is present.
- Haemodynamic monitoring.
- Vasopressors if the patient is hypotensive.
- Treatment of dysrhythmias (secondary to hypoxaemia, electrolyte imbalance, acidosis, and hypothermia).
- Monitoring of blood electrolytes and glucose levels.
- Fluid replacement guided by appropriate monitoring.
- Haemolysis may require blood transfusion.
- Monitor the core temperature, and rewarm as necessary (see Table 18.6, ➲ p. 493).

- Monitor urine output—haemolysis may cause haemoglobinuria and consequent acute kidney injury.
- Neurological observations—ischaemic cerebral damage and cerebral oedema may occur. Raised intracranial pressure should be reduced to maintain cerebral perfusion, and the patient should be closely monitored for seizures, with subsequent seizure management implemented (see ➔ p. 264).
- Insert a nasogastric tube for gastric decompression and to avoid aspiration.
- Antibiotic therapy is required if there is evidence of aspiration (e.g. mud, sand, or particulate matter on suction). Otherwise take specimens and treat as indicated.
- Metabolic acidosis may develop following intense peripheral vasoconstriction and hypoxaemia. Lactate levels rise as oxygen delivery to the tissues falls, but should improve as the patient is rewarmed and hypoxia is corrected.
- Physiotherapy.

Reference

3 Idris AH et al. Recommended guidelines for uniform reporting of data from drowning: the "Utstein style". *Resuscitation* 2003; **59**: 45–57.

Further reading

Soar J et al. European Resuscitation Council Guidelines for Resuscitation 2010 Section 8. Cardiac arrest in special circumstances: electrolyte abnormalities, poisoning, drowning, accidental hypothermia, hyperthermia, asthma, anaphylaxis, cardiac surgery, trauma, pregnancy, electrocution. *Resuscitation* 2010; **81**: 1400–33.

Hypothermia

Definition

A patient is considered to be hypothermic if they have a sustained core temperature below 35°C (mild, 32–35°C; moderate, 28–32°C; severe, < 28°C).

Causes

Environmental causes

- Immobility (e.g. due to coma, spinal injury, or in elderly).
- Submersion or immersion in cold water.
- Exposure or poor living conditions.

Secondary hypothermia

- Reduced metabolic rate caused by a primary metabolic disorder (e.g. hypothyroidism, hypopituitarism, malnutrition).
- Sepsis.
- Immediate post-operative.
- Erythroderma (generalized erythema and exfoliation).

Therapeutic

- Targeted temperature management following cardiac arrest (see ➲ p. 410) or traumatic brain injury (see ➲ p. 256).

Assessment findings

Table 18.5 summarizes the features of hypothermia.

- ECG changes—as the body temperature decreases, sinus bradycardia is followed by atrial flutter and fibrillation. The PR interval, QRS, and QT interval are prolonged. Atrial activity then ceases, and ventricular fibrillation is common at < 30°C, leading to asystole at < 28°C.
- Decreased cardiac output and blood pressure.
- Hypoxaemia due to hypoventilation and ventilation–perfusion mismatch.
- Respiratory acidosis due to increased CO_2 levels.
- Polyuria and electrolyte imbalance due to impaired tubular function and reduced responsiveness to antidiuretic hormone (ADH).
- Cerebral depression due to decreased cerebral blood flow.
- Metabolic acidosis due to increased levels of lactate and other metabolites.

Table 18.5 Features of hypothermia

Temperature	Assessment
> 33°C	Thermoregulatory mechanisms usually intact, marked shivering
< 33°C	Slowness and dysarthria
< 31°C	Loss of consciousness, pupillary dilatation, hypertonicity, life-threatening cardiovascular dysfunction
< 28°C	Rigor mortis-like appearance, impalpable arterial pulse, cessation of respiration

- Hyperglycaemia due to decreased insulin release, glucose metabolized from liver glycogen, or pancreatitis which may develop.
- Coagulopathy.

Management

- Airway management and oxygenation.
- Monitor core temperature.
  - Assess for ongoing hypothermia and impact of rewarming techniques to return patient to normothermia.
  - Consider targeted temperature management, maintaining therapeutic hypothermia if there has been a return to spontaneous circulation following cardiac arrest (see ➔ p. 410).
  - Ensure that the patient does not become hyperthermic as a result of rewarming therapy.
- Rewarming (see Table 18.6).
- ECG monitoring and detection of dysrhythmias.
  - In the event of cardiac arrest (and no evidence of other fatal disease), full resuscitation should continue until the patient is normothermic.
  - VF is resistant to defibrillation in the temperature range 28–30°C.
- Haemodynamic monitoring.
  - Vasodilation occurs as the patient is rewarmed, which may require large amounts IV fluids and vasoconstrictor.
- Monitor fluid status and provide warm IV fluids as required.
- Monitor urine output.
- Monitor blood glucose levels, electrolytes, and clotting profile.
- Neurological observations, including assessment of and treatment for seizures.

Table 18.6 Rewarming

Passive	Mild hypothermia	Rewarm slowly (0.5–1°C/h) Warm environment Reflective space blanket/warm air blanket Extra blankets Cover exposed skin (e.g. scalp) Remove wet clothes
Active	Moderate hypothermia	Heated humidified respiratory gases Warmed IV fluids Electrically heated mattress or pads
Core warming	Severe hypothermia	Rapid rewarming techniques (1–5°C/h) Gastric and bladder lavage with warmed fluids Peritoneal/haemodialysis Extracorporeal circuits

Complications following trauma

Hypovolaemic shock

See ➲ p. 175.

Compartment syndrome

This results from swelling, bleeding, or ischaemia within the fascial compartments of the limbs. The interstitial tissue pressure rises as the compartments are unable to expand. When this pressure exceeds that of the capillary bed, local ischaemia of nerve and muscle occurs. Rhabdomyolysis (see ➲ p. 281), permanent paralysis, or gangrene may result.

Features

- Pain.
- Tense swelling of the fascial compartment(s).
- Reduced sensation over the dermatomes supplied by the affected nerves.
- Absence of distal pulses (a late sign—may be irreversible damage).

Management

- Monitor the limbs for swelling, abnormal perfusion, temperature differences, and pain.
- Remove restrictive dressings.
- Needle manometry (pressures of > 20mmHg are abnormal).
- Fasciotomy.

Fat embolism

Fat macroglobules and marrow enter the systemic circulation from bone fractures (usually of the long bones and pelvis) and cause mechanical obstruction of vessels.

Features

- Hypoxaemia.
- Tachypnoea, tachycardia, and pyrexia.
- Hypotension and decreased cardiac output.
- Oliguria.
- Petechiae.
- Confusion, drowsiness, decerebrate signs, convulsions, or coma.

Management

- Supportive treatment.
- Supplementary oxygen or mechanical respiratory assistance to correct hypoxaemia.
- Maintain circulatory volume.
- Inotropic support.
- Renal support—CVVHD/dialysis.

Air embolism

This occurs when air leaks from the lungs directly into the pulmonary circulation and into the left side of the heart. It can occur in severe lung injury due to a bronchopulmonary vein fistula or from direct penetrating injury to the pulmonary veins. Major cardiovascular collapse follows, with associated hypoxaemia. Treatment consists of turning the patient on their left side in a head-down, feet-up position, and the air is aspirated from the left ventricle, followed by thoracotomy of the injured side.

Post-traumatic stress disorder (PTSD)

In addition to the physiological impact of trauma on the body, traumatic injury can significantly influence the mental well-being of the patient who has experienced the trauma, as well as that of their family. For the assessment and management of PTSD, see ➔ pp. 28 and 524.

Further reading

Aitken LM et al. Health status of critically ill trauma patients. *Journal of Clinical Nursing* 2014; 23: 704–15.

Chapter 19

End-of-life care

End-of-life issues in critical care

So far the chapters of this book have focused on active treatment and the prolongation of life in critical care. However, it is important to consider the significant mortality rate in critical care, as clearly not all critically ill patients will survive.

Death in critical care can be very complex and difficult for patients, families, and staff alike. It may happen very suddenly due to acute deterioration, or it may occur as a result of slow deterioration, failure to respond to treatments, or the decision to withdraw treatment.

Irrespective of this, it is important that patients facing death in critical care areas and their families should be treated with sensitivity, empathy, and compassion, as these are essential foundations for effective end-of-life care.

End-of-life care has received much criticism recently, and complaints about lack of individuality, compassion, and caring have led to a review of end-of-life care provision. In particular the Liverpool Care Pathway (LCP) has been criticized, largely due to inconsistent and incorrect interpretation of the framework. This has led to a perceived lack of public support for the pathway recommendations, and a recent review[1] highlighted the need to change the focus of end-of-life care to personalized care planning to ensure that patients' deaths are individualized.

Alongside this, critical care nurses also have to deal with a number of other complexities associated with end-of-life care. These include:

- the impetus to withdraw treatment
- transition of care from acute to palliative
- uncertainty in decision making
- support of conscious and unconscious patients
- support of families, relatives, and friends.

Reference

1 Neuberger J et al. *More Care, Less Pathway: a review of the Liverpool Care Pathway*. Department of Health: London, 2013.

Recognition of end of life

Recognition that a patient has reached the end of life can be a challenging concept in critical care settings. There are a number of objective criteria that may enhance the ability to predict the trajectory of severe illness, such as APACHE scoring and organ function or failure modelling. However, these tools are not always reliable.[2]

Some of the issues faced by the critical care team include:

- the complexity of the patient's condition
- unexpected or unpredictable death
- difficulty in recognizing when further intervention is futile
- difficulty in decision making
- lack of agreement:
  - between disciplines
  - within disciplines.

Although ultimately the responsibility with regard to decision making rests with the consultant in charge of the patient's care, the importance of a multidisciplinary approach to end-of-life issues cannot be over-emphasized.

Reference

2 Coombs MA et al. Challenges in transition from intervention to end of life care in intensive care: a qualitative study. *International Journal of Nursing Studies* 2012; 49: 519–27.

Decision making

In an attempt to improve end-of-life care, the General Medical Council (GMC) has issued medical staff with detailed guidelines relating to end-of-life decision making.[3]

These emphasize the need to be clear about exactly what decisions have to be made about treatment. They also provide guidance to facilitate decision making both in cases where the patient is conscious and has mental capacity and in cases where the patient is unconscious or is not deemed to have mental capacity.

The GMC suggests that in cases where the patient is deemed to have mental capacity:

- staff should keep the patient fully informed of their progress in language and terms that they can understand
- the patient should always be involved in the decision-making process, and should be provided with sufficient information to allow them to make an informed decision about the choices that relate to end-of-life care
- the patient can, if they choose, nominate another adult to act as an advocate for them should they be unwilling or unable to make a decision.

For patients who are not deemed to have mental capacity, decisions should be grounded in ethical principles. However, staff can review a number of issues that may enable decision making to occur. This includes reviewing whether:

- the patient has made an advance care plan
- the patient has previously appointed an advocate or granted a family member power of attorney.

If neither of these are available, decisions are normally based on bioethical principles (see Table 19.1), and should include discussion with:

- the medical team
- the nursing team
- allied health professionals
- the family, relatives, and friends.

It may also be helpful to use a decision-making model, such as the Morton and Fontaine model[4] (see Box 19.1). Decisions may relate to such issues as:

- ceilings of treatment
- withholding treatment
- withdrawal of treatment.

Table 19.1 Guiding bioethical principles

Non-maleficence	An obligation not to harm another person
Beneficence	An obligation to ensure that any care given is of benefit to the patient and promotes the welfare of the individual
Respect for autonomy	An obligation to respect the choices made by others if they are capable of self-determination
Justice	An obligation to be fair and equitable in the decisions made and distribution of care
Veracity	An obligation to be truthful
Fidelity	An obligation to ensure that commitments made to the patient are kept

Box 19.1 Model for ethical decision making

Prior to decision making there is a need to:
- identify all the appropriate people who need to be involved in the decision
- identify any ethical issues that may arise as a result of this and consult with others as needed
- analyse any problems using bioethical principles
- identify all of the alternatives and select the most appropriate one—it is important to be able to justify the choices made
- evaluate decisions made and reflect on these.

References

3 General Medical Council. *Treatment and Care Towards the End of Life: good practice in decision making*. General Medical Council: London, 2010.
4 Morton PG and Fontaine DK. *Essentials of Critical Care Nursing: a holistic approach*. Lippincott, Williams & Wilkins: Philadelphia, PA, 2012.

Advance care planning

Some patients who are admitted to critical care may have made advance decisions about their own care plan. This may be likely if the patient has a chronic condition or knows that their condition may deteriorate or become life-threatening. The Gold Standards Framework suggests that this enables patients to make choices in anticipation of deterioration in their condition.

Essentially advance care planning covers two main aspects:

- advance statement
- advance decisions.

Advance statement

An advance statement provides an indication of what the patient would like to happen to them. These statements are sometimes referred to as advance directives. It is important to note that such statements are not legally binding. However, they may be helpful in allowing critical care teams to understand the patient's preference for care, in the event that the patient is not able to make their preferences known.

Advance decision

An advance decision is a document that clarifies refusal of treatment that the patient does not wish to receive. For example, a patient with COPD may request that they receive non-invasive ventilation, but refuse invasive ventilation in the event of respiratory failure.

These decisions can be legally binding if they are correctly formulated. Correct formulation involves assessment of mental capacity to ensure that the patient was mentally able to make that decision at the time it was taken (www.goldstandardsframework.org.uk/advance-care-planning). Advance decisions may help to strengthen decision making, especially if someone has been previously granted lasting power of attorney.

Care of the dying patient

Recent reviews have highlighted the need for individualized care planning for patients who are dying. Although the emphasis remains on individualized care planning, there will be some commonalities in care for patients at the end of life.

The World Health Organization emphasizes the need for appropriate planning, and highlights the need to provide appropriate symptom control.[5] Neuberger and colleagues have highlighted the need for compassionate and patient-centred care.[6] This will of course include appropriate assessment of physical, psychological, and spiritual needs.

From a physical perspective this may encompass assessment and management of:

- effective and appropriate pain control
- promotion of comfort
- nausea and vomiting
- breathlessness
- secretion control
- incontinence and urinary retention
- restlessness and confusion
- hydration
- nutrition
- personal care needs.

From a psychological perspective this may encompass assessment and management of:

- stress
- anxiety
- fear
- the appropriate environment
- the desire and ability to discharge the patient home
- discontinuation of unnecessary interventions.

From a spiritual perspective this may encompass assessment and management of:

- spiritual needs
- spiritual beliefs
- the support systems available
- religious beliefs
- religious perspectives.

References

5 World Health Organization. *WHO Definition of Palliative Care.* ℘ www.who.int/cancer/palliative/definition/en

6 Neuberger J et al. *More Care, Less Pathway: a review of the Liverpool Care Pathway.* Department of Health: London, 2013.

Care of the relatives, family, and friends

The need for appropriate support for the relatives, family, and friends of patients at the end of life is a significant consideration. NICE has highlighted the need to ensure that relatives are offered:

- comprehensive holistic assessments in response to their changing needs and preferences
- holistic support appropriate to their current needs and preferences.[7]

NICE suggests that consideration is given to assessment and management of individualized needs.[7] This would include consideration of each individual's:

- physical needs
- psychological needs
- social needs
- spiritual needs
- cultural needs.

Acknowledgement of the importance of effective and clear communication with family members and assessment of individualized needs helps to promote effective family-centred care. Rocker and colleagues identified a number of positive influences on families during this difficult time.[8] Positive care factors included:

- being treated with respect and compassion
- being provided with sufficient information
- discussing sensitive issues such as withdrawal of treatment in a sensitive manner
- having conversations with members of the multidisciplinary team in a quiet place
- ensuring discussion about the patient's preferences
- feeling able to voice their concerns and worries
- feeling that their relative was comfortable and not suffering
- being offered pastoral and psychological support.

Issues that relatives found caused them most anxiety included:

- being given incomplete or conflicting information
- guilt about decisions made
- the nature of their role in the decision-making process.

References

7 National Institute for Health and Care Excellence (NICE). *End of Life Care for Adults*. QS13. NICE: London, 2011. ☞ www.nice.org.uk/guidance/qs13

8 Rocker G et al. *End of Life Care in the ICU: from advanced disease to bereavement*. Oxford University Press: Oxford, 2010.

Special end-of-life considerations: brainstem death testing

Brainstem death testing is normally associated with patients who have [illegible] acquired brain injury, e.g. head injury, subarachnoid [illegible] [illegible] with [illegible] [illegible] raised [illegible] pressure.

[illegible] brainstem death (BSD) [illegible] corresponds to the state in which the individual [illegible] irreversibly comatose:

- [illegible] ventilator [illegible]
- [illegible] to be [illegible] ventilated

[illegible] confirmation of [illegible] death [illegible] [illegible] only [illegible]

It is important to note that some countries, such as North America and Australia, [illegible] be tested. [illegible]

The number of patients who [illegible] [illegible]

- [illegible] brainstem death testing
- [illegible] must be [illegible] before [illegible]
- [illegible] performed [illegible]

Staff involved in brainstem death testing

[illegible] medical practitioners [illegible] registered with the GMC [illegible] one must be a consultant [illegible]

Criteria that must be met before testing

[illegible] irreversible [illegible] [illegible] must be considered:

- [illegible] sedatives, muscle [illegible]
- [illegible] [illegible]
- [illegible]
- [illegible]
- body temperature [illegible]

Brainstem death tests

[illegible] brainstem [illegible] [illegible] [illegible] dead [illegible]

Special end-of-life considerations: brainstem death testing

Brainstem death testing is normally associated with patients who have a serious acquired brain injury (e.g. head injury, subarachnoid haemorrhage, stroke). It can also be seen in patients with global stroke following prolonged hypoxia that has led to significant cerebral ischaemia and raised intracranial pressure.

In the UK, brainstem death (BSD) is considered to be a state in which the individual has simultaneously and irreversibly lost the:

- capacity for consciousness
- capacity to breath unassisted.

In the UK, confirmation of brain death correlates with confirmation of brainstem death, as the assessment is based on the principle that if the brainstem is dead this will lead to irreversible loss of consciousness and ability to breathe spontaneously.

It is important to note that some countries, such as North America and Australia, test for brain death, and this may require other investigations to be performed.

The number of patients who meet the criteria for brainstem death testing is decreasing. There are a number of factors that need to be taken into consideration before brainstem death testing can occur, and guidance is available relating to:

- staff who are able to undertake brainstem death testing
- criteria that must be met before such testing can occur
- the brainstem death tests that must be performed.

Staff involved in brainstem death testing

The guidance specifies that testing must be undertaken by two medical professionals. Both must have been registered with the GMC for at least 5 years, and one must be at consultant grade.

Criteria that must be met before testing

It is important to eliminate any reversible cause of loss of consciousness. Therefore consideration must be given to:

- the length of time since the last administration of sedative, muscle relaxant, or opiate analgesia
- the pharmacological half-life of the drug (for barbiturate-infused drugs this can be of the order of days)
- metabolic disorders
- electrolyte imbalances
- body temperature.

Brainstem death tests

The brainstem death tests aim to test the function of the brainstem. If any aspect of the test is positive, the patient is not brainstem dead. If all aspects of the first brainstem death test are negative, the patient is brainstem dead, but it is normal practice for a second medical doctor to repeat the tests.

Time of death is recorded as the time of completion of the first set of tests (this can be confusing for the family).

The brainstem death tests are listed in Table 19.2, and the procedure for an apnoea test is described in Box 19.2.

The equipment required for brainstem death testing includes the following:

- ophthalmoscope
- light source for pupil responses
- otoscope
- ice and kidney dish to collect iced water
- 50 mL syringe and quill
- gauze and cotton wool
- endotracheal catheter
- blood gas syringes (several).

In summary, a patient is considered to be brainstem dead if the tests identify that:

- both pupils are fixed and do not react to light
- there is no corneal reflex
- the oculo-vestibular reflex is absent
- there is no motor response to central pain sources
- there is no cough reflex
- there is no evidence of spontaneous ventilation.

When the brainstem death tests are complete the team will then discuss with the family:

- the option of organ donation if this is applicable (it is useful to consider early involvement of donor nurse specialists)
- the option of withdrawal of life-sustaining treatment.

Table 19.2 Brainstem death tests

Test	Area/cranial nerve tested
The pupils are fixed and do not react to an intense light source	Mesencephalon and cranial nerves II and III
There is no corneal reflex when the cornea is irritated with a cotton wool tip	Pons cranial nerves V and VII
The tympanic membrane is checked to ensure that it is intact. Ice-cold water is injected into each external auditory meatus. No eye movement is noted during instillation of iced water	Pons cranial nerves VII, II, IV, and VI
No motor response is noted by adequate stimulation (e.g. supraorbital pressure). Care must be taken to use a central painful source, as peripheral sources may elicit a spinal cord *reflex* or may not work in the presence of spinal cord injury	
There is no cough reflex to bronchial stimulation with a suction catheter	Medulla, cranial nerves IX and X

Box 19.2 Apnoea testing

This should only be performed once the brainstem death tests in Table 19.2 have been completed. The apnoea test involves the following steps:

- Increase the patient's FiO_2 to 1.0.
- Check the arterial blood gases.
- Once the patient's O_2 saturations are greater than 95%, the minute volume should be gradually decreased to allow a rise in PCO_2.
- It is necessary to ensure that the CO_2 level rises sufficiently to stimulate spontaneous ventilation (at least 6 kPa).
- Once the CO_2 level has risen and the pH has decreased, O_2 should be delivered via an endotracheal catheter and the patient should be observed for 5 min.
- After 5 min, blood gas analysis should be repeated to ensure there has been a minimum of 0.5 kPa rise in PCO_2 from the baseline.
- If there is no evidence of spontaneous respiration following this procedure, loss of respiratory drive is confirmed and the patient is reattached to the ventilator.

Special end-of-life considerations: organ donation (heart-beating donation)

Special end-of-life considerations: organ donation (heart-beating donation)

For patients who meet the criteria for brainstem death, heart-beating donation is an option for the patient's family to consider. This type of donation refers to the removal of organs, eyes, and tissue for the purpose of transplantation. The patient is taken to surgery and some organs are removed while the heart is still beating.

If the patient is a suitable candidate for organ donation it is usual practice to contact the nurse specialist from the organ donation team. It is preferable for contact to be made prior to the completion of brainstem death tests, but if this is not possible then it should occur as soon as the tests have confirmed brainstem death. Early referral to the team enables:

- assessment of the suitability of the candidate
- support of the family
- checking of the organ donor register.

The donor nurse specialist's role is to:

- make a detailed assessment of the potential for donation
- identify whether the patient is a suitable candidate for donation
- support the family
- stabilize the patient and prepare for donation
- coordinate the arrival of the transplant team
- provide aftercare for the patient.

Absolute contraindications for donation include:

- known or suspected Creutzfeldt-Jakob disease (CJD)
- known HIV disease.

Other contraindications may include:

- disseminated malignancy
- age > 70 years
- known active TB
- untreated bacterial sepsis.

It is usual practice for the doctor to contact the coroner (in England, Wales, and Northern Ireland)) or the Procurator Fiscal (in Scotland).

Special end-of-life considerations: organ donation (non-heart-beating donation)

[illegible]

Non-heart-beating donation

[illegible]

Tissue donation

[illegible]

Special end-of-life considerations: organ donation (non-heart-beating donation)

Most patients who die in critical care units may be eligible for non-heart-beating donation or tissue donation, and this is an important choice to be able to offer to the family.

Non-heart-beating donation

This can normally be considered if the patient's treatment is being withdrawn. The contraindications and absolute contraindications are the same as for heart-beating donation, but the process is slightly different, although it will still be coordinated by the nurse specialist for organ donation.

Because of the need to remove the organs as soon after certification of death as possible, the donor team needs to be ready in theatre before treatment is withdrawn.

It is usual for preparations for donation to be made first, and then the patient's treatment is withdrawn. The patient is observed for 5 min after cessation of cardiorespiratory function, and then death is certified by senior medical staff. The patient is immediately taken to theatre and the organs are retrieved by the team. The patient's family are able to see the patient in the initial period after death and then later, supported by the nurse specialist, following donation.

The nurse specialist for organ donation has a pivotal role in:

- organization
- coordination of the team
- support of the family before and after donation
- aftercare of the patient.

Tissue donation

Most patients who die in an intensive care unit can also be considered for tissue donation. This again involves the role of the nurse specialist for donation, but tissues are taken in the period after death in the mortuary.

The contraindications to tissue donation are listed in Box 19.3. It is necessary to liaise with the nurse specialist not only to coordinate the tissue donation after death, but also to support the family while the decision is being made.

Relatives are required to sign a lack of objection form which will also indicate which tissues may be taken. These may include:

- corneas
- heart valves
- bone
- skin.

Age restriction may occur with regard to donation of some tissues, and the medical staff will also need to obtain permission from the coroner or the Procurator Fiscal.

Box 19.3 Contraindications to tissue donation

- HIV infection
- Hepatitis C and hepatitis B
- Human T-cell lymphotropic virus
- Syphilis
- CJD
- CNS disorders of unknown aetiology
- Leukaemia
- Lymphoma
- Myeloma
- Alzheimer's disease or unexplained confusional states

Useful websites

www.organdonation.nhs.uk
www.nhs.uk/planners/end-of-life-care/Pages/End-of-life-care.aspx
www.gmc-uk.org
www.goldstandardsframework.org.uk/advance-care-planning

Transfer of the critical care patient

Transfer principles

The transfer of critical care patients can occur at various times throughout the admission period (e.g. following the initial stabilization of the patient, for diagnostic or interventional procedures, or for specialist treatment or repatriation). Other indications for patient transfer may be due to bed and staffing availability.

Critically ill patients are extremely vulnerable during transfer, and a high level of expertise is required in order to safeguard the patent from adverse events or near misses. Only experienced and well-trained critical care teams that are able to work together to manage the patient's condition and the potential deterioration of the patient should undertake transfers.

Recommendations from the Intensive Care Society[1] include competency-based training for all staff involved in patient transfers (i.e. ambulance crew, air medical crew, medical staff, operating department practitioner, nursing staff, and portering staff). The decision to transfer a patient must be made by the responsible consultant in consultation with colleagues from both the referring and receiving hospitals. All inter- and intra-hospital transfers should be audited, and any adverse event or near miss should be reported.

Although there are obvious differences between intra- and inter-hospital transfer (e.g. indication, duration, environment of transfer, availability of personnel, and equipment required), the main considerations when undertaking the preparation and execution of the transfer are similar. They mainly involve mitigating the associated risks (see Table 20.1).

Table 20.1 Risks involved in transferring the critical care patient

Potential risk	Examples
Technical complications	Displacement of airway Displacement of intravascular lines or drains Mechanical failure of equipment Power failure of equipment
Inadequate monitoring or therapy	Simplified monitoring/ventilators Interference due to motion
Pathophysiological deterioration	Increased ICP with supine positioning Hypotension or oxygen desaturation Rupture of fibrin clots Dislocation of unstable fractures
Inadequate personnel	Lack of competence Lack of additional support

Reference

1 Intensive Care Society. *Guidelines for the Transport of the Critically Ill Adult*, 3rd edn. Intensive Care Society: London, 2011.

Intra-hospital transfer

Intra-hospital transfer

This refers to transfers that take place within the hospital setting either as part of the admission or discharge process, or to enable surgery, specialist procedures, or diagnostic tests. Although the patient remains within the hospital, they are still exposed to high-risk and unfamiliar environments, and staff need to be mindful of this when undertaking the transfer (see Table 20.2).

Table 20.2 Preparing the critically ill patient for safe intra-hospital transfer

Preparation	Prior to transfer
Respiratory support	ABG and/or chest X-ray if necessary Intubate if there is potential for the patient to deteriorate. Insert nasogastric tube (aspirate and free drainage) Secure airway; check that the patient tolerates portable ventilator Chest physiotherapy, suction, nebulizers
Cardiovascular support	Establish access (triple-lumen central venous catheter) and arterial line Correct electrolyte or pH abnormalities Set up drug infusions with back-up syringe and pumps, and ensure that colloid and crystalloid infusions are available Insert urinary catheter If the patient is bleeding, carry cross-matched/O-negative/group-specific blood
Gastrointestinal support	Pause enteral feeding Pause unnecessary infusions (e.g. TPN, insulin)
Patient anxiety	Introduce self and team, and briefly discuss reasons for transfer, destination, journey time, and location of critical care unit
Pain control and sedation	Assess level of pain and need for increased analgesia or sedation during journey. Ensure that infusions and bolus drugs are available for journey
Pressure damage, wounds, or fractures	Assess pressure areas and avoid further pressure damage to vulnerable areas using pillows and/or pressure-relieving devices Ensure that fractures are stabilized prior to movement of patient Check that wound dressings are patent and unlikely to leak Protect cervical spine
Equipment or battery failure	Ensure that batteries are charged and check function of all equipment prior to moving

Relocation stress

Patients have reported experiencing negative physical and psychological responses to transfer. This is termed 'relocation stress', which occurs as a result of transfer from one environment to another. The key points to consider with regard to care of the patient include the process of transferring the patient, the information given, and the management of the patient post-transfer. Although the majority of patients report that relocation is a stressful experience, patients also regard transfer to a ward as a sign of improvement in their condition and relief from the stress of the critical care environment.

A significant factor in the patient experience is the abruptness of the transfer and the time of day at which it takes place. Preparation of the patient for transfer or discharge should begin early in the patient's admission. Both the patient and their significant others need to be informed of the process and timing of the transfer and the management of the patient's care post-transfer. Inadequate and poorly coordinated transfers must be avoided, so the following strategies should be considered.

- **Patient diaries** that are commenced on admission and maintained during critical care and post transfer can help to reorientate the patient and provide them with the opportunity to reflect on their care in terms of their progress and ongoing care needs.
- **Information** that is prepared using either local or national initiatives. For example, the Intensive Care Unit Support Teams for Ex-Patients (ICUsteps) was founded in 2005 by former patients, their relatives, and ICU staff to support patients and their families in their recovery from critical illness. ICUsteps have produced a range of literature, including *Intensive Care: a guide for patients and relatives* and *Guide to Setting up a Patients and Relatives Intensive Care Support Group*. The literature and further information are available from their website (http://icusteps.org). Information based on local or national initiatives may be available in a written or Internet-based format. Managing the expectations of patients and their significant others will help to reduce anxiety, especially with regard to the change in staff to patient ratio. Where possible the information should be individualized to the specific patient.
- **Timing** of transfers is important. They should avoid out-of-hours periods and not overburden the workloads of the receiving staff.
- **Acknowledgement** by critical care staff of the anxiety that transfer can generate for the patient is important, as is recognition of the signs of stress, and helping patients to learn methods of managing their anxiety.
- **Communication** between staff who are transferring and receiving the patient and communication with the patient and their significant other must be considered an essential component of every transfer. Debriefing following a transfer may help to identify points of good and poor practice.

Inter-hospital transfer

This refers to transfers that take place between critical care units for tertiary specialist care, or when a lack of critical care beds requires the patient to be transferred elsewhere.

Additional requirements for inter-hospital transfer

- Staff should be specifically trained and experienced.
- They should wear suitable clothing (for warmth and visibility).
- They should take with them a charged mobile phone containing the contact details of the referring and receiving hospitals.
- They should establish roles and responsibilities for the transfer and the level of experience within the transfer team.
- They should establish the route to the receiving hospital, the entry site, and the route from the entry site to the critical care unit.
- The trolley that is used to transport the patient and the equipment should be designed to withstand acceleration/deceleration forces and facilitate the mounting of equipment below the patient in order to maintain a lower centre of gravity and provide full access to the patient.
- The equipment should be designed for transport, so should be light, reliable, and with a battery life of more than 4 h.
- The equipment should be checked and calibrated prior to use, and fully charged.
- Monitoring should include ECG, blood pressure (intra-arterial blood pressure or non-invasive), temperature, SpO_2, and $ETCO_2$ if the patient is intubated.
- Adequate supplies of oxygen and medications should be prepared for the expected journey time, plus an extra 2 h (see Box 20.1).
- A transfer bag with additional equipment for emergency use may be available. Emergency equipment should include a full range of resuscitation drugs and apparatus for administration, a defibrillator, intubation equipment, and suction (see Box 20.2).
- The patient should be stable prior to commencement of the journey:
  - ventilation—ensure adequate ventilation or spontaneous breaths and gas exchange confirmed with ABG
  - cardiovascular—optimize blood pressure and heart rate
  - neurological—manage raised intracranial pressure.

Prior to commencement, the patient's family should be informed of the destination details, the approximate length of the journey, and the reasons for the transfer. It is not usual for the patient's family to be allowed to travel with the patient, due to vehicle insurance restrictions.

The receiving hospital should be informed of the patient's departure and estimated time of arrival.

Physiological effects of transfer

In addition to the physiological effects of speed, acceleration, and deceleration on the patient during and in the hours subsequent to the transfer, there are other environmental effects, including temperature, noise, light, vibration, and atmospheric pressure.

Box 20.1 Calculating oxygen cylinder duration for transfer

Modern transport ventilators have a continuous flow of gas in the circuit to allow for flow triggering of spontaneous breaths (terms used include 'bias flow', 'flow-by', or 'base flow'). This creates a small amount of gas consumption in addition to the patient's minute volume, and should be included in the calculation of how long a cylinder will last. The amount of continuous flow will vary according to the ventilator:

$$\text{oxygen flow rate} = FiO_2 \times (\text{minute volume} + \text{bias flow})$$

$$\text{e.g. } 0.50 \times (8.0 + 0.5\ \text{L/min}) = 4.25\ \text{L/min oxygen flow rate}$$

Using the oxygen flow rate and the volume of the cylinder it is then possible to determine the duration of the cylinder.

For BOC Integral Valve Cylinders the duration of the cylinder contents can be calculated to ensure that an adequate number of cylinders are taken for the patient transfer.[2]

Box 20.2 Transfusion of blood components during transfer

Blood components required during transfer are best commenced 15 min prior to the transfer in order to manage a potential transfusion reaction while the patient is in a stable environment. If the transfusion is only commenced in transit, all routine checks must be applied (i.e. check patient details against the blood component, and check that integrity, expiry date, and the blood group of the patient match the blood component). In addition, routine monitoring must be adhered to (i.e. baseline observations, observations 15 min from the start, and if the patient is stable, hourly observations until the end of the transfusion).

Blood components must be transported in a designated sealed transfer box. Once opened the full contents must be transfused within 4 h of breaking the seal (document this time). Traceability documentation must be returned to the referring hospital, and any unused components must be sent to the receiving hospital's Transfusion Laboratory.

Acceleration and deceleration will primarily affect the cardiopulmonary system. Acceleration will cause a drop in venous pressure and a corresponding drop in cardiac output. This reduction will also lead to a potential sympathetic response. In contrast, deceleration will increase venous pressure and cardiac output. This increase in filling pressure may not be accommodated, as the heart is unable to respond by increasing output, resulting in heart failure. Changes in heart rate occur when changes are maintained sufficiently for baroreceptor stimulus. A decrease in preload will lead to tachycardia, and bradycardia is associated with an increase in preload.

Acceleration for a patient in the upright position leads to less perfusion of the apices and more in the bases, resulting in a ventilation–perfusion mismatch. Therefore an increase in acceleration increases alveolar apical volume, which is unperfused, and causes an increase in basal shunt. In the supine position, acceleration towards the head means that the apical alveoli are stretched, whereas those at the bases are compressed. *The key is to optimize filling pressures.*

Indemnity information

The NHS Litigation Authority currently provides insurance for nurses for emergency transfers only (see NHS Risk Pooling Scheme). For planned transfers there is no formal cover. In order to increase or improve the cover currently available, nurses can obtain cover through a professional organization, arrange their own and seek reimbursement from their employing NHS trust, or set up a voluntary group personal accident scheme sponsored by the trust. Some NHS trusts have arranged commercial insurance cover for their employees.

Handover

Documentation should be maintained at all stages of the transfer. This should include details of the patient's condition, the reason for transfer, the names of the referring and accepting consultants, the patient's clinical status prior to transfer, and details of vital signs, clinical events, and therapy given before and during transfer. The patient's clinical notes and investigation results should accompany them, and copies should be retained by the receiving hospital.

A formal handover must be undertaken between the transfer team and the medical and nursing staff who will have responsibility for the patient. The handover should include a verbal and written account of the transfer and the patient's condition. The Intensive Care Society recommends the use of standardized transfer documentation.[3]

References

2 BOC Healthcare. *Medical Oxygen: integral valve cylinders (CD, ZD, HX, ZX)*. ℜ www.bochealthcare.co.uk/internet.lh.lh.gbr/en/images/504370-Healthcare%20Medical%20Oxygen%20Integral%20Valve%20Cylinders%20leaflet%2006409_54069.pdf

3 Intensive Care Society. *Guidelines for the Transport of the Critically Ill Adult*, 3rd edn. Intensive Care Society: London, 2011.

Further reading

Association of Anaesthetists of Great Britain and Ireland (AAGBI). *AAGBI Safety Guideline: inter-hospital transfer*. AAGBI: London, 2009.

Bench S et al. Effectiveness of critical care discharge information in supporting early recovery from critical illness. *Critical Care Nurse* 2013; **33**: 41–52.

Cullinane J and Plowright C. Patients' and relatives' experiences of transfer from intensive care unit to wards. *Nursing in Critical Care* 2013; **18**: 289–96.

Day D. Keeping patients safe during intrahospital transport. *Critical Care Nurse* 2010; **30**: 18–32.

Fanara B et al. Recommendations for the intra-hospital transport of critically ill patients. *Critical Care* 2010; **14**: R87.

Fludger S and Klein A. Portable ventilators. *Continuing Education in Anaesthesia, Critical Care & Pain* 2008; **8**: 199–203.

National Institute for Health and Care Excellence (NICE). *Rehabilitation after Critical Illness*. CG83. NICE: London, 2009. ℜ www.nice.org.uk/guidance/cg83

van Lieshout EJ and Stricker K. *Patient Transportation: skills and techniques*. European Society of Intensive Care Medicine: Brussels, 2011.

Chapter 21

Rehabilitation and discharge

Psychological impact of critical care

The experience of being a patient in a critical care unit, along with the recovery period afterwards, may result in the development of significant psychological disorders, such as delirium, depression, anxiety, or post-traumatic stress disorder. Early identification and management of psychological problems will help to improve the patient's quality of life and functional abilities after their recovery from critical illness.[1] See ➲ p. 28 for an overview of mental health assessment, ➲ p. 29 for mental capacity assessment, and ➲ p. 527 for non-physical dimensions of the critical care rehabilitation pathway.

Examples of strategies to help to reduce the psychological impact of critical care include patient diaries, follow-up clinics, support groups, and other online resources that involve sharing stories of patients' experiences. All of these types of interventions may be therapeutic for some people in helping to reduce the psychological impact of being critically ill, but may be unhelpful for others if they provoke anxiety or remind them too much of the negative aspects of their critical care stay.

Patient diaries

- These are used to help patients to make sense of their critical care experience and to reduce the psychological impact of critical illness on the patient's recovery.[1]
- There are a number of different types of diaries:
  - nurse led, with critical care nurses adding text and photos and facilitating the contribution of other healthcare professionals, family members, and patients to the diary
  - family led, with the family members taking full responsibility for the format and content of diary entries
  - patient led, if the patient is awake, well enough, and interested in keeping a diary
  - responsibility for the diary shared by healthcare professionals, family, and/or the patient.
- The legal, ethical, and professional implications of diary use in the critical care setting must be explored before introducing diaries to a critical care unit.

Follow-up

- Critical care outreach nurse follow-up on the ward after the patient has been discharged from the critical care unit.
- Critical care follow-up clinic which provides the patient with an opportunity to discuss their physical and psychological recovery with someone from the critical care team and receive ongoing support after being discharged home.
- There are a number of different types of critical care follow-up clinic:
  - nurse led by a critical care nurse and/or outreach nurse
  - physiotherapy led
  - medically led by an intensive care consultant
  - multidisciplinary in approach.

- Community-based support such as that provided by the patient's GP, psychologist, mental health team, occupational therapist, or social worker.

Support groups

- Some patients find meeting up with other people who have experienced being a critically ill patient is a supportive experience that has a positive effect on their psychological recovery.
- There are a number of different types of support group:
  - formal organizations (international, national, or local)
  - informal groups that meet in hospital or social settings on a regular or ad-hoc basis
  - patient-led groups, often with the involvement of family members of people who have been critically ill
  - healthcare professional-led groups, including regular support group meetings or one-off events (e.g. inviting service users to speak at a conference or teach students).

Online resources

- Online support for patients can be found on the ICUsteps[2] and Intensive Care Foundation[3] websites.
- A large collection of online video clips of patients talking about their critical care experience is freely available on the HealthTalkOnline[4] website.

References

1 Jones C et al. Intensive care diaries reduce new onset post traumatic stress disorder following critical illness: a randomised control trial. *Critical Care* 2010: **14**: R168.
2 ICUsteps. www.icusteps.org
3 Intensive Care Foundation. *Patients and Relatives*. www.ics.ac.uk/icf/patients-and-relatives
4 HealthTalkOnline. http://www.healthtalk.org/Intensive_care

Further reading

Peskett M and Gibb P. Developing and setting up a patient and relatives intensive care support group. *Nursing in Critical Care* 2009; **14**: 4–10.
Rock LF. Sedation and its association with posttraumatic stress disorder after intensive care. *Critical Care Nurse* 2014; **34**: 30–39.
Schandl AR et al. Screening and treatment of problems after intensive care: a descriptive study of multidisciplinary follow-up. *Intensive and Critical Care Nursing* 2011; **27**: 94–101.
Wake S and Kitchiner D. Post-traumatic stress disorder after intensive care. *British Medical Journal* 2013; **346**: f3232.
Williams SL. Recovering from the psychological impact of intensive care: how constructing a story helps. *Nursing in Critical Care* 2009; **14**: 281–8.

Critical illness rehabilitation

Guidance for rehabilitation of patients who have been critically ill has been provided by NICE,[5] and will be briefly summarized here (Tables 21.1 and Table 21.2 list the physical and non-physical dimensions to consider throughout the rehabilitation process). Rehabilitation should be started while the patient is still in the critical care unit, and continued on the ward and then at home after hospital discharge (see Figure 21.1 on ➲ p. 529 for an overview of this rehabilitation care pathway continuum, and ➲ p. 524 for further information about the psychological impact of critical illness).

Key principles of care[5]

- Ensure that the short-term and medium-term rehabilitation goals are reviewed, agreed, and updated throughout the patient's rehabilitation care pathway.
- Ensure the delivery of the structured and supported self-directed rehabilitation manual, if applicable.
- Liaise with primary or community care for the functional assessment at 2–3 months after discharge from critical care.
- Ensure that information, including documentation, is communicated as appropriate to any other healthcare settings.
- Give the patient the contact details of the healthcare professional(s) on discharge from critical care, and again on discharge from hospital.

Information and support[5]

- During the critical care stay, provide information about the patient's illness, interventions and treatments, equipment used, and any short-and/or long-term physical and non-physical problems if applicable. This information should be communicated more than once.
- Before the patient is discharged from critical care, or as soon as possible after their discharge from critical care, give them information about:
  - the rehabilitation care pathway, and, if applicable, emphasize the information about possible physical and non-physical problems
  - the differences between critical care and ward-based care, and the transfer of clinical responsibility to a different medical team
  - sleeping problems, nightmares, and hallucinations, and readjustment to ward-based care, if applicable.
- Before the patient is discharged home or to the community, give them information about:
  - their physical recovery (based on the goals set, if applicable) and how to manage activities of daily living
  - diet and any other continuing treatments
  - driving, returning to work, housing, and benefits (if applicable)
  - local support services
  - general guidance for the family or carer about what to expect and how to support the patient at home.
- Give the patient their own copy of the critical care discharge summary.

Table 21.1 Physical dimensions[5]

Physical problems	Weakness, inability/partial ability to sit, rise to standing, or walk, fatigue, pain, breathlessness, swallowing difficulties, incontinence, inability/partial ability to self-care
Sensory problems	Changes in vision or hearing, pain, altered sensation
Communication problems	Difficulties in speaking or using language to communicate, difficulties in writing
Social care and equipment needs	Mobility aids, transport, housing, benefits, employment and leisure needs

Table 21.2 Non-physical dimensions[5]

Anxiety, depression, and post-traumatic stress-related symptoms	New or recurrent somatic symptoms, including palpitations, irritability, and sweating; symptoms of derealization and depersonalization; avoidance behaviour; depressive symptoms, including tearfulness and withdrawal; nightmares, delusions, hallucinations, and flashbacks
Behavioural and cognitive problems	Loss of memory, attention deficits, sequencing problems, deficits in organizational skills, confusion, apathy, disinhibition, compromised insight
Other psychological or psychosocial problems	Low self-esteem, poor or low self-image and/or body image issues, relationship difficulties, including those with the family and/or carer

Reference

5 National Institute for Health and Care Excellence (NICE). *Rehabilitation after Critical Illness*. CG83. NICE: London, 2009. ℛ www.nice.org.uk/guidance/cg83 (Reproduced with permission.)

Further reading

Grap MJ and McFetridge B. Critical care rehabilitation and early mobilisation: an emerging standard of care. *Intensive and Critical Care Nursing* 2012; **28**: 55–7.

Rehabilitation care pathway

Figure 21.1 shows the rehabilitation process as set out by the NICE guidelines on critical illness rehabilitation.[6]

Reference

6 National Institute for Health and Care Excellence (NICE). *Rehabilitation after Critical Illness*. CG83. NICE: London, 2009. ↗ www.nice.org.uk/guidance/cg83

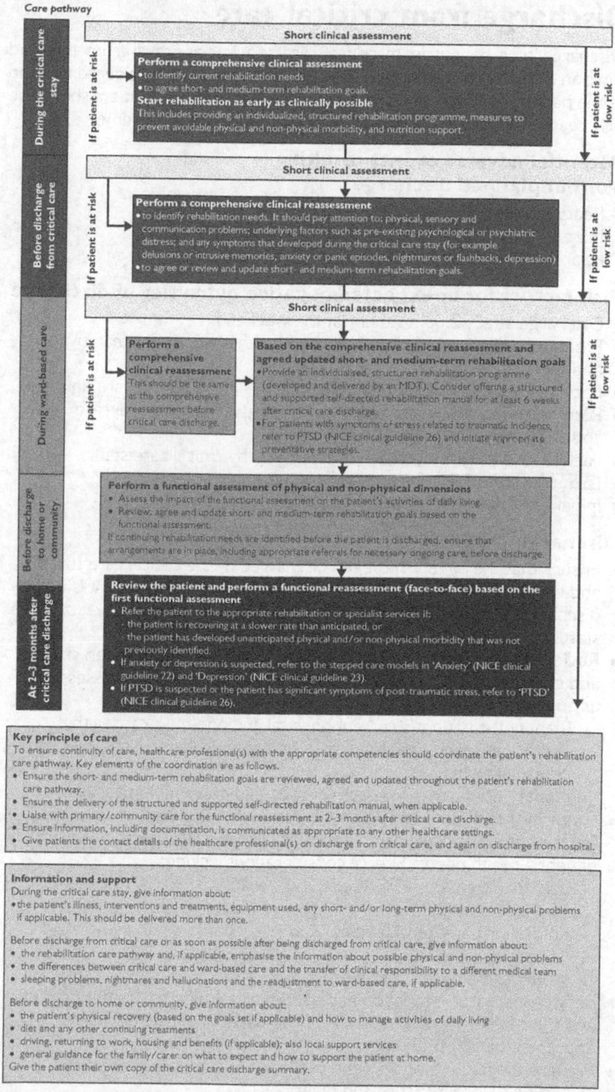

Figure 21.1 Rehabilitation care pathway. (Reproduced with permission from National Institute for Health and Care Excellence (2009) *CG83 Rehabilitation after Critical Illness*. London: NICE. Available from http://guidance.nice.org.uk/CG83)

Discharge from critical care

Discharge of a patient from critical care requires approval from the lead clinician (e.g. the critical care consultant), and should be considered as soon as the patient no longer requires critical care services. The patient should be fully ready for discharge and transferred out at an optimum time.

Potential adverse events resulting from unplanned discharge

- Readmission to critical care.
- Increased mortality.
- Poor experience for the patient and their family.

Risk factors for unexpected negative outcomes of discharge

- Discharge after 22.00 hours or at the weekend.
- Premature discharge dictated by need for the bed, rather than by patient readiness.
- Poor communication and teamworking within the critical care unit.
- Poor communication and teamworking between the critical care unit and the ward.
- Lack of critical care outreach or follow-up by critical care staff.
- Lack of a step-down facility.
- Initial illness severity.

Discharge process

- Ensure that the patient has been discharged by the critical care team and remains ready for discharge (the area to which the patient is being discharged should be appropriate to the patient's current Level of Care status).
- Review the rehabilitation care pathway if one has already been started, and complete a short, comprehensive, or functional clinical assessment as appropriate (see ➲ p. 529).
    - Identify the patient's current physical and non-physical health needs and specific treatments to be continued after discharge from critical care.
    - Identify risk factors for deterioration and preventive measures.
- Confirm that the area to which the patient is being discharged is ready for the patient and will be able to safely provide all aspects of the patient's health needs. Special considerations include:
    - pain management—PCA, epidural
    - tracheostomy
    - enteral or parenteral feeding
    - IV therapy
    - wounds, drains, or ostomies.
- Provide discharge education and psychological support for the patient and their family (for a discussion of the patient-centred discharge approach, see ➲ p. 531).
- Prepare the patient, equipment, medications, and documentation according to local practice and protocols.

- Refer the patient to other services as appropriate (e.g. critical care outreach, site manager, physiotherapist, occupational therapist, speech and language therapist, dietitian, social worker).
- Transfer the patient out of critical care, providing a systematic handover to the nurse taking over care of the patient.

Patient-centred discharge

- Involve the patient and their family throughout the decision-making process in relation to discharging the patient from critical care.
- Provide reassurance and support for the patient and their family before, during, and after discharge.
- If the patient remains in critical care due to a lack of available ward beds, do not continue to provide Level 3 care. For example:
  - Care for the patient according to their current level of acuity.
  - Stop unnecessary continuous monitoring, such as ECG, arterial blood pressure, and CVP monitoring.
  - Monitor observations as frequently as would be done on the ward for the patient's current status.
  - Encourage the patient to be as independent as possible with regard to personal hygiene needs and eating and drinking.
  - Encourage mobilization as appropriate for the patient's condition.
- Provide the patient with a patient discharge summary written in a way that the patient and family can easily understand, using lay terminology.[7,8]
  - Delirium and memory loss during the critical care stay can cause distress and impede psychological recovery after discharge. A patient discharge summary may help the patient to understand what happened to them during their critical care stay.
  - White and colleagues[9] have provided a freely available online discharge summary training resource for critical care healthcare professionals, which also includes a patient discharge summary template.

References

7 Bench S, Day T and Griffiths P. The effectiveness of written and/or verbal critical care discharge information to support early critical illness recovery: a narrative critical review. *Critical Care Nurse* 2013; **33**: 41–52.

8 Bench S et al. Providing critical care patients with a personalized discharge summary: a questionnaire survey and retrospective analysis exploring feasibility and effectiveness. *Intensive & Critical Care Nursing* 2014; **30**: 69–76.

9 White C, Bench S and Hopkins P. *Critical Care Patient Discharge Summary Training Pack.* ℘ www.icusteps.org/assets/files/ccpatient-discharge-pack.pdf

Index

I

Q

R

S

T

U

V